How to...
collected articles from
BSAVA **companion**

Published by:

British Small Animal Veterinary Association
Woodrow House, 1 Telford Way, Waterwells
Business Park, Quedgeley, Gloucester GL2 2AB

A Company Limited by Guarantee in England.
Registered Company No. 2837793.
Registered as a Charity.

A catalogue record for this book is available from the British Library.

ISBN   978-1-905319-50-3

The publishers, editors and contributors cannot take responsibility for information
provided on dosages and methods of application of drugs mentioned or
referred to in this publication. Details of this kind must be verified in each case
by individual users from up to date literature published by the manufacturers or
suppliers of those drugs. Veterinary surgeons are reminded that in each case
they must follow all appropriate national legislation and regulations (for example,
in the United Kingdom, the prescribing cascade) from time to time in force.

Printed in India by Imprint Digital
Printed on ECF paper made from sustainable forests

Contents

Contributors

Nick Bexfield BVetMed PhD DSAM DipECVIM-CA MRCVS
*European Specialist in Small Animal Internal
Medicine*
Department of Veterinary Medicine,
University of Cambridge, Madingley Road,
Cambridge CB3 OES

Matt Brash BVetMed CertZooMed MRCVS
Ark Vets, Givendale House, Givendale
Pocklington, York YO42 1TT

Kevin Eatwell BVSc(Hons) DZooMed(Reptilian)
DipECZM(Herp) MRCVS
Exotic Animal and Wildlife Service,
Royal (Dick) School of Veterinary Studies,
University of Edinburgh, Hospital for Small
Animals, Easter Bush Veterinary Centre,
Midlothian EH25 9RG

Allison German BVSc MSc PhD MRCVS
Department of Infection Biology, Institute of
Infection and Global Health, University of
Liverpool, Leahurst, Chester High Road,
Neston, Wirral CH64 7TE

Gillian Gibson VMD DipACVIM MRCVS
Axiom Veterinary Laboratories,
The Manor House, Brunel Road,
Newton Abbot, Devon TQ12 4PB

Mark Goodfellow MA VetMB CertVR DSAM
DipECVIM-CA MRCVS
Davies Veterinary Specialists,
Manor Farm Business Park,
Higham Gobion, Hertfordshire SG5 3HR

David Gould BSc(Hons) BVM&S PhD DVOphthal
DipECVO MRCVS
*RCVS & European Specialist in Veterinary
Ophthalmology*
Davies Veterinary Specialists,
Manor Farm Business Park,
Higham Gobion, Hertfordshire SG5 3HR

Nicki Grint BVSc DVA DipECVAA MRCVS
School of Veterinary Science,
University of Bristol, Langford House,
Langford, Bristol BS40 5DU

Danièlle Gunn-Moore BSc BVM&S PhD FHEA
MACVSc MRCVS
RCVS Specialist in Feline Medicine
Royal (Dick) School of Veterinary Studies,
University of Edinburgh, Hospital for Small
Animals, Easter Bush Veterinary Centre,
Midlothian EH25 9RG

Georgie Hollis BSc
Intelligent Wound Care and The Veterinary
Wound Library, The Old Hall Cottage,
93 Back Street, Garboldisham,
Diss IP22 2SD

Laura Holm BVM&S CertSAM MRCVS
Anderson Moores Veterinary Specialists,
The Granary, Bunstead Barns, Poles Lane,
Hursley, Winchester, Hampshire SO21 2LL

Karen Humm MA VetMB CertVA DipACVECC FHEA
MRCVS
Department of Veterinary Clinical Sciences,
The Royal Veterinary College,
Hawkshead Lane, North Mymms,
Hatfield, Hertfordshire AL9 7TA

Rosanne Jepson BVSc MVetMed PhD DipACVIM
MRCVS
Department of Veterinary Clinical Sciences,
The Royal Veterinary College,
Hawkshead Lane, North Mymms,
Hatfield, Hertfordshire AL9 7TA

Mike Jessop BVetMed MRCVS
Ash Veterinary Surgery, Aberdare Road,
Merthyr Tydfil, Mid Glamorgan,
Wales CF48 1AT

Victoria Johnson BVSc DVR DipECVDI MRCVS
*RCVS & European Veterinary Specialist in
Diagnostic Imaging*
Vet CT Consultants in Telemedicine,
St Johns Innovation Centre, Cowley Road,
Cambridge CB4 0WS

Peri Lau-Gillard DrMedVet CertVD DipECVD MRCVS
European Specialist in Veterinary Dermatology
Cave Veterinary Specialists, George's Farm,
West Buckland, Nr Wellington TA21 9LE

Philip Lhermette BSc(Hons) CBiol MSB BVetMed MRCVS
Elands Veterinary Clinic, St John's Church, London Road, Dunton Green, Sevenoaks, Kent TN13 2TE

Janet Littlewood MA PhD BVSc DVR DVD MRCVS
RCVS Recognised Specialist in Veterinary Dermatology
Veterinary Dermatology Referrals,
2 Waterbeach Road, Landbeach,
Cambridge CB25 9FA

Brigitte Lord BVetMed(Hons) CertZooMed MRCVS
RCVS Certified in Zoological Medicine
Exotic Animal and Wildlife Service,
Royal (Dick) School of Veterinary Studies,
University of Edinburgh, Hospital for Small Animals, Easter Bush Veterinary Centre,
Midlothian EH25 9RG

Mark Lowrie MA VetMB MVM DipECVN MRCVS
RCVS & European Veterinary Specialist in Neurology
Davies Veterinary Specialists,
Manor Farm Business Park,
Higham Gobion, Hertfordshire SG5 3HR

Lisa Milella BVSc DipEVDC MRCVS
European Veterinary Specialist in Dentistry
The Veterinary Dental Surgery,
53 Parvis Road, Byfleet, Surrey KT14 7AA

Carmel Mooney MVB MPhil PhD DipECVIM-CA MRCVS
Veterinary Clinical Studies Section,
School of Veterinary Medicine,
University College Dublin, Belfield,
Dublin 4, Republic of Ireland

Elizabeth Mullineaux BVM&S DVM&S CertSHP MRCVS
Secret World Wildlife Rescue,
Highbridge, Somerset TA9 3PZ

Kate Murphy BVSc(Hons) DSAM DipECVIM-CA PGCert(HE) MRCVS
European Veterinary Specialist in Small Animal Internal Medicine
Bath Veterinary Referrals,
Rosemary Lodge, Wellsway BA2 5RL

Gerry Polton MA VetMB MSc(Clin Onc) DipECVIM-CA(Onc) MRCVS
RCVS & European Veterinary Specialist in Oncology
North Downs Specialist Referrals,
Friesian Building 3&4, The Brewer Street Dairy Business Park, Brewer Street, Bletchingley, Surrey RH1 4QP

Roger Powell MA VetMB DipRCPath DipACVP FRCPath MRCVS
PTDS, Unit 2a, Manor Farm Business Park,
Higham Gobion, Hertfordshire SG5 3HR

Alasdair Renwick BVMS DSAS(Orth) MRCVS
East Neuk Veterinary Clinic, Netherton Estate,
Station Road, St Monans, Anstruther,
Fife KY10 2DW

Kirsty Roe BVSc CertSAM DipACVIM MRCVS
American Specialist in Small Animal Internal Medicine
Willows Veterinary Centre and Referral Service,
Highlands Road, Shirley, Solihull,
West Midlands B90 4NH

Richard Saunders BSc BVSc MSB CBiol CertZooMed DipZooMed(Mammalian) MRCVS
Bristol Zoological Gardens Veterinary Department, Clifton, Bristol BS8 3HA

Chris Shales MA VetMB CertSAS DipECVS MRCVS
RCVS & European Specialist in Small Animal Surgery
Willows Veterinary Centre and Referral Service,
Highlands Road, Shirley, Solihull,
West Midlands B90 4NH

Susana Silva DVM CertSAM DipECVIM-CA MRCVS
European Specialist in Veterinary Internal Medicine
Vets Now Referrals Swindon, Unit 10,
Berkshire House, Shrivenham Road,
County Park, Swindon SN1 2NR

Andrew Sparkes BVetMed PhD DipECVIM MRCVS
International Society of Feline Medicine,
Taeselbury, High Street, Tisbury,
Wiltshire SP3 6LD

Kit Sturgess MA VetMB PhD CertVR DSAM CertVC MRCVS
RCVS Recognised Specialist in Small Animal Medicine
Vet Freedom Ltd, PO Box 343, Brockenhurst, Hampshire SO41 1BW

Nuala Summerfield BSc BVM&S DipACVIM DipECVIM-CA MRCVS
RCVS, American & European Specialist in Veterinary Cardiology

Simon Tappin MA VetMB CertSAM DipECVIM-CA MRCVS
RCVS & European Veterinary Specialist in Internal Medicine
Dick White Referrals, Station Farm, London Road, Six Mile Bottom, Cambridgeshire CB8 0UH

Kathleen Tennant BVetMed CertSAM CertVC FRCPath PGCAP MRCVS
Diagnostic Laboratories, Langford Veterinary Services, University of Bristol, Langford House, Langford, Bristol BS40 5DU

Angelika von Heimendahl MScAgr BVM(Berlin) DipECAR MRCVS
European Specialist in Small Animal Reproduction
Veterinary Reproduction Service, 27 High Street, Longstanton, Cambridge CB24 3BP

David Walker BVetMed(Hons) DipACVIM MRCVS
RCVS & American Specialist in Small Animal Internal Medicine
Anderson Moores Veterinary Specialists, The Granary, Bunstead Barns, Poles Lane, Hursley, Winchester, Hampshire SO21 2LL

Penny Watson MA VetMD CertVR DSAM DipECVIM MRCVS
Queen's Veterinary School Hospital, University of Cambridge, Madingley Road, Cambridge CB3 0ES

Dick White BVetMed PhD DSAS DVR DipACVS DipECVS FRCVS
RCVS, American & European Specialist in Small Animal Surgery, RCVS Specialist in Veterinary Oncology and ACVS Founding Fellow in Surgical Oncology
Dick White Referrals, Station Farm, London Road, Six Mile Bottom, Cambridgeshire CB8 0UH

John Williams MA VetMB LLB CertVR DipECVS FRCVS
European Specialist in Small Animal Surgery
Northwest Surgeons, Delamere House, Ashville Point, Sutton Weaver, Cheshire WA7 3FW

Foreword

One of the joys of being a vet is the practical aspects of the work and the ability to 'do' things. So, it is a great pleasure for me to write the Foreword for this excellent collection of **companion** articles.

The 'How to' series of articles have been a must read every time **companion** arrives at our practice. Each has precise step-by-step instructions and excellent illustrations. These have now been produced in a single publication as an easy reference booklet.

The articles in this collection cover a wide range of subjects at various different levels from the 'How to... Choose a cat urinary catheter' to the more complex, but vital, 'How to... Select and carry out a gastropexy procedure'. The photos and illustrations are of high quality, which is essential when trying to learn or refresh your knowledge of a technique or subject.

This booklet will be of useful guide to almost all vets, but will be of particular value to the practitioner. I see this publication not being kept in the practice reference library but the 'Prep' room for quick and instant reference and will become well thumbed.

I would like to thank all the authors and the BSAVA team assisting them from behind the scenes for all their work and congratulate them on an excellent publication.

Mark Johnston
BVetMed MRCVS

BSAVA President 2012–13

Introduction

It is with great pleasure that I write the Introduction to this collection of 'How to...' articles, which have featured in **companion**, the BSAVA membership magazine over the last 4 years. When **companion** was first devised we wanted to include CPD articles that would offer comprehensive, accurate, contemporary advice to BSAVA members in an easy-to-read, approachable format. Rather than wading through pages of prose we wanted to produce well illustrated, concise articles that could be read in a coffee break but that would fully appraise the reader of the pertinent points of a given topic, and thus the 'How to...' was born.

Consistently one of the most appreciated and best features in **companion**, we have gathered together some of the best 'How to...' articles from the last few years into this easy-to-refer-to book. Articles have been revised and updated by the authors where necessary, so they remain as current as the originals were. Hopefully this collection will become a well thumbed addition to your practice shelf, which can be added to with each new edition of **companion**.

Mark Goodfellow
MA VetMB CertVR DSAM DipECVIM-CA MRCVS

Editor, **companion**
August 2012

How to...

Place an oesophagostomy tube

by Nick Bexfield and Penny Watson

When to consider nutritional support

Special nutritional support (i.e. a change to a high-calorie, high-protein diet and/or assisted (tube) feeding) should be considered in cases of:

- **Recent weight loss:** Has the dog or cat lost >10% of its bodyweight not due to dehydration or obvious fluid shifts (e.g. diuresis)?
  - This is relevant even in obese animals: weight loss in an obese, sick animal will predominantly be attributed to loss of lean body mass rather than fat and this is undesirable. Weight loss and anorexia in an obese cat are particularly worrying because of the risk of hepatic lipidosis.
- **Partial or complete anorexia for >3 days:** Has the dog or cat eaten <85% of its calculated resting energy requirement (RER) for the last 3 or more days?
- **Animal in very catabolic state or at risk of overt malnutrition:**
  - Does the animal have: severe burns; draining sepsis, such as pyothorax or septic peritonitis; malabsorption or protein-losing enteropathy; or nephropathy?
  - If so, is it receiving enough calories and/ or protein?
  - Is there an obvious loss of weight or lean body mass to suggest it is not?

Routes of enteral support

There are a few important general rules for feeding hospitalised animals:

1. IF THE GUT WORKS, USE IT (applies to the vast majority of our patients).
2. If only PART of the gut works, use THAT part of the gut.
3. When feeding enterally, use the simplest route possible which avoids stress to the animal.
4. Appetite stimulants are NOT very effective acutely and are best reserved for when the patient has been discharged home and is recuperating.

There are a number of advantages of feeding animals enterally, which is why every effort should be made to feed animals in this way. **Note:** Before nutritional interventions are initiated, the patient must be stable cardiovascularly and have had any fluid, electrolyte and acid–base abnormalities addressed.

There are many enteral feeding methods available to the practising veterinary surgeon, ranging from oral or force-feeding to a number of tube-feeding methods. When using any syringe- or force-feeding method, it is important to ensure that the animal is receiving a significant amount of its daily caloric requirements. If it is not, or if it is becoming stressed by the procedure, some sort of feeding tube should be placed.

The choice of tubes includes:

- Naso-oesophageal
- Oesophageal
- Gastrostomy (placed at laparotomy or as a percutaneous endoscopic gastrostomy (PEG))
- Jejunostomy.

The feeding route selected for a particular animal is based on the following decision-making process. Jejunostomy tubes are used only if there is a specific contraindication to placing a tube more proximally in the gastrointestinal tract.

The decision-making process

- **Is the feeding tube going to be required long term?** If so, consider gastrostomy/ PEG or oesophagostomy tube and NOT naso-oesophageal tube.
- **Is there a specific contraindication to one or more tube types?** For example, a naso-oesophageal tube would be contraindicated in nasal disease; both oesophagostomy and naso-oesophageal tubes are contraindicated where there is oesophageal disease (such as megaoesophagus or oesophagitis).
- **Is there an anaesthetic risk that makes tube placement under anaesthesia an unacceptable hazard?** If so, naso-oesophageal tube placement should be considered as it does not require a general anaesthetic. This could be used as a temporary measure until the animal is well enough for a general anaesthetic and more long-term tube placement.
- **What types of diet does the patient require?** Naso-oesophageal tubes require

liquid diets, whereas gastrostomy and oesophagostomy tubes are of a wider bore and so a greater range of gruel diets can be used.

It is extremely important to include the owner in the decision-making process, as they must be willing and able to provide the necessary nutrition if the animal is to be able to go home. Many owners can handle the three or four feedings per day that are typically required for oesophagostomy or PEG tubes.

Oesophagostomy tubes offer advantages to practitioners over PEG tubes. Oesophagostomy tubes can be placed without specialized equipment or expertise. In addition, whilst they require anaesthesia for proper placement, the amount of time required is much shorter than for other procedures. For these reasons, these tubes are a useful method of providing enteral nutrition in the practice setting.

Oesophagostomy tubes should **not** be placed in animals with the following conditions:

- Comatose, recumbent or dysphoric animals at risk of aspiration
- Persistent vomiting – the tube may be expelled or retroflexed into the nasopharynx
- Oesophagitis or severe oesophageal dysfunction (e.g. megaoesophagus).

Cellulitis is the major complication seen after oesophagostomy tube placement. Oesophageal stricture formation and fistula formation are possible but very rare.

Placement technique

The equipment you will need is listed in Figure 1. General anaesthesia is required. The patient is placed in right lateral recumbency, and lateral and ventral aspects of the neck prepared aseptically over an area from the angle of the jaw to the shoulder.

- Oesophagostomy tube (red rubber tube, standard polyurethane feeding tube or silicone feeding tube):
  - Cats: 10–14 Fr; 23 cm long
  - Dogs: 14–24 Fr; 40 cm long
- Long curved forceps, e.g. Rochester–Carmalt
- No. 15 or 20 scalpel blade and holder
- 25 mm wide adhesive tape
- Non-absorbable suture material, needle and needle-holders
- Sterile dressing to cover the tube site
- Light bandage for the neck
- Cotton wool or soft swabs
- 4% chlorhexidine gluconate or 10% povidone–iodine
- 70% surgical spirit
- 1 sterile fenestrated skin drape

Figure 1: Equipment required for oesophagostomy tube placement

TECHNIQUE

1. Insert the curved forceps through the mouth and into the oesophagus, to the mid-cervical region.
2. Turn the tip of the forceps laterally and use the scalpel to make a 5–10 mm skin incision over the point of the tips.

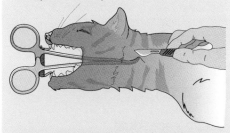

3. Bluntly dissect through the subcutaneous tissues and make an incision into the oesophagus over the tips of the forceps.
4. Push the tips of the forceps outwards through the incision to the external surface.
5. Measure the oesophagostomy tube from this point to the 7th intercostal space (distal oesophagus) and mark the tube with a piece of adhesive tape.

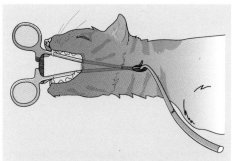

6. Open the tips of the forceps and grasp the distal end of the feeding tube.

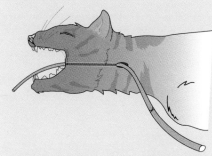

7. Draw the end of the feeding tube through the oesophagostomy incision and rostrally into the pharynx to exit the mouth.
8. Disengage the tips of the forceps, curl the tip of the tube back into the mouth and feed it into the oesophagus.

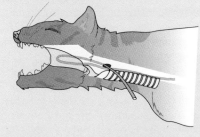

9. Visually inspect the oropharynx to confirm that the tube is no longer present in the oropharynx.
10. The tube should slide easily back and forth a few centimetres, confirming that it has straightened.

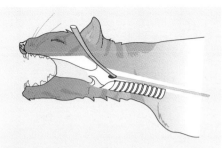

$$RER \text{ (kcal)} = 70 \times \text{bodyweight (kg)}^{0.75}$$
OR
$$RER \text{ (kcal)} = 30 \times \text{bodyweight (kg)} + 70$$

To convert kcal (Cal) to kilojoules (kJ) multiply by 4.185

Figure 2: Formulae for calculating the resting energy requirement

11. Secure the tube by placement of a "Chinese finger-trap"/"Roman Sandal" suture.
12. Take a thoracic radiograph to confirm correct tube placement: the tip of the tube should be in the distal oesophagus, not the stomach. If the tube does have an integral radiodense marker, iodinated (not barium) contrast medium can be instilled into the tube to aid visualisation.
13. Cover the tube site with a sterile dressing and place a soft padded loose neck bandage.

Meeting energy requirements

Determining the exact energy requirements of individual patients is unfeasible in clinical practice as it would require some form of direct or indirect calorimetry. A more practical and sensible approach is to calculate the patient's resting energy requirement (RER), which corresponds to the number of calories per day it needs to meet basic needs. This is a very rough estimation and may need adjusting in the long term, depending on patient weight loss or gain. Recent studies show, perhaps surprisingly, that there is not a great increase in energy requirement associated with trauma, sepsis or major surgery in dogs. Therefore, the RER is now used as the 'baseline' energy recommendation for hospitalized dogs and cats, regardless of the disease or surgery. A number of equations are used to estimate RER; the simplest are shown in Figure 2.

The RER can then be divided by the caloric density of the diet to calculate the amount to be fed. It is worth noting that EU petfood labelling regulations prohibit the inclusion of the caloric density of diets on the tin or bag, but the information can be obtained from product guides or by contacting the manufacturer.

The RER should be viewed as a starting point and the amount fed adjusted upwards (if continued weight loss is apparent) or downwards (if the patient cannot tolerate this amount, e.g. it vomits).

Meeting protein requirements

If using a balanced dog or cat diet, protein requirements are typically met when the calculated calories are fed. However, as a general guideline, estimated protein requirements for hospitalized dogs and cats are:

- Dogs: 5–7.5 g protein per 100 kcal fed
- Cats: 6–9 g protein per 100 kcal fed.

Feeding schedule

Note that calculated food intake should not be given immediately on the first day but introduced gradually over 2–3 days to allow the animal's metabolism and gastrointestinal tract the time to adapt. This is particularly important if using feeding tubes (Figure 3). The stomach's capacity may reduce by up to 50% after as little as 48 hours of anorexia. In addition, reduced gastric tone and

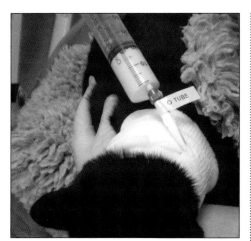

Figure 3: An anorexic cat being fed through an oesophagostomy tube. Courtesy of Rachel Lumbis

emptying are features of anorexia, along with changes in gastrointestinal flora and metabolic changes, all of which need time to adapt to the new diet.

- Feeding can commence as soon as the patient has recovered from general anaesthesia.
- The daily requirement should be divided into multiple (5 or 6) feeds per 24-hour day.
- *Before and after feeding each time*, the tube should be flushed with small amounts (5–10 ml) of lukewarm tap water.
- The food should be warmed to body temperature and injected over several minutes.

- If the animal shows regurgitation, vomiting or diarrhoea after feeding, reduce the amount fed in each meal and check that the food fed is warm and iso-osmolar.

Tube care and removal

Once a day, the neck wrap and sterile dressing should be removed and the stoma cleaned using cotton wool or gauze swabs soaked in 4% chlorhexidine gluconate or 10% povidone–iodine. If oozing of purulent liquid suggests infection, an antibiotic ointment can be applied. A new sterile dressing is then applied and the neck wrap replaced.

The oesophagostomy tube can be removed when it is no longer required; unlike a gastrotomy tube there is no minimum length of time an oesophagostomy tube must have been in place prior to removal. To remove the tube, take off the dressing, remove the suture and pull the tube gently out. The stoma site will close rapidly once the tube is removed, but skin sutures can be placed if preferred.

Acknowledgements

The line diagrams in this article have been reproduced from the *BSAVA Guide to Procedures in Small Animal Practice*, edited by Nick Bexfield and Karla Lee. The diagrams were drawn by Samantha Elmhurst BA Hons (www.livingart.org.uk) and are printed with her permission. ■

How to...

Investigate and treat
a feather plucking parrot

by Kevin Eatwell

Feather plucking, feather picking and self-trauma are commonly presented in clinical practice. Many owners will present a bird looking for a quick resolution to a problem that has existed for many years. Yet unless these cases are investigated thoroughly to identify any underlying factors leading to the plucking, presumptive treatment is likely to fail.

The causes for feather plucking broadly fall into two categories: either a psychological problem that has resulted from captivity; or a specific illness leading to the damage. What the clinician must do first is identify any problems by reviewing the clinical history, physical examination and diagnostic testing. These findings should be evaluated in context of the feather plucking to associate them directly with the problem. At this stage therapy can begin, depending on the diagnosis. In urgent cases remedial therapy may be required whilst achieving a diagnosis. Common causes associated with feather plucking are listed in Figure 1.

- ■ **After wing clipping**
- ■ Air sacculitis
- ■ Allergic disease (inhaled or food)
- ■ **Behavioural problems**
- ■ Chlamydophilosis
- ■ Cloacal disease
- ■ Excessive allopreeening from another bird
- ■ Folliculitis (bacterial or fungal)
- ■ Heavy metal toxicity
- ■ Hepatic disease
- ■ Hypocalcaemia
- ■ Neoplasia
- ■ Nutritional disorders
- ■ Painful focus
- ■ Parasitic disease
- ■ **Poor socialisation**
- ■ Proventricular dilatation disease
- ■ **Reproductive activity**

Figure 1: Differential diagnosis list for causes of feather plucking (most common in bold)

What clinical signs may be seen?

The external appearance of a pet parrot is usually of importance to the owner, but despite this some owners fail to present a bird until the clinical signs are severe. The pattern of feather change or damage may lead the clinician to suspect particular conditions and it is important to identify the exact nature of the feather damage. Feather plucking can be seen when the bird is physically removing feathers, preventing regrowth of an area and leading to alopecia (Figure 2). In contrast, feather pickers or chewers traumatise feathers; these can be clearly evident on examination but are not plucked. A third group can self-traumatise areas leading to intense pain, blood loss, alopecia and scarring. In these cases urgent intervention is required.

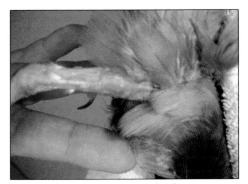

Figure 2: This Patagonian conure has been selectively plucking feathers on the legs. This can indicate underlying reproductive disease and inappropriate pair bonding of a parrot to its owner

What are the important questions to ask during a consultation?

It is critically important to evaluate the bird's history as a whole. Many factors, ranging from skin irritation or desiccation through to inadequate nutrition, can predispose to feather damage. Thus a thorough husbandry review is indicated and all predisposing factors should be eliminated. General husbandry advice s hould be given (and followed) in all cases of birds with feather damage (Figure 3).

It is important to discuss the bird's socialisation with the owners in detail. Parrots generally perceive their owners as parental figures when young, siblings when adolescent, and as mates and competitors when adult. Inappropriate pair bonding may be seen, with the bird becoming fixated on one individual and aggressive to other people. Signs seen may include mating postures or regurgitation, for example.

The anatomical site where the bird has damaged the feathers is important. The distribution of feather damage may suggest a painful focus in the area and may be centred over a wing clip (Figure 4), the proventriculus, the ovary, the air sacs, the liver or vent, for

- Improve the diet and avoid fatty foods. A complete pelleted diet should be offered, along with some fresh fruits and vegetables.
- Provide the bird with access to either natural or artificial UV-b light. Birds can see into the UV spectrum and this facilitates natural behaviour and helps prevent hypocalcaemia (which is a particular problem in grey parrots).
- Ensure the bird is not exposed to an excessive photoperiod; 12 hours of light a day is sufficient for most equatorial species.
- Avoid any inhaled toxins such as tobacco smoke, PTFE (from non-stick frying pans) or deodorants.
- Spray or mist the bird daily with warm water.
- Improve the bird's socialisation with multiple owners and consider training the bird to stimulate it.
- Never get the wings clipped.

Figure 3: General husbandry advice for owners

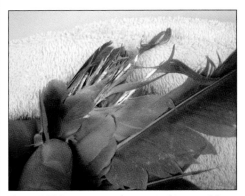

Figure 4: This grey parrot has started traumatising the feathers at a site of a previous wing clip. This can progress to self-trauma of the skin of the wing tip, requiring amputation

example. It is important to identify where the feather damage started, as it can spread over a wider area over time as clinical signs progress.

Having worked out the site of the damage, you then need to find out if the owner is witnessing any inappropriate behaviour such as excessive grooming, plucking or even pain responses from the bird. If so, this may associate the damage with the presence of the owner and it may be that the bird is seeking attention from its owners, which they probably will be giving and hence rewarding the behaviour. Conversely, other birds may damage themselves when the owners are absent.

You also need to identify if any previous treatment has been administered by the owner or other veterinary surgeons prior to visiting you. Some of these treatments may have been inappropriate. There may have been some diagnostic tests performed previously as well, the results of which may be useful.

How can I investigate the causes of feather plucking?

Every clinician you speak to will have a different list of diagnostic procedures they perform and each plan is, of course, tailored to each individual case. The important factor is to prioritise diagnostics and aim to get as much information as possible to rule out as many of the underlying factors quickly and economically.

Whilst screening for infectious disease is important (there are PCR tests for psittacine beak and feather disease (PBFD), polyoma virus and *Chlamydophila*), the importance of such results has to be taken in context. What is the real likelihood of an adult grey parrot, housed in isolation for a number of years, with perfect head feathers, having been exposed to PBFD? Although a *Chlamydophila* PCR may be positive, is there significant pathology (liver or air sac disease) leading to plucking over the keel? Instead of rushing in with specific testing, looking at the bird's health status as a whole may yield more useful results.

Author's suggested investigatory procedure

■ The bird should be anaesthetised and a full blood profile taken. This is useful to rule out hypocalcaemia, liver disease, renal disease,

low proteins and also to check for signs of systemic infection such as a monocytosis or toxic activity within the white cell lines. For example, if the bird had PBFD then a low white cell count may be seen. In contrast, significant *Chlamydophila* infection will elevate the white cell count and there may be signs of liver damage on the profile.

■ Radiography is important and two views should be taken, a lateral and a ventrodorsal. These can be useful to look for signs of proventricular enlargement or for radiodense foreign bodies such as heavy metals. Chronic joint disease causing a painful focus may also be seen in older birds.

■ The next step to consider is laparoscopy (Figure 5). This, although invasive, provides far more information about the bird's health status. The clinician can evaluate the air sacs, liver, heart, proventriculus, lungs, kidneys, gonads (and hence reproductive status), spleen, intestines and cloaca. This essentially rules out or diagnoses many of the potential underlying factors leading to feather plucking. At this point, if a number of common medical conditions have been eliminated, remedial hormonal therapy may

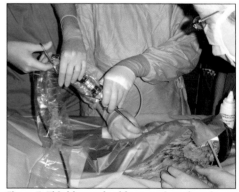

Figure 5: This blue and gold macaw is undergoing laparoscopic biopsy as it has hepatomegaly which may be related to its poor feather quality

be indicated, if an active gonad (and hence likely excessive pair bonding) was identified on laparoscopy.

- Should these tests fail to lead to a diagnosis then investigation of primary skin disease should follow. Detailed examination of the skin and feathers is important and should be undertaken while the bird is anaesthetised. If any areas are of concern, then diagnostic samples can be taken. Fret marks can be seen where feather growth has been disrupted due to a poor diet or PBFD. Changes in pigmentation of feathers, which can become black or pink plumage depending on species, can occur with liver disease.

Skin scrapes can be examined for ectoparasites in areas of hyperkeratosis. Abnormally thickened blood feathers can be removed and the pulp examined cytologically for 'pulpitis'. Diff Quik staining can reveal bacteria or heterophillic inflammation. Alternatively a skin biopsy sample can be taken (including a quill feather) and sent for histopathology. This is of particular importance where ulceration, nodules or signs of chronic disease are seen. Neoplastic conditions are also on the differential list in these cases (Figure 6).

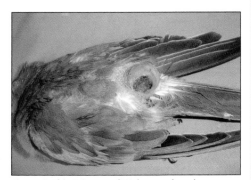

Figure 6: This Princess of Wales parakeet has a uropygial gland tumour that requires surgical removal. A collar will need to be placed to prevent damage to the granulating surgical wound created

Culture of skin lesions can also be performed. The techniques used mirror that used for mammalian skin disease.

Caution is to be advised when interpreting skin tests, as many cases of 'pulpitis' or inflammation can be due to secondary opportunistic infections as a consequence of the feather plucking. Treatment of theses conditions with antibiotics and analgesics may help to control feather plucking, but the underlying cause should always be thoroughly evaluated.

- Specific diagnostics may be indicated for an individual case: e.g. PBFD or *Chlamydophila* PCR; crop biopsy if proventricular dilatation disease is suspected; or blood lead or zinc levels if heavy metal toxicity is suspected. A full faecal analysis may also be required if endoparasitic disease is suspected.
- If all medical conditions have been excluded it suggests that there is a behavioural element to the problem and remedial behavioural therapy can be undertaken.

How should a severe case be managed?

If the bird is at risk of causing significant self-trauma then remedial action may need to be undertaken urgently for humane reasons. This may necessitate: a collar to be placed to prevent self-trauma; analgesia for pain control; debriding, cleaning and dressing wounds; and antibiotics if the wounds are infected. However these are not standalone solutions, and a thorough review of husbandry and clinical history are indicated alongside a diagnostic plan. There is little point in collaring a bird and providing psychotropic drug therapy without confirming this is 100% necessary.

Other birds may start performing self-trauma as a result of a painful focus. This can be seen in birds that have been wing clipped and that have subsequently damaged the end of their wing, impairing feather regrowth. In severe cases amputation of the wing tip is required. Another common site of self-trauma is the keel. Birds incapable of flight can jump off high perches or the top of the cage when scared. The landing is rough, leading to a 'split keel' as the bird hits the ground. Osteomyelitis is possible in these lesions and surgical treatment is generally indicated.

How should treatment be tailored?

Improving husbandry and treating any specific condition identified is important. Damaged feathers may require removal under anaesthesia (Figure 7) or imping (grafting of donor feathers on to damaged feather shafts). Analgesia is important during the regrowth phase as the bird may become overly pruritic as a large number of follicles all grow at once. Topical treatments may be used but should be limited to products specifically marketed for birds. Topical steroids are generally contraindicated.

What prognosis should I give?

In many chronic cases resolution is difficult and at best the condition is managed. The

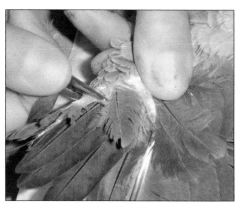

Figure 7: This grey parrot is having severely traumatised feathers removed under anaesthesia to facilitate new growth

owner requires total commitment to the case. It can take many months to improve a bird's condition and these cases require a primary clinician to be in charge of case progression. Consideration should be given to refer to an RCVS specialist for a complete evaluation of the case, diagnostic evaluation and subsequent management. The BSAVA *Manual of Psittacine Birds* provides more details on the diagnosis and treatment of psychological problems and skin disease in parrots. ∎

How to...

Approach the anorexic cat

by Allison German

C ats will often present at the veterinary surgery with loss of appetite. Feeding is a focal interaction for owners with their cats, so refusal of food can be very distressing. Cats also tend to be non-demonstrative when they are ill, so anorexia is often the first presenting sign of a wide number of disease processes (Figure 1). The cat who communally feeds *ad libitum* may have pronounced anorexia and weight loss before a problem is noticed by the owner.

Appetite is controlled by a wide spectrum of neurotransmitters and involves multiple

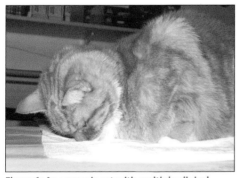

Figure 1: An anorexic cat with multiple clinical problems at the time of presentation, including hepatic lipidosis, glomerulonephropathy, hypokalaemia and thiamine deficiency. Note the neck ventroflexion and weakness. This cat was managed with an oesophagostomy tube and made a steady recovery after 6 weeks of supportive care

centres in the brain. It responds to the action of the autonomic nervous system on peripheral and central receptors. Satiety occurs during the absorptive phase after food ingestion when nutrients become available from the gastrointestinal tract. Hunger occurs during the post-absorptive phase when energy is derived by gluconeogenesis from stored nutrients. The 'hunger' or 'feeding' centre' is located in the lateral hypothalamic nuclei. It is modulated by a 'satiety centre' in the ventromedial hypothalamic nuclei.

Anorexia is defined as a loss or lack of appetite. Anorexia may be **partial** or **complete** and is recognised in two forms:

- **True anorexia** occurs due to a decreased appetite, where the animal has **no interest in food**. This can be secondary to various systemic diseases, pain, neoplasia, neurological diseases reducing cerebral arousal, or cranial trauma. Chemotherapeutics causing nausea and opioids inhibiting the orexigenic (appetite-stimulating) network can also inhibit or reduce appetite. Animals receiving total parenteral nutrition (TPN) may mimic an absorptive state, decreasing hunger and promoting satiety. True anorexia can be subdivided into primary and secondary anorexia. **Primary anorexia** can occur with central neurological disorders affecting the satiety centre. Secondary anorexia occurs due to the influence of a disease process on the cytokine, endocrine or neurological control of appetite. **Secondary anorexia** is the most common cause of anorexia in cats

■ **Pseudoanorexia** occurs secondary to conditions that do not directly affect the appetite centre. Thus, the animal **will still have a central drive to eat but this is overridden by another factor**. Such conditions include: environmental stress (change in housing/family members/ furniture) or psychological distress (fear, anxiety); diet change or poor palatability; anosmia; upper respiratory tract/nasal disease reducing the ability to smell; lower respiratory tract disease causing difficulties in breathing; swallowing dysfunction (lingual, pharyngeal, oesophageal, neurological); and oral pain (tooth root abscess, fractures, periodontal disease, neoplasia, oral foreign body).

More recently, the term **hyporexia** has been introduced, to describe a reduction in rather than a complete loss of appetite.

The **clinical examination** can help define a tighter differential list by: assessment of any physical abnormality; observation of behaviour; assessment of the ability to smell; palpation to investigate pain; assessment of dental health; and evaluation of the respiratory tract. The possibility of systemic disease should be investigated, particularly if the cat has fever, pale mucous membranes, abdominal discomfort, orthopaedic pain, masses, respiratory abnormalities or a cardiac murmur. Ocular examination is important when considering infectious diseases (FeLV, FIV, toxoplasmosis, FIP) and lymphoma.

The **diagnostic work-up** will be directed by the clinical findings. This may entail a complete blood count, biochemistry panel, urinalysis, feline pancreatic lipase immunoreactivity (fPLI), cobalamin and virus screening; more complicated cases may require diagnostic imaging, cytology/ histopathology or more advanced procedures (depending on indication) such as bone marrow biopsy and exploratory coeliotomy. In the majority of cases, the cause of anorexia can be identified through a thorough clinical examination and minimum database. A minimum of packed cell volume, total protein and electrolyte measurements should be repeated once the cat is rehydrated and at regular intervals for monitoring.

Bodyweight and body condition score (BCS) should be recorded on admission and then daily (twice daily for more critical patients). Bodyweight alone does not give information on body condition and will be affected by faecal mass (anorexic cats are often dehydrated and constipated) and effusion volume (the long-term anorexic patient will be protein-deficient and prone to effusion development, particularly following rehydration). BCS is measured on either a 5 point (Edney and Smith, 1986) (Figure 2) or 9 point (Laflamme *et al.*, 1994) scale.

Intervention

Feeding an anorexic patient prevents malnutrition. Malnutrition compromises the immune system, delays healing, decreases hepatic detoxification and increases intestinal permeability. Ensuring adequate nutrition thus enhances recovery rates and reduces morbidity and mortality. Intervention should occur early, once fluid and electrolyte imbalances have been corrected. Current advice is to intervene when weight loss is above 10% (including in obese patients) or when there has been partial (<85% calculated energy requirements) or complete anorexia for more than 3 days. In addition, those patients in a catabolic state (burns, severe inflammation, major surgery or trauma) require nutritional support.

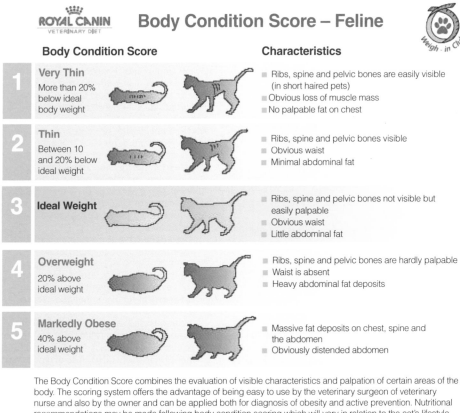

Figure 2: Royal Canin 5 grade body condition scoring system. Modified from Edney and Smith, 1986.
Reproduced with permission from Royal Canin, Crown Pet Foods Ltd., UK

Management is based on identifying and treating the underlying cause. Some general treatment goals follow.

- The patient should be rehydrated and reassessed. Sometimes, once fluid balance has been restored, the cat will eat.
- Electrolytes should be supplemented as indicated from regular monitoring, particularly potassium.

Serum potassium	Amount to add to 250 ml 0.9% NaCl
<2 mmol/l	20 mmol
2–2.5 mmol/l	15 mmol
2.5–3 mmol/l	10 mmol
3–3.5 mmol/l	7 mmol
	5 mmol represents the minimum daily requirement in anorexic cats

- Adequate analgesia, for example sublingual buprenorphine 0.01–0.02 mg/kg q6–12h, should be provided for cats in any painful condition. Recognising pain in cats can sometimes be difficult. If in doubt as to whether a patient would benefit from analgesia, a therapeutic trial can be instituted and behaviour monitored to see whether analgesia results in improvement.
- Cats that have been anorexic for 3 days or more should have a feeding tube placed (see below). Timely nutritional support is essential, to prevent both malnutrition and the development of hepatic lipidosis, which is becoming more widely recognised in the United Kingdom.
- Appetite stimulants should be avoided until the underlying disease has been identified and treated. If a feeding tube is in place there is no need to worry about nutritional status, as the cat is adequately supported without stimulants.
- In nauseous cats with systemic disease, it is best not to tempt the patient to eat until it is stabilised and recovering. Offering food items early in disease can contribute to food aversion and make it more difficult to get the cat eating. Once the cat is feeling better, it will often start eating voluntarily.
- Using feline facial pheromone fraction F3 (Feliway) in the cattery can help reduce anxiety.

Tempting a cat to eat should be done with small food items, which can be warmed to enhance smell. Syringe feeding cats can be stressful and lead to food aversion so, in this author's opinion, is best avoided. Sometimes placing food in the mouth or on the lips can stimulate the cat to eat, but this method is only suitable for cats that are stable and improving, as again this can encourage food aversion and heighten stress. Some cats respond well to food hides; other cats prefer company and encouragement to start eating.

APPETITE STIMULANTS*

- **Cyproheptadine** (Periactin): An antihistamine with serotonin antagonistic effects. 0.1–0.5 mg/kg orally q8–12h. Therapeutic levels are reached after approximately 3 days. Some owners report cats that become anorexic again if the dose is suddenly stopped, so tapering treatment should be considered. Reported side effects include lethargy or agitation.
- **Mirtazapine** (Zispin): An adrenergic and serotonergic anti-depressant that acts as an appetite stimulant and anti-emetic. The soluble form can be administered through feeding tubes, but should not be given orally. 1.875–3.75 mg per cat q72h. Reduce dose by 30% in cats with renal or hepatic compromise. Monitor blood pressure as can cause hypertension.
  - [**Diazepam**: A benzodiazepine used as an appetite stimulant, anticonvulsant, anxiolytic and skeletal muscle relaxant. 0.5–1 mg/kg slow i.v. Use of diazepam is not advised as an appetite stimulant due to the risk of fulminant hepatic necrosis.]
  - [**Prednisolone** is sometimes recommended as an appetite stimulant; however it is not suitable for this purpose. Prednisolone can mask some diseases and make them more difficult to diagnose and treat in the longer term (e.g. lymphoma). Rather than inappropriate use of prednisolone, the underlying disease should be identified and treated and appetite stimulated by other means.]
  - [**Nandrolone** is sometimes given as an appetite stimulant, although there is limited supportive evidence. It is a testosterone with anabolic and anti-catabolic actions. 1–5 mg/kg i.m., s.c. q21days. Maximum dose of 20–25 mg for the cat. It may cause hepatotoxicity.]

ANTI-EMETICS*

- **Maropitant** (Cerenia): 0.5 mg/kg s.c. q24h.
- **Metoclopramide**: 1–2 mg/kg constant rate infusion; protect from light.
- **Mirtazapine**: 3.75 mg per cat every 3 days.
- **Chlorpromazine**: 0.1–0.5 mg/kg s.c. or i.m. q8–12h (for intractable vomiting). May cause sedation and hypotension.

Getting a cat to eat within a hospital environment can be difficult due to the limitations of space and food placement. For anorectic long-stay patients, large cages are preferable. Utilising vertical space in the cage environment with platforms or boxes can help wellbeing, but may not be practical if the cat is on intravenous fluids. Cats prefer wide shallow ceramic bowls that are placed at a distance from their litter tray and from their water. Offering a patient only the appropriate prescription diet may be counterproductive. In the short term, the aim is to get the cat eating; a switch to an appropriate diet can be done at home once the cat is stable.

Feeding tube placement

Feeding tubes enable enteral nutrition, involving use of all or part of the gastrointestinal tract. Enteral nutrition is preferable to parenteral ('intravenous feeding') as enterocytes derive 50% of their nutrients directly from the intestinal lumen. If the enterocytes are starved, the intestinal mucosa becomes hypoplastic and hypofunctional, with increased permeability. Furthermore, parenteral nutrition is technically challenging, requires good asepsis and should be reserved for malabsorption syndromes, acute severe pancreatitis and severe persistent vomiting.

Practically, enteral nutrition is suitable in most situations and can be achieved in a number of ways. When choosing the method of enteral nutrition delivery, the site of tube placement should depend on the anticipated duration of support and the site of the disease (tubes should be placed distal to the problem area).

Short-term support

- **Naso-oesophageal (NO) tube (Figure 3)**. Use for patients without oral, nasal, pharyngeal or oesophageal disease and that are not vomiting. The advantages are that placement of an NO tube is quick and

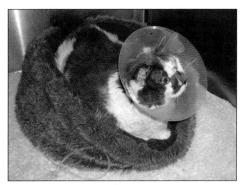

Figure 3: Naso-oesophageal tube in a cat diagnosed with multifocal alimentary lymphoma, FIV infection and hepatic lipidosis. Naso-oesophageal tubes can be used for short-term support, as in this case, for a few days at home before euthanasia

easy, and does not require anaesthesia or sedation in most cases. However, NO tubes are only suitable for a short duration of use, diet choice is limited by what can pass through the narrow tube diameter, and some cats do not tolerate the positioning of the tube around their face.

Longer-term support

- **Oesophagostomy tube (Figure 4)**. Very useful and well tolerated in cats. Suitable for cats with oral and nasal disease but not

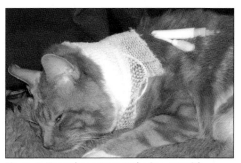

Figure 4: Oesophagostomy tube in a cat with vestibular disease, secondary to polyp surgery and total bulla osteotomy. Foley catheters can be used if there are no appropriate oesophagostomy tubes available

those with vomiting or oesophageal disease. A wide-bore tube can be used, making feeding easier. The tube is comfortably bandaged at the neck and does not affect the whiskers or grooming as much as the naso-oesophageal tube.

- **Gastrostomy tubes** are most practical for long-term feeding (such as in hepatic lipidosis) and are suitable for prolonged use (12 months or more). Tubes can be placed surgically or endoscopically (PEG). Gastrostomy tubes are contraindicated in gastroduodenal disorders, especially where persistent vomiting is present.
- **Jejunostomy/enterostomy tubes (Figure 5)** are rarely indicated and require placement by an experienced surgeon. Consider use in gastric disorders where small intestinal function remains normal. As the stomach is bypassed, food is not mixed and stored appropriately, so the patient is more prone to complications such as vomiting, diarrhoea and abdominal pain. Similarly, continuous infusions are required to trickle food into the intestine.

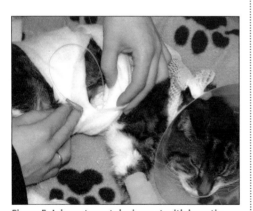

Figure 5: Jejunostomy tube in a cat with hepatic lipidosis, vomiting and severe malnutrition. The tube attaches to a syringe driver for continuous food infusion. These tubes require intensive management. This cat was supported for 4 weeks until it started eating voluntarily

Feeding guidelines

How much should I feed?

Food requirements are based on energy, as this is the most important factor. Calculation of energy requirements is controversial in both human and veterinary patients. For critical care patients, the daily requirements are best calculated from estimated resting energy requirement (RER). The main controversy involves how much this RER differs in critical illness. Correction factors used to be applied, but there is no validation for these factors. A better approach is to work with RER and monitor the patient's weight and body condition and adjust the intake as necessary. For cats that have not fed for a prolonged period, slowly introduce feeding over a 3-day period, starting at 1/3 RER divided into multiple small meals. This is particularly important in hepatic lipidosis and severe malnutrition cases, to help avoid refeeding syndrome (where metabolic and fluid disturbances occur within 4 days of reinstituting feeding).

OPTIONS FOR CALCULATING RER
RER (kcal) = 70 x (current bodyweight in kilograms)$^{0.75}$ OR   For animals >5 kg: RER(kcal) = 30 x BW_{kg} +70   1 kJ = 4.185 kcal

What diet do I choose?

Use any tasty food to get the cat interested initially. Ask the owner for the cat's preferences. For tube feeding, it is best to use a commercial diet as these will satisfy energy, protein and micronutrient requirements. A high-energy, high-protein, easily digestible diet is recommended, although this may be manipulated depending on the underlying disease. Liquid enteral diets (such as Fortol) are best for small-diameter feeding tubes. Larger-bore tubes can carry liquidised prescription diets. As enteral diets are low residue, there will be little faecal matter produced, although the cat should be monitored closely and hydration kept optimal to ensure against constipation.

How long should I tube feed?

- Patients should be supported until their voluntary intake is >85% of maintenance requirements.
- Gastrostomy and enterostomy tubes must remain in place for at least 7–10 days to allow a seal to form with the abdominal wall.

- Oesophagostomy and gastrostomy tubes can be managed on an out-patient basis, allowing owners to feed their cat at home. This is particularly useful for cats with hepatic lipidosis, chronic kidney disease or those with severe rostral trauma. ■

*Editor's note: Readers are reminded that not all drugs described are authorized for use in this species. Veterinary surgeons should adhere to the prescribing cascade when choosing drugs for use 'off licence'.

How to...
Utilise blood products
in small animals

by Gillian Gibson

Blood component therapy

Initial blood collection, using a suitable anticoagulant and collection system, yields whole blood containing red blood cells (RBCs), white blood cells (WBCs) and platelets suspended in the liquid plasma portion. Historically whole blood has been most often administered to small animal patients, often collected at the time of need. However, blood components can be separated using variable-speed temperature-controlled centrifuges, according to standard blood banking protocols.

Advantages of component therapy include:

■ Specific replacement therapy – only giving the patient what is needed and reducing the risk of transfusion reactions
■ One unit of donated blood can be used to help more than one patient
■ Maximises the storage life of blood products.

The production of components is limited by the availability of specialist equipment and skills (e.g. referral hospitals with in-house blood banks) but, following recent legislative changes, licensed UK pet blood banks are now able to provide components for more widespread use.

The components of whole blood most often used in veterinary transfusion medicine are RBCs and plasma products. RBCs contain haemoglobin, which is necessary for oxygen transport from the lungs to the rest of the body. RBC transfusions provide the recipient with an additional red cell mass and consequently increased oxygen-carrying capacity. Plasma products are a source of coagulation factors and various plasma proteins that may be used to replace them in states of deficiency. Platelet products are not readily available and will not be discussed here. Figure 1 summarises the properties and uses of different blood products.

Blood product preparation

To prevent microbial contamination of any of the component products, a closed collection system must be used, and the transfer of the components from the collection bag to the individual satellite storage bags is achieved by a system of integrated tubing (Figure 2). In these closed systems there is no exposure of the collection bag or its contents to air prior to administration, other than when the needle is uncapped to perform venepuncture at collection.

The collection and processing of blood components following appropriate guidelines provides a supply of products with little risk of microbial contamination and maximal storage

Blood component	Constituents/ properties	Storage	Indications
Red blood cell products			
Fresh whole blood (FWB)	RBCs, platelets, coagulation factors and plasma proteins all present and functional	Must be used within 8 hours of collection	Thrombocytopenia or thrombocytopathia causing severe uncontrolled or life-threatening haemorrhage; anaemia with concurrent coagulopathy
Stored whole blood (SWB)	RBCs and plasma proteins, but not functional platelets or coagulation factors	Stored at 1–6°C for approximately 28 days; depends on anticoagulant used	Anaemia with concurrent hypoproteinaemia
Packed red blood cells (PRBCs)	Red blood cells	RBCs separated from plasma, stored at 1–6°C for 20 days; or extended to 35 days with use of appropriate preservative	Clinically symptomatic euvolaemic anaemia (e.g. IMHA, non-regenerative anaemia)
Plasma products			
Fresh frozen plasma (FFP)	All plasma coagulation factors, including labile coagulation factors V and VIII, and plasma proteins	Separated from PRBCs and frozen within 8 hours of collection; stored at −20°C for up to 1 year*	Acquired or inherited coagulopathies (e.g. inherited factor deficiencies, vitamin K deficiency, vitamin K antagonist intoxication, DIC, severe liver disease)
Stored frozen plasma	Some vitamin K dependent factors, albumin and globulin	FFP >1 year of age, or plasma not frozen within 8 hours, or FFP that has been thawed and refrozen. Many useful clotting factors and anti-inflammatory proteins will have been lost. Stored at −20°C for 5 years*	Vitamin K deficiency, vitamin K antagonist intoxication, hypoproteinaemia (colloidal support)
Cryoprecipitate (CPP)	von Willebrand factor, factor VIII, factor XIII, fibrinogen and fibronectin	Extracted from FFP. Stored at −20°C for up to 1 year*	Replacement therapy for deficiencies of von Willebrand factor, factor VIII (haemophilia A) or fibrinogen
Cryosupernatant/ Cryo-poor plasma	Many clotting factors, including vitamin K-dependent factors II, VII, IX and X, other anticoagulant and fibrinolytic factors, albumin and globulin	Produced from a unit of FFP by separation from CPP. Stored at −20°C for up to 1 year*	Coagulopathies or hypoproteinaemias not requiring supplementation of the CPP components

Figure 1: Summary of blood component properties, storage requirements and indications for use. (*from date of collection)

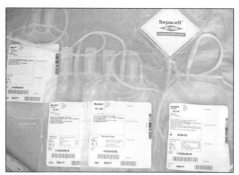

Figure 2: Closed collection system used for blood component processing

times. Plasma is separated from the RBCs by centrifugation; the red cells separate to the bottom of the collection unit and the plasma can be removed and stored separately (Figure 3). The prepared units are sealed with a handheld clip sealer or heat sealer prior to storage.

If blood is collected into an open system, one in which there is one or more additional sites of potential bacterial contamination during blood collection or processing, all components must be used within 24 hours. Using syringes with added anticoagulant to collect blood is an example of an open system.

Storage of blood products

RBCs are refrigerated
- Temperature is maintained at 1–6°C, checked daily with a refrigerator thermometer.
- A dedicated household refrigerator is often suitable, as long as there is low in and out traffic (e.g. it is not used for storing frequently used products such as vaccinations).
- Store upright.

Plasma products are frozen
- Temperature is maintained at –20°C or below, checked daily with a thermometer to ensure maintenance of adequate storage conditions.
- A dedicated household freezer may suffice, but the temperature within the freezer may vary depending on the storage compartment and it is therefore important to check the temperature in each compartment.
- When the plasma is still liquid, an elastic band is placed around the middle of the bag to create an indentation ('waist') during freezing. The band is removed once the unit is frozen hard. Loss of this waist in a stored frozen plasma unit suggests that the unit

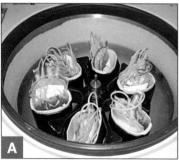
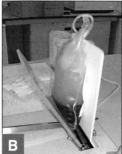
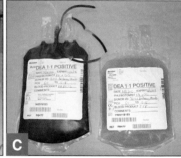

Figure 3: Separation of plasma and PRBCs. (A) Collection bags in a specialised variable-speed temperature-controlled centrifuge. (B) Following centrifugation, the plasma component is gently separated from the RBCs by gentle pressure. The plasma is transferred to a separate empty storage bag that is connected to the original blood collection bag by integral tubing. (C) Plasma and PRBCs are stored separately and may be used for different patients

has thawed and refrozen, which could compromise the plasma quality.
- Care should be taken not to drop the frozen plasma units as they are vulnerable to cracking.

Choosing the appropriate blood product for the patient

RBC products

RBC products may be indicated in any anaemic patient, regardless of the cause of anaemia (haemorrhage, haemolysis or impaired erythropoiesis) if they will benefit from an additional red cell mass and hence increased oxygen-carrying capacity.

There is no precise packed cell volume (PCV) below which RBC transfusion should be administered. Consideration of a number of factors, including volume status, rate of onset of anaemia, ongoing losses and patient clinical condition, must influence the decision to transfuse. General guidelines are offered below.

PCV

- Almost all patients with a PCV ≤12% would benefit from a transfusion.
- Any patient with a PCV ≤20% should be considered a transfusion candidate.
- Some patients with a PCV >20% may benefit from an RBC transfusion (e.g. acute haemorrhage with ongoing blood loss).
- Chronic anaemia is typically better tolerated than acute anaemia due to compensatory mechanisms.

Volume status

- Animals with a reduced red cell mass but a normal intravascular volume (euvolaemic anaemia) may benefit from an RBC transfusion but not require the volume of accompanying plasma; therefore a PRBCs transfusion would be recommended.

Examples would be animals with immune-mediated haemolytic anaemia (IMHA) or a non-regenerative anaemia.
- In animals with volume depletion as a consequence of acute haemorrhage (hypovolaemic anaemia), a whole blood transfusion or the combination of appropriate components (e.g. PRBCs plus plasma) would be recommended.

Clinical signs

Clinical signs are the most important factor in deciding when to administer an RBC transfusion. The following signs suggest that the patient may benefit from additional oxygen-carrying support:

- Tachypnoea
- Tachycardia
- Bounding or poor peripheral pulses
- Pallor
- Collapse
- Lethargy or weakness
- Decreased appetite.

Plasma products

Plasma products are most commonly used to treat inherited or acquired coagulopathies. Plasma is of little benefit in hypoproteinaemic patients, and other modes of therapy (synthetic colloids, nutritional support) are recommended.

Administration of blood products

Blood types are determined by species-specific inherited cell surface antigens. Incompatibility between species or individuals may result in transfusion reactions or neonatal isoerythrolysis. A more in-depth discussion regarding blood types and cross-matching may be found in the BSAVA Manual of Canine and Feline Emergency and Critical Care, 2nd edn. However, these general guidelines should be followed:

Canine

- Blood type of donor and recipient should be assessed prior to transfusion.
- If it is not possible to type the recipient, ideally a DEA 1.1-negative donor should be used.
- DEA 1.1-negative recipients should only receive DEA 1.1-negative RBCs.
- DEA 1.1-positive recipients may receive either DEA 1.1-negative or DEA 1.1-positive RBCs.

Feline

- Incompatibility transfusion reactions can be fatal.
- Blood type of donor and recipient must **ALWAYS** be assessed prior to transfusion.
- Type A cats should *only* receive type A blood or plasma.
- Type B cats should *only* receive type B blood or plasma.
- Type AB cats may receive either type AB (preferable) or type A (acceptable) blood and ideally only type AB plasma.

Cross-match recommendations

Cross-matching should be carried out:

- Prior to first transfusion in cats
- When the recipient has previously been transfused (>4 days prior)
- When there is history of a transfusion reaction
- If the patient's transfusion history is unknown.

Figure 4 provides a description of an abbreviated in-house slide cross-match method that may be used in an emergency situation if laboratory services are not available.

Route of administration

- Blood products are usually administered intravenously.

---

1. Collect blood into an EDTA tube from recipient and donor.
2. Centrifuge tubes to settle the RBCs, remove the supernatant and transfer to a clean, labelled glass or plastic tube.
3. For each donor prepare 3 slides labelled as major, minor and recipient control.
4. Place 1 drop of RBCs and 2 drops of plasma on to each slide according to the following:
   - Major cross-match = donor RBCs + recipient plasma
   - Minor cross-match = recipient RBCs + donor plasma
   - Recipient control = recipient RBCs + recipient plasma.
5. Gently rock the slides to mix the plasma and red cells and examine for haemagglutination after 1–5 minutes (presence of agglutination indicates incompatibility); recipient control agglutination will invalidate results.

Figure 4: Abbreviated slide cross-match procedure

- If venous access is not possible (e.g. neonatal patient) the intraosseous route may be used.
- Blood products should not be given intraperitoneally.

Filter

An in-line filter is required for all products with a maximum size of 170–260 µm; this is usually incorporated within a standard blood infusion set.

- Filtration removes any small blood clots and particles that could be harmful if infused into the recipient.
- Microaggregate filters of 18–40 µm are available and can be placed in line when infusing small volumes of product or blood collected in syringes (Figure 5).

Dose

The amount of product to be given greatly depends on the product type, indication for administration, and desired response in the patient. A useful formula to calculate the

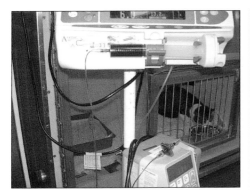

Figure 5: Example of a paediatric blood filter that may be used in line with small blood transfusions

amount of whole blood required for transfusion is noted in Figure 6. In general most patients will receive:

- Whole blood: 10–22 ml/kg
- PRBCs or FFP: 6–12 ml/kg.

Volume (ml) =

85 (dog) or 60 (cat) x bodyweight (kg) x
[(desired PCV – actual PCV) / donor PCV]

Figure 6: Formula for calculating the volume of whole blood required for transfusion

Product quality inspection

- Stored RBC products should be examined for any discoloration of the cells or suspension fluid (e.g. brown or purple) and the presence of clots, as these changes may indicate bacterial contamination, haemolysis or other storage lesions.
- Plasma bags should be examined for evidence of thawing and refreezing (disappearance of the waist), and cracking or tearing of the bag.

Preparation

- Stored RBC products need not be warmed prior to use, unless they are being given to very small animals or neonates.

- PRBCs stored without an added preservative may be resuspended or co-administered with 100 ml of physiological saline to decrease viscosity and improve flow (Figure 7).
- Frozen plasma products are gently thawed in a warm water bath. The plasma bag should be placed inside a sealed plastic bag prior to immersing in the water bath to protect the injection ports from possible microbial contamination.

Method and rate of administration

- Blood products are most commonly infused by gravity flow, although infusion pumps validated for the administration of products may also be used (Figure 7).

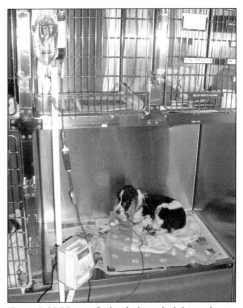

Figure 7: PRBC transfusion being administered to a dog. Note the use of a specialised blood infusion set that allows co-administration of physiological saline. When a preservative has been added to the PRBCs prior to storage, co-administration with saline is not required. An intravenous fluid pump validated for the administration of red cells is being used in this case

- Small volumes (<100 ml) are often delivered by syringe driver or slow, intermittent, small-volume bolus injections (see Figure 5).
- Animals should not receive any food or medications during a transfusion.
- To prevent incompatibility reactions, only 0.9% saline may be simultaneously administered through the same catheter as a blood product.
- All infusions should be completed within 4 hours.

The **rate** of administration is dependent on the cardiovascular status of the patient, and care should be taken when infusing patients with risk of volume overload (e.g. cardiovascular disease, renal failure).

- During the first 20 minutes use an infusion rate of 0.25–1.0 ml/kg/h.
- If the transfusion is well tolerated, the rate is increased to deliver the remaining product over 4 hours.
- NOTE: If the patient is at risk of volume overload, do not exceed 3–4 ml/kg/h.

Monitoring the transfusion patient

The patient's vital signs should be measured prior to (baseline) and every 15–30 minutes during, as well as 1, 12 and 24 hours following the transfusion. These include:

- Attitude
- Rectal temperature
- Pulse rate and quality
- Respiratory rate and character
- Mucous membrane colour and capillary refill time.

Any change in plasma or urine colour indicative of haemolysis may be significant and should be noted. Blood samples to reassess PCV or clotting times are usually obtained at some time point after completion of the transfusion, unless deterioration of the patient requires otherwise. Repeating these

parameters provides an assessment of efficacy as well as helping to determine whether a further transfusion is required.

Transfusion reactions

Any undesired side effect noted as a consequence of a blood product transfusion is considered a transfusion reaction. Reactions are classified as immunological, non-immunological and delayed. Prompt recognition and treatment of potential adverse transfusion reactions is essential.

RBC incompatibility reactions (immunological) may cause acute haemolysis and can be life-threatening.

Signs may include:

- Pyrexia
- Tachycardia
- Tachypnoea
- Weakness
- Salivation/vomiting
- Diarrhoea
- Haemoglobinaemia
- Haemoglobinuria.

Non-haemolytic immunological reactions are acute allergic/anaphylactic reactions, signs of which include:

- Oedema
- Erythema
- Pruritus
- Urticaria
- Vomiting
- Dyspnoea.

Non-immunological transfusion reactions may often be avoided by rigorous donor screening and adherence to blood banking protocols. Such reactions include:

- Anaphylactoid (often a consequence of rapid infusion rate)
- Volume overload

- Transmission of infectious disease
- Hypocalcaemia (secondary to excessive citrate anticoagulant)
- Polycythaemia and hyperproteinaemia (excessive volume of blood product administered)
- Dilutional coagulopathy
- Microbial contamination (signs may be similar to acute haemolytic reaction)
- Hyperkalaemia, acidosis, hyperammonaemia, hypophosphataemia (storage lesions)
- Air embolus.

Treatment of acute transfusion reactions

1. **Stop transfusion:**
   a. In case of allergic/anaphylactic reaction, if reaction subsides may restart transfusion at 25–50% of previous rate
   b. If signs of acute haemolytic reaction, do not continue with transfusion.
2. Donor and recipient blood type, product type and expiration date should be confirmed, and a cross-match may be performed (if not done prior to transfusion).
3. Treat any clinical signs of shock, including fluid therapy.
4. Antihistamines:
   a. Chlorpheniramine: maximum recommended dose 0.5 mg/kg q12h (dogs and cats)
      i. Dogs: small to medium, 2.5–5 mg/dog i.m. q12h
      ii. Dogs: medium to large, 5–10 mg/dog i.m. q12h
      iii. Cats: 2–4 mg/cat orally q12h.
   b. Diphenhydramine 1–2 mg/kg i.m. q12h (dogs and cats).
4. Corticosteroids: Dexamethasone 0.5–1.0 mg/kg i.v.
5. Monitor for development of fluid overload.
6. Monitor for development of hypotension or oliguria.

7. Administer H2 blockers, colloids, dopamine and/or aminophylline as needed.
8. Samples of both donor and recipient blood should be evaluated for haemolysis, and saved for microbial culture and infectious disease testing if required.
9. Broad-spectrum antibiotics may be administered if bacterial contamination is suspected.

Delayed haemolytic reactions may be recognised by an unexpected decline in the PCV or by jaundice developing at some time 2–21 days post-transfusion. These often do not require any specific therapy.

Finally

It is important to note on the patient's file that it has received a blood product transfusion, and to make the owner aware that this information should be passed along to other veterinary surgeons that may be caring for their pet in the future. ■

REGISTERS AND BANKS

The Animal Blood Register (**www.animalbloodregister.com**) is a national donor database for UK pets, and Pet Blood Bank (**www.petbloodbankuk.org**) is a not for profit charitable organisation offering a full range of transfusion products. These organisations give veterinary surgeons in practice previously unattainable access to lists of matched donors and to blood products respectively. This freedom from the necessity for individual practices to health screen and cross-match local donors and be proficient in blood collection allows the use of blood products more widely than has previously been possible.

See the *BSAVA Manual of Canine and Feline Haematology and Transfusion Medicine* and *BSAVA Manual of Canine and Feline Emergency and Critical Care* for useful information.

How to...
Unravel the mystery of
feline alimentary lymphoma

by Mark Goodfellow

L ymphoma is the most common cancer in the cat, comprising a heterogeneous group of neoplasms that arise from the lymphoreticular cells of the lymph nodes, spleen, bone marrow and elsewhere in the body. Classically lymphoma was regarded as a disease of the young feline leukaemia virus (FeLV)-positive cat but, as understanding of this disease has grown and the prevalence of FeLV has reduced, a marked change in signalment, presentation and aetiopathogenesis of lymphoma in cats has come to be recognised.

FeLV as a cause of lymphoma in the 1960s to 1980s

Feline leukaemia virus was the most common cause of haemopoietic tumours of the cat during the 1960s–1980s, when 60–70% of feline lymphoma cases were associated with FeLV antigenaemia. At this time the mean age of cats diagnosed with lymphoma was 2–5 years and the most common presentations were the (T cell) mediastinal and/or multicentric forms of the disease.

Development of lymphoma is a direct consequence of FeLV infection. The virus 'hijacks' the cellular organelles and, following random insertion of viral DNA (provirus) into host DNA, new virus particles are budded from the cell membrane. After initial infection, FeLV spreads to the bone marrow and infects

haemopoietic stem cells. Provirus is randomly inserted into the host DNA. An insertion of viral DNA next to a host gene (most commonly *myc*) that codes for cellular proliferation may ultimately lead to neoplasia. The association with FeLV antigenaemia is so strong that it has been suggested that cats infected with FeLV are 60 times more likely to develop lymphoma than are their FeLV-negative counterparts. Overall a quarter of FeLV-positive cats are expected to develop lymphoma during their lifetime.

Why is lymphoma more common nowadays when we vaccinate for FeLV?

Over the past 20–30 years a profound change has occurred in viral status, presentation, signalment and anatomical sites affected by lymphoma in cats. This change appears to coincide temporally with the widespread use of FeLV diagnostic assays, FeLV vaccination and other preventive regimes associated with a reduction in the prevalence of FeLV infection in the feline population.

So perhaps it is not unexpected that a decline in the prevalence of FeLV has been mirrored by a decline in prevalence of FeLV-associated lymphoma. Overall, however, the prevalence of feline lymphoma appears to be increasing, possibly due to an increase in our ability to identify affected cats and/or due to an increase in the relative frequency of the abdominal forms. At present it is unclear which of these is most likely or if it is a combination.

It should be noted that use of sensitive diagnostic techniques such as PCR have clouded the picture somewhat. We now know that cats that have been infected with FeLV at some point during their lifetime will have FeLV proviral DNA incorporated into their genome, and will be positive on PCR, even if they are FeLV-negative on ELISA (i.e. they are not antigenaemic). Whether subsequent development of lymphoma later in life is as a result of this provirus is unclear. But, given that PCR demonstrated FeLV provirus in 25% of cats with intestinal lymphoma that were seronegative for FeLV antigen by ELISA, the virus may still be playing an important, if hidden, role in the pathogenesis of feline lymphoma.

There is a growing body of evidence that lymphoma may be associated with, or the endpoint of, chronic inflammation. Serial histological documentation of worsening inflammatory bowel disease (IBD) in cases that subsequently develop intestinal lymphoma supports this hypothesis as does IBD in other regions of the gut in cats diagnosed with alimentary lymphoma.

Finally, the role of environmental factors is beginning to be recognised. Exposure to cigarette smoke is a risk factor for developing lymphoma in humans and the same appears to be true in cats. Cats exposed to environmental tobacco smoke are 2.4 times more likely to develop lymphoma than their smoke-free counterparts. If they have been exposed to tobacco smoke for >5 years, the risk increases to 3.2 times. Exposed cats are also more likely to develop the alimentary form of the disease. Thus, it may be that human lifestyle has not only resulted in disease in our pet cats but also has contributed to the changed pattern of lymphoma presentation over the past 30 years.

Presentation of the cat with lymphoma

The cohort of affected animals now differs markedly from those affected in the 'FeLV era': the median age of cats diagnosed with lymphoma is now 11 years and only a minority (8–14%) of these older cats are FeLV-positive. Whilst all anatomical forms of lymphoma still occur, the alimentary form is by far the most common.

The anatomical forms traditionally associated with FeLV antigenaemia, such as mediastinal lymphoma, still occur, and in a distinct group of young FeLV-positive individuals the traditional presentations are still most common, but this group is clearly separate from the older affected majority.

Given that alimentary lymphoma is the most prevalent form and that its treatment is (unlike other feline lymphoma) tailored specifically to the histological grade, the remainder of this article will deal with this presentation alone. However, the majority of points regarding investigation and therapy remain valid, irrespective of the site of the disease.

Alimentary lymphoma – a disease of the older cat

As noted above, gastrointestinal lymphoma has become the most common anatomical presentation (32–72%) and occurs most frequently in older (median 11 years) FeLV-negative cats. The disease usually results in segmental or generalized thickening of the small intestine. The stomach, caecum and colon are rarely affected, but lymphoma is still the most common gastric tumour in cats. In most cats with intestinal lymphoma, the mesenteric lymph nodes are involved. No breed predilection has been identified. As discussed above, cats with intestinal lymphoma have a low incidence of FeLV antigenaemia but a role for prior FeLV infection may be suggested by a positive PCR result.

Presentation

Cats with alimentary lymphoma usually present with a chronic history of anorexia and weight loss of several months' duration. Vomiting and diarrhoea are present in less than half of cases and other uncommon clinical signs include lethargy, weakness, polydipsia, polyuria, pica, and abdominal swelling. Clinical examination may reveal thickened bowel loops or an abdominal mass, but will yield normal results in many cats with alimentary lymphoma.

Diagnostic clues

The most common clincopathological finding is hypoalbuminaemia, which occurs in approximately half of patients. Other noteworthy abnormalities include anaemia (non-regenerative or regenerative), elevation in liver enzymes and hypocobalaminaemia. Elevations in liver enzymes are suggestive of neoplastic lymphoid infiltration into the hepatic parenchyma although normal liver enzyme concentrations do not exclude this possibility. As in other circumstances, hypocobalamin-aemia results from distal small intestinal disease. As in all forms of feline lymphoma, and in contrast to canine lymphoma, hypercalcaemia is rare.

Unfortunately abdominal radiography often yields normal or non-specific findings, such as a reduction in intra-abdominal contrast, dilation of small intestinal lumen or the presence of an ill-defined soft tissue opacity which might be a mass. In contrast, abdominal ultrasonography is very useful and may identify mesenteric lymphadenopathy, a thickened intestinal wall (Figures 1 and 2), disruption of intestinal wall architecture and bowel hypomotility or ileus. These ultrasonographic features are not unique to lymphoma but can be distinct from those seen in inflammatory bowel disease (in which intestinal wall layering is usually preserved), or intestinal adenocarcinoma (in which focal

eccentric intestinal luminal narrowing usually occurs without associated lymphadenopathy). Unfortunately normal ultrasonographic findings do not rule out a diagnosis of alimentary lymphoma.

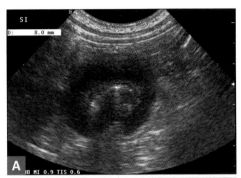

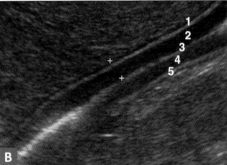

Figure 1: (A) Transverse ultrasonogram showing a thickened loop of intestine with complete loss of layering. This appearance is typical of, but not specific for, intestinal lymphoma.
(B) Ultrasonographic appearance of the normal small intestinal wall. 1 = lumen (containing mucus); 2 = mucosa; 3 = submucosa; 4 = muscularis; 5 = serosa. Reproduced from *BSAVA Manual of Canine and Feline Abdominal Imaging*

Species	Duodenum	Remainder of small intestine
Cat	2.4 ± 0.51 mm (range 1.3–3.8 mm)	2.09 ± 0.37 mm (range 1.6–3.6 mm)

Figure 2: Normal small intestinal widths in the cat. (Newell *et al.*, 1999)

To biopsy or not to biopsy? That is the question

Cytological examination of fine needle aspirates of mesenteric lymph nodes or thickened intestinal wall, retrieved under ultrasound guidance, can be sufficient to achieve a diagnosis particularly of lymphoblastic lymphoma. However, the treatment choices and prognosis for cats with alimentary lymphoma are dependent on tumour grade. Grading, and diagnosis, particularly of lymphocytic lymphoma, is achieved by histopathological examination of a biopsy specimen. This may be procured by endoscopy or laparotomy.

Endoscopy (Figure 3) has the obvious advantages of being non-invasive and requiring no post-procedure convalescence, but samples obtained are superficial and there is a risk of missing submucosal (often high-grade) disease. Furthermore, an endoscope is unable to reach the jejunum and the majority of the ileum, where most lymphoma lesions are located.

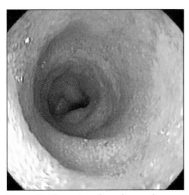

Figure 3: Alimentary lymphoma does not have a pathognomonic appearance, so biopsy is required to achieve a diagnosis and grade the disease

Laparotomy (Figure 4) has the advantage of allowing full-thickness intestinal biopsy and, in addition, allows specimens of the liver, mesenteric lymph nodes and pancreas to be

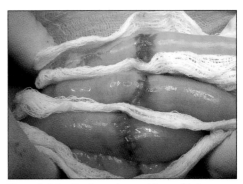

Figure 4: Intestine loops layered for multiple intestinal biopsy, 'stack and snip'. Biopsy samples have been taken from the duodenum, jejunum and ileum

obtained, even in the absence of gross lesions. Laparotomy has the disadvantage that chemotherapy must be delayed for 10–14 days after surgery to prevent dehiscence or delays in wound healing. It is noteworthy that attempted resection of apparently focal alimentary lymphoma has not been correlated with increased or decreased survival times.

In general, tumour stage does not appear to be predictive of outcome in cats with lymphoma. The cost and invasiveness of complete staging should therefore be weighed against the benefit of the additional information gained. However, it should be remembered that these older patients may have comorbidities that can influence prognosis and treatment choices. Thus, as a minimum, all patients in which lymphoma has been confirmed should have had a complete haematology, serum biochemistry and urinalysis profile performed, in addition to determination of FeLV and FIV status prior to undertaking definitive lymphoma treatment.

Treatment choice is dictated by the histological findings

Feline alimentary lymphoma is categorised histologically into one of three grades: low-grade (lymphocytic or small cell), intermediate or high-grade (lymphoblastic or large cell). This classification guides treatment choices and is indicative of prognosis. As discussed above, inflammatory bowel disease may be a precursor to intestinal lymphoma and, on occasion, immunohistochemical stains are required to differentiate the two. This distinction is of profound clinical and prognostic relevance, as cats with inflammatory bowel disease may have a significantly better prognosis than those with alimentary lymphoma if treated appropriately.

Treatment protocols are distinct for the different forms of feline alimentary lymphoma. **High-grade** (lymphoblastic, immunoblastic or large cell) lymphoma is treated with conventional CHOP- or COP-based protocols. The COP protocol (cyclophosphamide, vincristine and prednisolone) is often associated with adverse gastrointestinal effects (vomiting, diarrhoea, anorexia) but these are usually manageable with supportive treatment. Both vincristine and cyclophosphamide are myelosuppressive and thus haematology must be performed weekly initially and treatment withheld if neutropenia develops. Thankfully cyclophosphamide rarely causes sterile haemorrhagic cystitis in cats.

Addition of doxorubicin to create a CHOP protocol is of questionable benefit in the case of high-grade feline alimentary lymphoma. Based on a small number of studies, average remission rates are no better than using a COP-type protocol but those cats who do respond appear to survive longer. Doxorubicin, whilst not cardiotoxic to cats, is profoundly nephrotoxic and its use necessitates frequent monitoring of renal function; furthermore, it is often associated with the adverse effects documented above. At present we are unable to identify those cats that are more likely to benefit from the addition of doxorubicin to their cytotoxic regime and the decision of whether to add this drug is made on a case-by-case basis. Overall, only 20–30% of these patients achieve full remission, and median survival times are 2–3 months only.

Low-grade, lymphocytic alimentary lymphoma has a good prognosis, with 60–70% of cats achieving complete remission and median survival time of 17–25 months. Those cats that achieve complete remission may live considerably longer than this median survival. Given the more slowly progressive nature of their disease a more tempered cytotoxic protocol is appropriate based on chlorambucil, an alkylating agent, and prednisolone. Adverse reactions to chlorambucil are rare but can include gastrointestinal toxicity, myelosuppression and hepatotoxicity. Haematology and serum biochemistry should be performed weekly for the first month of treatment and every 3 months thereafter.

Intermediate-grade intestinal lymphoma is treated with a COP- or CHOP-type protocol. In these patients addition of doxorubicin may be of benefit, but this is based on factors above and beyond survival advantage alone (expense, toxicity and clinician experience). Unfortunately, apart from histological grade there are few other prognostic indicators to help the clinician and client to make treatment choices. Initial response to treatment is correlated with overall survival and this suggests that until our understanding of prognostication of this disease improves, a treatment trial should be considered in all cats.

Supportive care plays a vital role in maintenance of quality of life when treating alimentary lymphoma. Oral appetite stimulants such as cyproheptadine can be useful in increasing voluntary food intake. As previously mentioned, these patients may benefit from cobalamin supplementation as deficiency results in anorexia. Anti-emetics may aid control of nausea and vomiting, which may result from the disease itself or as a consequence of therapy.

What does the future hold?

In summary, the pattern of lymphoma in cats has changed over the past three decades, with the majority of patients now presenting in older age with previously uncommon anatomical forms unrelated to FeLV antigenaemia. One such form, alimentary lymphoma is now the most common presenting form of lymphoma and its histological grade is strongly predictive of response to treatment and prognosis. This separation of lymphoma into subcategories with differing behaviours, treatments and prognosis is likely to become the norm as we better understand this complex and diverse disease. No longer does one protocol or prognosis suit all and 'personalised' treatment protocols, devised on a case-by-case basis, as are the aim of human oncology practice, are within the grasp of the veterinary surgeon.

Acknowledgements

This article previously appeared in an alternate form in Bristol Vet School's *Feline Update* and is reprinted and modified with their permission. ◼

SELECTED CHEMOTHERAPY PROTOCOLS USED BY THE AUTHOR FOR CATS WITH ALIMENTARY LYMPHOMA

CHOP protocol

- Cyclophosphamide* 200 mg/m^2 i.v./p.o., weeks 2, 7, 13, 21
- Vincristine (Oncovin) 0.7 mg/m^2 i.v., weeks 1, 3, 6, 8, 11, 15, 19, 23
- Prednisolone 2 mg/kg p.o. q24h for 28 days; then 1 mg/kg p.o. q48h until relapse or adverse steroid effects, in which case taper dose and discontinue
- Doxorubicin 25 mg/m^2 i.v., weeks 4, 9, 17, 23

COP protocol

- Cyclophosphamide* 300 mg/m^2 i.v./p.o. q21days
- Vincristine (Oncovin) 0.75 mg/m^2 i.v. q7days for 4 weeks then every third week
- Prednisolone 2 mg/kg p.o. q24h for 1 week; then 5 mg p.o. q48h until relapse or adverse steroid effects, in which case taper dose and discontinue

Chlorambucil and prednisolone protocol (for lymphocytic alimentary lymphoma (low grade) only)

- Chlorambucil 2 mg/cat p.o. q48–72h
- Prednisolone 10 mg/cat/day p.o. q24h until relapse or adverse steroid effects, in which case taper dose and discontinue

*25 mg cyclophosphamide tablets suitable for cats are available. Seek advice from the VMD

There are various COP- and CHOP-style protocols and the reader is advised always to seek advice from a veterinary oncologist prior to undertaking treatment with an unfamiliar protocol. Doxorubicin and vincristine are vesicants and must be delivered through an intravenous cannula placed cleanly on the first attempt

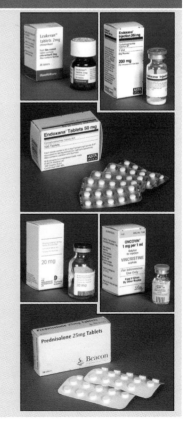

How to…
Use a **direct ophthalmoscope**
by David Gould

I n theory, the direct ophthalmoscope is simple to use. It provides an upright, magnified and real image. Its primary use is for examination of the ocular fundus, although it also allows magnified examination of anterior ocular structures, including the vitreous, lens, anterior segment, ocular surface and eyelids.

In practice, however, many veterinary surgeons lack confidence when using a direct ophthalmoscope. This is in part due to perceived difficulties in distinguishing normal from abnormal findings. In addition, there is unfamiliarity with the instrument itself. The aim of this article is to summarise the main features of a direct ophthalmoscope and to review its use in clinical practice.

Choice of model

There are a number of manufacturers of direct ophthalmoscopes, including Welch-Allyn, Neitz and Keeler. Rechargeable or battery options are available. The choice of direct ophthalmoscope is primarily one of personal preference, and as such it may be helpful to 'road test' a few models prior to purchase.

Key features

Figure 1 shows the observer and patient aspects of a typical direct ophthalmoscope head.

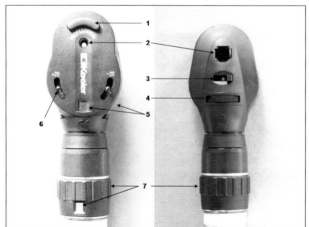

Figure 1: Observer and patient aspects of a direct ophthalmoscope head.
1 = brow rest; 2 = eyepiece/ illumination mirror and dust cover; 3 = filter settings; 4 = aperture settings; 5 = flywheel/ lens magazine; 6 = quick-step swing (+/– 20D); 7 = rheostat

Its main features include the following:

- A brow rest – the head of a direct ophthalmoscope is ergonomically designed to fit comfortably against the observer's orbital rim. Whenever a direct ophthalmoscope is in use, the brow rest should always be in contact with the observer's brow. Compare looking through the eyepiece of the ophthalmoscope with looking through a keyhole; the closer you get, the greater the field of view
- An eyepiece – in which lenses of varying strengths (dioptres) can be inserted by means of a flywheel
- Filters – to supply white, red-free and cobalt blue light
  - White light is used for most applications
  - Red-free light (which appears green in colour) is designed to filter out red light, allowing the examiner to distinguish retinal haemorrhage from pigment. Blood appears black under the red-free light; pigment brown
  - Cobalt blue enhances fluorescence after application of fluorescein dye
- Variable aperture settings – the variety of settings depends on the model, but may include wide, intermediate and narrow beam, graticule and slit beam (Figure 2)
  - A wide beam is most commonly used in practice, and maximises the field of view through the ophthalmoscope
  - A narrow beam is useful for small pupils, to reduce light reflection from the iris
  - The graticule can be used to roughly size a fundic lesion by comparing it to the size of the optic nerve head
  - The slit beam is useful for determining whether a fundus lesion is a depression (e.g. coloboma, optic disc cupping) or an elevation (e.g. retinal detachment, optic disc swelling). It can also be used to assess anterior chamber depth, and to identify aqueous flare
- A lens magazine – this provides lenses of varying focusing powers, usually by means of a flywheel
  - Zero dioptres (0D) is the default lens setting, assuming that both examiner and patient are emmetropic (i.e. have normal eyesight)
  - Positive dioptre lenses (typically +1 to +20D) are typically represented by black or green numbers and allow the examiner to focus progressively anteriorly, usually in single dioptre steps
  - Negative dioptre lenses (–1 to –20D) are typically represented by red numbers and allow the examiner to focus progressively posteriorly, usually in single dioptre steps. They are used for identifying optic disc cupping or colobomata
  - Some models have an additional 'quick step' swing of ± 20D. This is not used commonly in clinical veterinary practice, although the +20D lens can be useful when examining the eyelids, where it provides approximately 2X magnification. This can aid visualisation of small eyelid lesions such as distichia or ectopic cilia

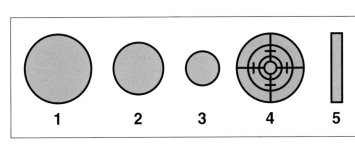

Figure 2: Aperture settings for a direct ophthalmoscope.
1 = wide angle;
2 = intermediate angle;
3 = small angle;
4 = graticule;
5 = slit

■ A light source and rheostat – the light source is reflected out of the eyepiece towards the patient, directly along the direction of view, by means of a mirror within the eyepiece. The rheostat allows variation in light intensity.

Distant direct ophthalmoscopy

This technique is mostly used for identifying cataracts, and for distinguishing cataract from age-related nuclear sclerosis. However, it will identify any opacity in the visual axis. This includes mucus and hairs on the cornea, corneal ulcers and other corneal lesions, and opacities within the vitreous.

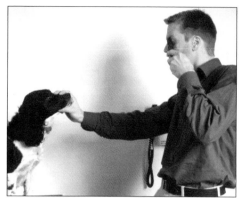

Figure 3: Distant direct ophthalmoscopy

■ Set the ophthalmoscope lens magazine to zero dioptres (0D), stand an arm's length away from the patient and look at the tapetal reflection through the ophthalmoscope (Figure 3). Remember to use the brow rest. Any opacities will appear black against the tapetal reflection (Figure 4).
■ You can localise lesions within the eye using the technique of parallax: whilst viewing the opacity through the ophthalmoscope, move to the left and then to the right and observe whether the opacity appears to move with you or against you. Anterior opacities (e.g. corneal lesions, anterior capsular cataracts) will appear to move in the opposite direction to you, whilst posterior opacities (e.g. posterior cataracts, vitreal opacities) will appear to move in the same direction.

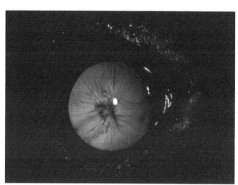

Figure 4: With distant direct ophthalmoscopy, cataracts appear dark when viewed against the bright tapetal reflex

Close direct ophthalmoscopy

Close direct ophthalmoscopy is primarily used to examine the ocular fundus. It provides around 15X magnification but at the expense of a small field of view (around 5–10 degrees). The small field of view means that performing a thorough fundus examination can prove challenging. Some tips to aid visualisation are as follows:

■ Before you use it to examine a patient, check that the ophthalmoscope is in good working order. Switch it on, turn the rheostat to maximum, set the lens magazine to zero dioptres (0D) and set the aperture to the wide angle setting. A bright, circular beam of light should be emitted (sometimes the flywheel can catch midway between lenses, cutting off a portion of light, or the dust cover may partly obstruct the light beam). Look through the eyepiece, ensuring that the brow rest is used. The view through the ophthalmoscope should be clear – use it to look around the room

- Apply a mydriatic eye drop to dilate the pupil of the patient prior to examination. Tropicamide 1% is effective within around 10 minutes, has a maximum effect around 30 minutes and lasts 2–3 hours. Atropine should be avoided, especially in cats, in which it induces excess salivation
- Perform ophthalmoscopy in a darkened room to minimise light reflection
- Set the rheostat to low or mid intensity when examining the fundus – using a low intensity of illumination will maximise patient comfort and cooperation
- Use the brow rest
- Get close to the patient ('looking through a keyhole'). The ophthalmoscope should be around 1–2 cm from the patient's eye. Ideally, use your right eye to examine the patient's right eye, and your left eye to examine the patient's left eye. This will help to avoid obstruction of view by the patient's nose (Figure 5)
- Try to perform an organised examination of the fundus:
  1. Identify the optic nerve head. In most patients it is located marginally below the midline, and slightly medial. If the optic nerve head appears out of focus then rotate the lens magazine clockwise or anticlockwise in single dioptre steps until the image becomes clear. Assess size, shape and colour of the optic nerve head, and compare left and right sides. Note that there is significant normal variation in the dog, less so in the cat
  2. Examine the superficial retinal blood vessels. In general, the venules are wider and darker than the arterioles. The normal canine fundus contains 15–20 arterioles and 3–5 venules that drain into a venous circle on the optic nerve head (Figure 6). In the feline fundus, three major pairs of arterioles and venules emerge from the edge of the optic nerve head (Figure 7). In the dog, there is considerable normal variation in the degree of blood vessel tortuosity, much less so in the cat

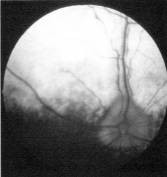

Figure 6: The normal canine ocular fundus

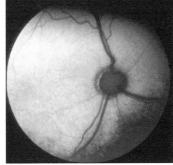

Figure 7: The normal feline ocular fundus

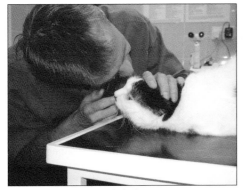

Figure 5: Close direct ophthalmoscopy

3. Examine the tapetal fundus, located dorsal to the optic nerve head. Using a low intensity of illumination will allow easier identification of abnormalities such as tapetal hyper- or hyporeflectivity

4. Examine the dark non-tapetal fundus, located ventral to the optic nerve head. Abnormalities may include areas of hypo- or hyperpigmentation

- Remember that the small field of view through the ophthalmoscope means that a thorough fundus examination takes some time
- If you are myopic or hyperopic (short- or long-sighted, respectively) then adjusting the lens magazine to your prescription will allow you to use the ophthalmoscope without having to wear your glasses. For example, if you are –2D myopic then adjust the lens magazine to –2D
- Attempting an ophthalmic examination on a patient under general anaesthetic is seldom rewarding. Rotation of the globes under anaesthesia makes intraocular visualisation particularly difficult. A combination of patience and gentle restraint is usually sufficient to allow ophthalmoscopy in the vast majority of patients.

Examining anterior ocular structures

The direct ophthalmoscope can also be used to examine structures anterior to the retina, by utilising the positive dioptre setting on the lens magazine. Approximate settings for examining structures of the canine eye are as follows:

- Posterior lens: +8D
- Anterior lens: +12D
- Cornea and eyelids: +20D

Summary

The direct ophthalmoscope is a versatile piece of equipment that is perhaps underused in general veterinary practice. As well as using it for detailed fundus examination, it is also helpful for identification and localisation of opacities in the visual axis, most notably cataracts. In addition it allows magnified examination of structures anterior to the retina, including the lens, cornea and eyelids. Familiarising yourself with the functions of your direct ophthalmoscope, and regular practice with its use, should increase your confidence in examining eyes and in diagnosing ophthalmic abnormalities. ■

How to…
Place local anaesthetic blocks
in small animals

by Nicki Grint

Local anaesthetic blocks are potentially the most effective form of analgesia for many small animal surgeries, but are also the most underused. For most of the blocks described in this article, all that is needed is a syringe, a needle, local anaesthetic and a knowledge of the appropriate anatomy. No specialist equipment is required but nerve location equipment can be used to guide perineural injections of local anaesthetics, as long as a motor nerve accompanies the sensory branch.

Local anaesthetic blocks can be used to augment analgesia whilst the animal is under a general anaesthetic; less of the volatile agent will be needed to maintain anaesthesia, and in general the anaesthetic episode will be 'smoother'. Alternatively, local anaesthesia can be used in sedated or conscious animals to allow minor surgical procedures or manipulations to be performed. Local anaesthetics are the only class of analgesics that completely block pain sensations, and are thus the only true 'analgesics'. In contrast, all the other drugs we consider 'analgesics', e.g. opioids and non-steroidal anti-inflammatory drugs (NSAIDs), are technically 'hypoalgesics' as they reduce pain sensations to a tolerable level.

Local anaesthetic drugs block pain because they stop the nerves conducting the pain signals and so work on the transmission part of the pain pathway. Local anaesthetics, when used in combination with other analgesic drug groups, e.g. opioids, NSAIDs, ketamine and alpha 2-adrenergic agonists, play a major role in **multi-modal analgesia**. This concept uses drugs that work at different parts of the pain pathway to provide more effective analgesia, whilst utilising smaller doses of drugs and therefore limiting their side effects.

To stop the transmission of the electrical impulses along nerves, local anaesthetics block the sodium channels in the nerve fibres. Both sensory and motor nerves may be affected, so areas of the body can be desensitised but the animal may temporarily lose function and movement of that part of the body if the motor nerves are affected.

Local anaesthetic drugs
Examples of local anaesthetic drugs include lidocaine, bupivacaine, ropivacaine, mepivacaine and procaine. Local anaesthetics are subdivided into two groups depending on their chemical structures; lidocaine, bupivacaine, mepivacaine and ropivacaine all belong to the *amide-linked* group, which undergo hepatic metabolism. Procaine belongs to the *ester-linked* group; these drugs are broken down in the blood by enzymes.

The most commonly used in small animal practice are lidocaine and bupivacaine.

Drug	Dose range	Onset	Duration
Lidocaine	2–4 mg/kg	10 min	1–2 hours
Bupivacaine	1–2 mg/kg	20–30 min	2.5 – 6 hours
Ropivacaine	0.1–2 mg/kg	2–20 min	2–6 hours
Procaine	6 mg/kg	10 min	30 min

Figure 1: Dose ranges of commonly used local anaesthetic drugs

Lidocaine has a short onset of action (5–10 minutes) but also lasts a short time (up to 1 hour), whilst bupivacaine has a longer onset (30 minutes) and duration (6–8 hours) of action. Combining lidocaine and bupivacaine together produces a fast onset block which has a relatively long duration. Maximum doses of the drugs are listed in Figure 1; however, many local blocks will also have a maximum volume of injectate. The volumes suggested in the following text are appropriate for an average sized doliocephalic dogs, and should be reduced appropriately according to the size of the dog or cat.

When performing any of these blocks, aspiration to check for blood after needle insertion but prior to local anaesthetic injection should always be performed, as local anaesthetics (with the exception of lidocaine in certain circumstances) should never be given intravascularly. Intravenous administration or overdose of local anaesthetics can cause cardiotoxic (peripheral vasodilation, hypotension, decreased myocardial contractility and arrythmias) or neurotoxic (sedation, disorientation, ataxia, convulsions) side effects.

Head blocks

Many of these blocks can be used for dental procedures, mandibular and maxillary surgery. If masses are being removed from the skin on the head or gums, this type of block will provide excellent analgesia, but instead of injecting around the mass, which may disseminate tumour cells, the injection site is remote from the surgery site. When deciding which block is appropriate in a given case, it should be remembered that only structures rostral to the injection site will be desensitised. The infraorbital and the mental nerve blocks may not desensitise teeth, unless the needles are inserted into the canals. However, the teeth will be blocked if the more caudal blocks (maxillary and mandibular) are performed.

Infraorbital nerve block

- The infraorbital foramen is midway between the rostrodorsal border of the zygomatic arch and the canine root tip (Figures 2 and 3).

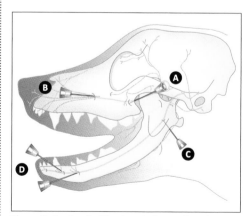

Figure 2: Anatomical landmarks for performing maxillary (A), infraorbital (B), mandibular (C) and mental nerve blocks (D) in dogs

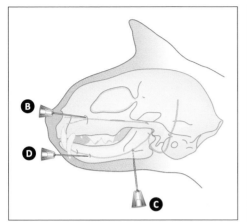

Figure 3: Anatomical landmarks for performing infraorbital (B), mandibular (C) and mental nerve blocks (D) in cats

- Local anaesthetic injected here will block the upper lip and nose (nasal planum and roof of nasal cavity), and skin rostroventral to the infraorbital foramen.
- Maximum volume 3 ml.

Maxillary nerve block

- Local anaesthetic injected into the pterygopalatine fossa, between the rostral alar foramen and the maxillary foramen (entrance to the infraorbital canal).
- The nerve is blocked by inserting a needle under the rostral portion of the zygomatic arch directing it to the maxillary foramen (see Figure 2).
- Blocks the nose (nasal planum and most of bridge of nose), upper lip, upper teeth, palate and maxilla.
- Maximum volume 3 ml.

Mental nerve block

- This nerve is blocked where the middle mental nerve exits from the middle mental foramen (see Figures 2 and 3). The middle mental foramen is biggest in dogs, and carries the largest of the mental nerves.

- Blocks the lower lip/chin rostral to site of block. (Not teeth.)
- Maximum volume 2 ml.

Mandibular (inferior alveolar) nerve block

- To block this nerve, palpate the lip of the mandibular foramen. Insert the needle percutaneously at the lower angle of the jaw, and advance it against the medial side of the mandible and direct it towards the foramen. Often the needle can be guided as you can feel the foramen and nerve from inside the mouth on the medial surface of the mandible.
- Local anaesthetic deposited here will block lower teeth, mandible, skin and mucosa of lower lip.
- Maximum volume 2 ml.

Retrobulbar block

The retrobulbar block is very useful for ocular surgery. The retrobulbar block involves injecting local anaesthetic behind the globe and will block cranial nerves II, III, IV, V (ophthalmic and maxillary branches) and VI. So as well as desensitising the globe, lids, conjunctiva, and much of the upper face, it will block the extraocular muscles and therefore produce a central eye. Some eyelid tone may remain from palpebral (cranial nerve VII) innervation.

There is a chance that the globe can be punctured when executing this block so it is best to reserve its use for surgeries when enuculeation is planned. Even in these cases, a retrobulbar block is contraindicated if tumour or overt infection is the reason for enucleation, as the needle may disseminate tumour cells or infection to the back of the eye. Retrobulbar injections may produce traction on the optic nerve and therefore the technique is often avoided in shallow orbited cats, whose optic nerves (both in the injected eye and the contralateral one) may be compromised by this tension.

- The needle is inserted at 10 o'clock and 5 o'clock sites. A slightly curved 21–23 G needle is used and the tip of the needle should be 'bounced off' the orbit until the tip sits behind the globe.
- Maximum volume 5 ml.
- Aspirate not just to check for blood but also for cerebrospinal fluid.

Auriculotemporal and great auricular nerve block

Blocking the auriculotemporal and great auricular nerve (Figure 4) desensitises the inner surface of the auricular cartilage and the external ear canal. This block is ideal for ear surgeries such as total ear canal ablation.

- The auriculotemporal nerve is blocked by inserting a needle rostral to the vertical ear canal and directing it towards the base of the 'V' formed by the caudal aspect of the zygomatic arch and the vertical canal.
- The great auricular nerve is blocked by inserting a needle ventral to the wing of the

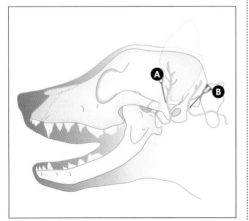

Figure 4: Anatomical landmarks for performing auriculotemporal (A) and great auricular (B) nerve blocks in dogs

atlas and caudal to the vertical ear canal, and directing it parallel to the vertical canal.

- An alternative to this block is a 'splash' block where local anaesthetic is squirted down the ear canal during surgery or injected around the surgical site prior to closure.

Limb blocks

As orthopaedic surgery becomes more and more commonplace in general practice, most aspects of limbs can be desensitized with one of the following blocks.

Intra-articular analgesia

This is a simple local anaesthetic block which can be done before or after any surgery involving a joint, including arthroscopy. As with all local anaesthetic blocks, it must be done in a strictly aseptic manner to avoid introducing infection into the joint. Current recommendation is that this is performed as a 'one-off shot' rather than as a continuous infusion.

As with all analgesia, pre-emptive administration is best, and so ideally the drug should be injected before surgery (often this can be performed once a joint tap has been performed, using the same needle left in place). Alternatively it can be injected at the end of surgery just before the joint is closed – just make sure not to flush with saline immediately afterwards. Bupivacaine is used as the local anaesthetic of choice, but in animals with chronic joint disease morphine can also be added to the local anaesthetic. In such cases of chronic joint inflammation, synovial opioid receptors are upregulated, and morphine should improve the quality and the duration of the analgesia.

Ring block

Local anaesthetic agents can be injected to encircle the area of interest, e.g. a distal limb. It is vital that local anaesthetic **without** adrenaline is used, otherwise the blood supply to the distal area could be compromised. The solution of local anaesthetic may be diluted to provide a more convenient volume to inject, and reduce the risk of causing toxicity. It is important not to inject through inflamed or infected tissue as this may disseminate infection and will be less effective due to the altered pH of the tissue.

IVRA

IVRA stands for 'Intravenous regional analgesia' and is often used to desensitise distal limbs. Only lidocaine (without adrenaline) should be used with this technique, as it is the least cardiotoxic of the local anaesthetics. Local anaesthetic is injected distal to a tourniquet which is in place to keep the lidocaine in a discrete area (including the surgical site). The local block works for as long as the tourniquet is in place, as the drug doesn't return to the liver to be metabolised. The tourniquet, however, should not be left in place for more than 60–90 minutes. An added bonus of this technique is that if you exsanguinate the limb, there will be a bloodless field for surgery.

1. Clip and prepare the area of interest and place an i.v. catheter (facing away from the heart).
2. Exsanguinate the limb from the toe upwards by wrapping some cohesive bandage starting at the toe, tying a tourniquet at the top, and then unwinding the bandage from the toe upwards.
3. Inject lidocaine into the catheter (up to 4 mg/kg and flush), then the catheter can be removed.
4. Wait 5 minutes before you start surgery.
5. Don't remove the tourniquet until at least 15 minutes after the local anaesthetic is injected. If removing earlier than this, monitor the ECG for PR and QRS prolongation and resulting arrhythmias.

Digital nerve block

This block is useful for any pad or digital surgery, including digit amputation. It is particularly useful with sedation to suture pads, and without sedation to pull torn nails. Insert a short needle in the gap between the digits. This will need to be done in the interdigital space either side of the affected digit. After aspiration to check for blood, a maximum volume of 0.5 ml can be injected either side.

Saphenous, common peroneal and tibial nerve blocks

Blocking these nerves (Figure 5) will provide analgesia for surgeries and injuries distal to the stifle.

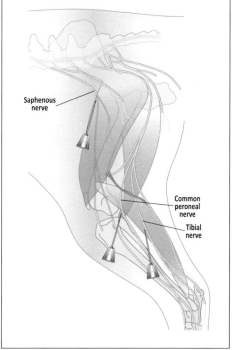

Figure 5: Anatomical landmarks for saphenous, common peroneal and tibial nerve blocks in dogs (median view)

- The saphenous nerve (branch of femoral nerve) is palpated in the femoral triangle on the medial aspect of the thigh. Pulsation of the artery can help guide needle placement, which should be aimed cranial to the artery.
- The common peroneal nerve (branch of the sciatic nerve) is blocked by injecting distal to the fibular head.
- The tibial nerve (branch of the sciatic nerve) is blocked by placing a needle deep to the medial and lateral heads of the gastrocnemius.

Radial, ulnar and median nerve blocks

Blocking these nerves will desensitise the distal forelimb.

In the cat, blocking the medial, ulnar and radial nerves will desensitise the forepaw (Figure 6).

- The radial nerve can be blocked by injecting local anaesthetic subcutaneously dorsomedial to the carpus, proximal to the joint.
- The medial and ulnar nerves are blocked by injecting medially and laterally to the accessory carpal pad on the palmar surface of the paw.

Blocking the radial, ulnar, median and musculocutaneous nerves (Figure 7) in the dog will desensitise the forelimb distal to the elbow.

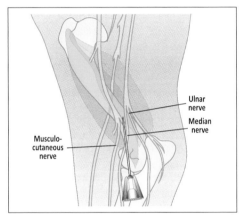

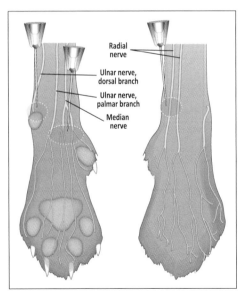

Figure 6: Anatomical landmarks for performing nerve blocks of the distal branches of the radial, ulnar and median nerves in cats. Shaded areas within dotted lines show areas to be blocked

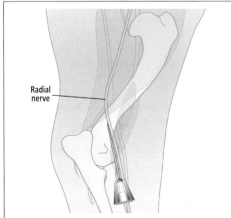

Figure 7: Anatomical landmarks for performing radial, ulnar, median and musculocutaneous nerve blocks in dogs

- The radial nerve is blocked by injecting proximal to the lateral epicondyle of the humerus and directing between the brachialis and lateral head of the triceps.
- The ulnar, medial and musculocutaneous nerves are blocked by injecting proximal to the medial epicondyle of the humerus and directing between biceps brachii and the medial head of the triceps.

Brachial plexus block

Blocking the nerves of the brachial plexus will provide excellent analgesia for some forelimb surgeries and fracture repairs. The traditional brachial plexus (axillary) block, injecting approximately 10–15 ml of local anaesthetic (for a 25 kg dog) into the axillary space at the level of the point of the shoulder (Figure 8) blocks the lower forelimb, but not the shoulder or the proximal humerus.

The paravertebral brachial plexus technique produces a more complete blockade, including more proximally. Local anaesthetic is injected so that the nerves of the brachial plexus are blocked as close as possible to the intervertebral foraminae (Figure 9).

1. Shift the scapula caudally to expose the large transverse process of the sixth cervical vertebra and the first rib.
2. Block the ventral branches of C6 and C7 as they cross the dorsal surface of the transverse process of the sixth cervical vertebra. This is done by inserting a needle dorsal to the process and directing it to the caudal and cranial margins.
3. Block the ventral branches of C8 and T1 on the lateral surface of the first rib by directing the needle to the cranial and ventral border of the dorsal part of the first rib.

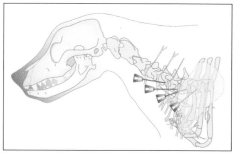

Figure 9: Anatomical landmarks for performing paravertebral blockade of the brachial plexus in dogs (dotted line shows normal anatomical position of the scapula)

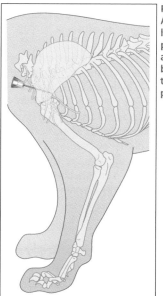

Figure 8: Anatomical landmarks for performing axillary blockade of the brachial plexus in cats

Pneumothorax is a potential complication of both of these brachial plexus blocks and aspiration to check for air should be performed before each injection. Bilateral blocks should be avoided due to potential blockade of the phrenic nerve.

Thoracic blocks

Intercostal nerve block

Intercostal nerve blocks are a useful analgesic adjunct for lateral thoracotomy surgeries, but also can be used to good effect to provide pain relief for rib fractures and for chest tube placements.

- The intercostal nerves are closely associated with the caudal borders of the ribs.
- There is much overlap of innervation of the chest wall, so that at least 2 'segments' cranial and caudal to the intercostal site/s where analgesia is needed should be blocked (Figure 10).
- Use a 23–25 G, ⁵⁄₈–1 inch needle.

1. Aiming perpendicular to the body wall, slide the needle through the skin, off the caudal border of the rib, and proximal to the 'wound'.
2. Aim as near to the intervertebral foramen as possible (i.e. as high up the intercostal nerve as possible, so as to block most of its branches).
3. Aspirate, to check that the needle tip isn't in a vascular part the of the neurovascular bundle.
4. Use ¼–1 ml per site, depending upon the animal's size.

Interpleural analgesia

Interpleural analgesia is also useful after thoracotomy, or for lateral thoracotomy or sternotomy. Local anaesthetic is instilled down the chest drain whilst the animal is still under anaesthesia, and then the animal is rolled so that the drug bathes the affected area (as long as the animal's ventilation is not compromised by that position). Interpleural anaesthesia can also provide pain relief for animals with indwelling chest drains. Analgesia of cranial abdominal organs and cranial mammary glands is also produced when local anaesthetics are injected inter-pleurally, due to the stellate ganglion in the thorax providing innervation to these organs.

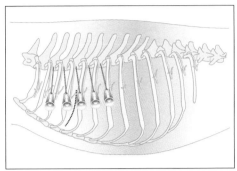

Figure 10: Anatomical landmarks for performing intercostal nerve blocks in dogs (dotted line shows position of surgical incision)

- Can be effected by instilling local anaesthetic down an indwelling chest drain.
- Otherwise, a catheter may be placed into the pleural space either percutaneously, or under direct view, for example before closure of a thoracotomy incision.

Wound soaker catheters

These are useful after large surgeries such as mammary strips and forequarter amputations, but the catheters can be implanted in any closed incision to provide excellent postoperative local analgesia. They are loosely tacked into place in the subcutis before skin closure, and then secured to the skin using a roman sandal suture. They can be removed easily by pulling once the roman sandal suture is cut. Local anaesthetic is diffused through the catheter after injecting it through a bacterial filter system (which is included in the catheter set), and can be injected in bolus doses or as a continuous rate infusion by attaching the catheter, via an extension set, to a syringe driver.

Conclusion

Local anaesthetic techniques are the only form of true analgesia where all pain sensations are blocked, rather than just reducing pain down to a tolerable level. When making an analgesic plan for any surgery, a local anaesthetic technique should be considered to contribute to multi-modal analgesia, as many anatomical sites can be 'blocked'. When used in conjunction with general anaesthesia, the anaesthetic will generally be smoother, with less volatile agent needed for maintenance. Alternatively, local blocks can be used in sedated animals or some animals whilst conscious to facilitate minor surgical manipulations or investigations.

Acknowledgements

The line diagrams in this article have been reproduced from the *BSAVA Manual of Canine and Feline Anaesthesia and Analgesia, 2nd edition*, edited by Chris Seymour and Tanya Duke-Novakovski. The diagrams were drawn by Samantha Elmhurst BA Hons (www. livingart.org.uk) and are printed with her permission. Thanks also to Emma Love and Rob Lowe for assistance with the manuscript. ■

How to...

Choose a cat
urinary catheter

by Danièlle Gunn-Moore

ifferent urinary catheters are needed for different tasks. While a short stiff catheter will be most useful at clearing a urethral obstruction, a longer softer one will be needed if it is to be left *in situ*.

Selecting a urinary catheter for unblocking the urethra of a tom cat

1 Anaesthetise the cat (the author prefers this to heavy sedation as it ensures the urethra is as relaxed as possible).

2 When possible, catheterise the bladder without first decompressing it as cystocentesis significantly increases the risk of urine leakage into the abdomen. However, if decompression prior to catheterisation is essential, perform cystocentesis using a fine-gauge butterfly needle attached to a three-way tap and syringe rather than a needle directly attached to a large syringe (reducing the risk of hand tremor and needle tip movement causing bladder trauma). Remove as much urine as is feasible.

3 Perform a rectal examination to feel for urethral stones, trauma, neoplasia or swellings (e.g. muscle spasm, bruising).

4 Clip and aseptically prepare the perineum.

5 Fully extrude the cat's penis (if possible) and examine it for signs of trauma, swelling or inflammation. Small uroliths (stones) or tightly packed urine-sand can become lodged in the very tip of the penis and can often be massaged out with gentle manipulation.

6 Select a non-traumatic, ideally open-ended, urethral catheter (Figures 1, 2 and 3) and lubricate it well with sterile lubricating jelly. Occasionally it is necessary to use a catheter with a very small aperture, e.g. the sheath of a 22-gauge intravenous catheter, or even a lachrymal catheter.

- **Standard (Jackson-type) Tom cat catheters** are often very useful for this purpose as they are easy to handle, stiff and inexpensive. However, most have side holes rather than being open-ended, so where the obstruction is very near the penis tip it may not be possible to get the catheter holes sufficiently far into the urethra to allow flushing with saline. In addition, they often require repeated application of lubricant and the rough edges of the side holes can be very traumatic.
- **Slippery Sam, Fioniavet and short Cook's catheters** are very useful for clearing distal penile obstructions as they are open ended and atraumatic.

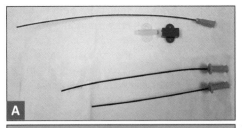

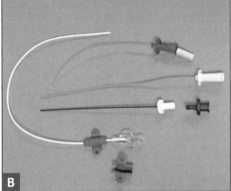

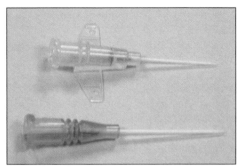

Figure 3: An intravenous catheter (with its stylet removed) can be used to unblock urethral obstructions that occur very close to the penis tip

Figure 1: Urethral catheters. From the top to the bottom: (A) Cook catheters: 3.5 F, 25 cm long (adjustable); 3.5 F, 14 cm long; 3.5 F, 10 cm long. (B) Standard (Jackson-type) Tom cat catheter (3 F, 10 cm long); Slippery Sam catheter (3 F, 11 cm long); Mila EZGO (Interurethral UC 310 3.5 F, 25 cm long (adjustable), plus its securing clip – if the clip is not available, secure the wings of the catheter to the insertion tube with sutures)

7 Advancing the catheter after clearing an obstruction – position the catheter within the penis tip, then hold the base of the penis and pull it caudally and dorsally. This acts to straighten out the urethra and allows for easier and less traumatic catheterisation. Urethral trauma is likely to occur if you do not do this, particularly when excessive force is applied.

8 The catheter should be gently advanced whilst flushing with sterile saline, which acts to distend the urethra and to flush obstructing material either back along the catheter and out of the penis tip or into the bladder (i.e. retrograde hydropulsion). Never use Walpole's solution, it is highly irritant and will cause severe inflammation of the mucosal lining of the urethra and bladder.

9 Urethral massage per rectum and retrograde hydropulsion using saline may assist in flushing urethral stones or debris back into the bladder. Urethral massage per rectum can also help to relax urethral muscle spasm.

10 Once the catheter has been advanced into the bladder, the bladder should be gently decompressed until it is empty, and then flushed with saline until the retrieved fluid runs clear. It should then be left empty.

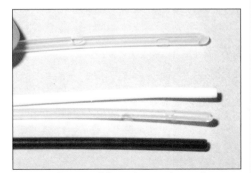

Figure 2: Close up of the catheters shown above demonstrating side holes (standard catheters) and open-ends (Mila EZGO and Slippery Sam)

Selecting an indwelling urinary catheter

If a catheter is to be left *in situ* it should be of a length sufficient to just reach into the bladder, and it should be made of soft non-traumatic material. The ideal position for the tip of an indwelling urinary catheter is just within the bladder, typically at the level of L6. All catheters move while in situ and the movement of the tip is most marked and likely to cause irritation: if the catheter is too short it will cause irritation within the proximal urethra, while if it is too long it will irritate the bladder wall (and can even cause perforation).

11

- **Standard (Jackson-type) Tom cat catheters are not suitable for this purpose** as they are too short and are made from very stiff plastic that typically has multiple side holes. These side holes have rough edges and since in most cats they end up sitting within the proximal urethra they can cause severe irritation and inflammation at this site, and may even result in perforation or stricture formation. In addition, these catheters tend to be too fine to fit snugly in the urethra so some cats will urinate around the catheter and this may lead to perineal staining and scalding.

- **Slippery Sam catheters are better suited as they are much less traumatic and are open ended.** However, they are typically only 11 cm long so they sit in the proximal urethra of larger cats, and while they are typically much less irritant than Jackson catheters, this is still not to be recommended. These catheters come with soft hubs, which while much more comfortable for the cat, can be rather fiddly to attach to the closed collection system. Occasionally, the hub can become detached from the catheter.

- **The Mila EZGO (Interurethral UC 310, 25 cm long, 3.5 F) from Direct Medical Supplies and the Cook's 25 cm long catheter** are currently the author's preference as they are soft and atraumatic, and the catheter's length can be determined by measuring it against the cat (then positioning the wings at the appropriate length on the catheter with the purpose-designed clip, or with a suture). The Mila catheter (Figure 4) is so soft it can be difficult to pass along the urethra until after the obstruction has been fully removed and the urethra has been flushed clean with saline. However, its passage can be made easier if it is stored in the freezer (it becomes stiffer when cold) and it is recommended that it is flushed with saline as it is advanced.

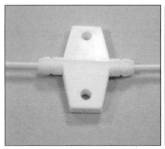 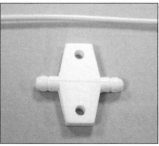 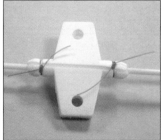

Figure 4: The Mila EZGO catheter has wings which can be separated from the catheter tube then repositioned at the appropriate length on the catheter once it has been measured against the cat. The two pieces are then attached together with a suture at each end of the wings

12 Secure the catheter to the cat by suturing it to the prepuce and attach a sterile extension line and closed-collection system. Tape the collection system to the tail so the tension is removed from the prepuce.

13 Fit the cat with an Elizabethan collar.

14 Monitor urine output and ensure the IV fluid input matches post-obstructional diuresis, and contains sufficient potassium.

15 Leave the catheter in place for 2–4 days (judge by the amount of blood within the urine).

16 Do not give antibiotics unless absolutely essential. (Giving antibiotics while a urinary catheter is in place risks selecting for resistant bacterial clones.) It is better to start antibiotics on removal of the catheter, preferably with those selected according to results of bacterial culture and sensitivity of the urine.

Ideally, give a spasmolytic (e.g. prazocin 0.5–1.0 mg/cat orally q8–12h) while the catheter is in place (to reduce the risk of the catheter causing urethral irritation and spasm) and for a further 1–2 weeks, as needed.

Catheters for female cats

1 To catheterise a female cat use a well lubricated **Jackson Tom cat catheter or Slippery Sam catheter**, insert it into the cat's vulva, then pull the vulva caudally and dorsally. This acts to straighten out the urethra and allows for easier and less traumatic catheterisation. Slide the tip of the catheter along the floor of the vulva and into the urethra.

2 Flush the bladder with sterile saline to remove debris, crystals, blood clots, etc.

3 It is very rarely necessary to leave an indwelling catheter in a female cat, but if it is use a suitably sized **soft Foley catheter** or, possibly, the **Mila EZGO** (as above; measure to ensure correct positioning to just within the bladder and suture the wings to the vulva). The standard long cat catheters (e.g. 4 F/1.3 mm 30.5 cm long catheter) are too stiff and because their length is not adjustable they tend to irritate the bladder wall where they loop round and lie in contact with it. Even more so than in males, standard catheters tend to be too fine to fit snugly within the wider female urethra leading to urination around the catheter and perineal staining or scalding. ■

How to...
Approach a dog with pale mucous membranes

by Laura Holm and Kit Sturgess

When presented with a patient with mucous membrane pallor, decisions made in the first few hours are critical.

Differential diagnoses for membrane pallor are:

- Anaemia
- Hypovolaemia/shock
- Poor cardiac output/high sympathetic tone.

Clearly these conditions have widely differing treatment strategies and prognoses, and rapid distinction is vital. Through implementation of the algorithm presented in Figure 1, this article aims to guide the reader towards achieving a working diagnosis from which rational therapy can be initiated. For each KEY POINT in the algorithm there is a corresponding explanatory text box.

Anaemia is defined as a reduction in red cell mass, usually measured as a reduction in packed cell volume (PCV), haematocrit, haemoglobin concentration or red blood cell count. Red cell count has usually fallen significantly before a patient will show pallor of the gums. Patients will frequently not show clinical signs of anaemia until it is moderate to severe (Figure 2), although the rate at which the anaemia develops does influence the point at which clinical signs become evident. For example, in chronic disease states, the PCV can fall into the mid teens or lower before

signs are evident, whereas animals with acute blood loss or haemolysis can often be severely compromised with PCVs above 25%. In dogs, a PCV below 6–7% is usually terminal. Further, the cause of the anaemia (e.g. bleeding neoplasm) or the effects of haemolytic anaemia (e.g. hyperbilirubinaemia) may also contribute to the clinical signs.

There are numerous potential causes for anaemia, so a thorough history, physical examination and investigation should be undertaken. It is essential to follow a logical approach to investigations to ensure that they are undertaken in the appropriate order and potential causes of the anaemia are not overlooked. The most common presenting signs for anaemic animals are lethargy, inappetence, and mucous membrane pallor.

KEY POINT: HISTORY

Valuable information may be gained through obtaining a full and thorough history, which may aid in rapid differentiation of the possible causes of pallor and, in particular, anaemia.

- **General health** (appetite/thirst/energy/bodyweight/vomiting/diarrhoea) – Many chronic diseases can cause anaemia, e.g. renal disease and the 'physiological' anaemia seen with hypothyroidism.
- **Description of clinical signs** – Examples of things that might help to differentiate the

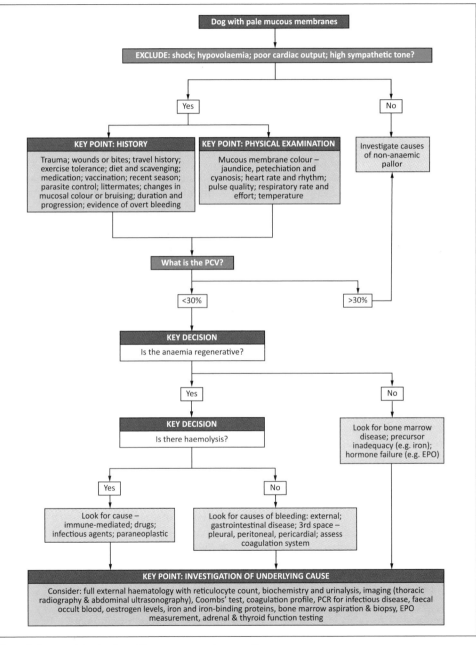

Dog with pale mucous membranes

EXCLUDE: shock; hypovolaemia; poor cardiac output; high sympathetic tone?

Yes

No

KEY POINT: HISTORY

Trauma; wounds or bites; travel history; exercise tolerance; diet and scavenging; medication; vaccination; recent season; parasite control; littermates; changes in mucosal colour or bruising; duration and progression; evidence of overt bleeding

KEY POINT: PHYSICAL EXAMINATION

Mucous membrane colour – jaundice, petechiation and cyanosis; heart rate and rhythm; pulse quality; respiratory rate and effort; temperature

Investigate causes of non-anaemic pallor

What is the PCV?

<30%

>30%

KEY DECISION

Is the anaemia regenerative?

Yes

No

KEY DECISION

Is there haemolysis?

Look for bone marrow disease; precursor inadequacy (e.g. iron); hormone failure (e.g. EPO)

Yes

No

Look for cause – immune-mediated; drugs; infectious agents; paraneoplastic

Look for causes of bleeding: external; gastrointestinal disease; 3rd space – pleural, peritoneal, pericardial; assess coagulation system

KEY POINT: INVESTIGATION OF UNDERLYING CAUSE

Consider: full external haematology with reticulocyte count, biochemistry and urinalysis, imaging (thoracic radiography & abdominal ultrasonography), Coombs' test, coagulation profile, PCR for infectious disease, faecal occult blood, oestrogen levels, iron and iron-binding proteins, bone marrow aspiration & biopsy, EPO measurement, adrenal & thyroid function testing

Figure 1: Approach to the dog with mucous membrane pallor

Parameter	Value, and severity of anaemia			
	Severe	Moderate	Mild	Reference
Packed cell volume (PCV) (%)	15	23	30	37–55
Red blood cell count (RBCC) (x1012/l)	2.0	3.5	4.8	5.0–8.5
Haemoglobin (Hb) (g/dl)	4.5	7.5	10.0	12.0–18.0

Figure 2: Grading of anaemia. Note: haematocrit is a derived parameter (from red cell number x mean cell volume) and approximates to PCV. Red cell swelling will artificially increase the haematocrit. If there has been a delay in processing (e.g. a postal sample), or the sample has undergone haemolysis, then haemoglobin is a more reliable assessment of anaemia than is haematocrit

above causes would be: presence/absence of coughing, weight loss, lethargy, fainting, observed bleeding, e.g. haematuria or dark urine, melaena, haematemesis, epistaxis, swellings or abdominal distension.

- **Any known trauma?** – This could suggest either shock/hypovolaemia or blood loss anaemia as a cause for pallor. Include any unexplained wounds/bites/injuries, e.g. snake bite, which can cause disseminated intravascular coagulation (DIC).
- **Duration and progression of clinical signs?** – Chronic anaemia may have a more waxing/waning history.
- **Current/recent medication?** (including herbal and human products) – For example, drugs for pre-existing cardiac disease, or drugs that may be associated with gastric ulceration, bone marrow suppression, reduced platelet function or haemolysis (e.g. non-steroidal anti-inflammatories, antibiotics, chemotherapy agents, anti-fungal agents).
- **Exercise tolerance?** – Has there been a general decline recently, suggesting either development of chronic anaemia or cardiovascular disease causing poor output (e.g. dilated cardiomyopathy)?
- **Is the patient being given an unusual diet, likely to eat foreign objects or scavenge?** – For example, diets with significant amounts of onion or garlic; ingestion of zinc in batteries, rodenticides or paracetamol.

- **Colour of skin, mucous membranes, bruising or overt bleeding?** – The owner may have detected jaundice, pallor, cyanosis, petechiation or ecchymosis. If so, when/for how long?
- **Previous/current neoplastic disease?** – For example, lymphoma, testicular tumours or haemangiosarcoma. Many types of neoplasia can be implicated in immune-mediated (IMHA) or microangiopathic haemolytic anaemia, thrombocytopenia, oestrogen-induced bone marrow suppression and DIC.
- **Recent vaccination?** – Vaccination has been weakly associated with an increased incidence of immune-mediated haemolysis and/or thrombocytopenia in the months following vaccination.
- **Recent season?** – There can be a hormonal role in immune-mediated haemolysis. High oestrogen levels can induce bone marrow suppression and thrombocytopenia.
- **Travel** – Many European/exotic infectious diseases can cause anaemia.
- **History of littermates?** – Inherited anaemias or coagulopathies.
- **Evidence of parasites?** – Fleas can directly cause anaemia if the burden is very heavy, especially in puppies. Many tick-borne diseases result in anaemia but are still rarely encountered in the UK.
- **Previous blood transfusion?** – Possible transfer of parasites causing anaemia; delayed transfusion reactions?

In addition to narrowing a differential list based on the facts gleaned from the owner, the clinical examination provides further information to allow prioritisation of differential diagnoses. Often there is sufficient information gained on clinical examination to allow differentiation of anaemia from other cases of pallor.

- **Mentation** – Animals with chronic anaemia may be better adapted than animals with acute anaemia (they can be walking around apparently quite happily with a PCV of <10%). Chronic anaemia is more likely to be non-regenerative, so this helps with narrowing the list of possible differentials. Animals may appear distressed due to the sensation of dyspnoea (e.g. with oedema or effusions resulting from cardiac disease; haemothorax), or due to pain from injuries leading to shock; hypoxaemia is also described as being painful in its own right in people. They may be more obtunded in states of severe shock or terminal anaemia.
- **Mucous membrane colour (Figure 3):**

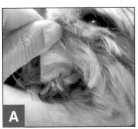
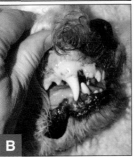

Figure 3: (A) Mucosal pallor. (B) Mucosal pallor, jaundice and petechiation

1. **Jaundice** can indicate liver disease or haemolysis – *but not all haemolytic anaemias are jaundiced at presentation.*
2. **Identification of petechiation or ecchymoses** would point towards an investigation for thrombocytopenia/ thrombocytopathy, or other coagulopathy such as von Willebrand's disease or vasculopathy.
3. **Cyanosis** indicates severe hypoxaemia, usually secondary to pulmonary disease or a right–left shunting cardiac defect. A pure anaemia will not cause cyanosis. If the haemoglobin is <5 g/dl cyanosis will not be visible.

- **Heart rate/rhythm** – Tachycardia and arrhythmias can be present with shock, cardiac disease, or anaemia.
- **Presence/absence/grade of heart murmur** – If a murmur has not been documented on previous health checks, then a new-onset murmur may be haemic in origin and should resolve on treatment of the anaemia.
- **Pulse quality** – Pulses tend to be bounding but easily compressible with anaemia and early (compensated) shock. Note, however, that in compensated shock, mucous membranes are often dark pink rather than pale. Pulses can be poor with cardiac disease, severe hypovolaemia or more advanced shock.
- **Respiratory rate and effort** – Animals with cardiac disease, shock or anaemia may all be tachypnoeic and/or hyperpnoeic. Dyspnoea may be more common in cardiac disease associated with pulmonary oedema, but animals heading towards terminal stages of shock can also be dyspnoeic.
- **Temperature** – Pyrexia can indicate infectious, immune-mediated or neoplastic disease and can also be present with pain. Subnormal temperature is more common with cardiac disease/shock. The colour of stool on the thermometer should be noted

(e.g. black could indicate melaena; orange could indicate haemolysis or liver disease).

■ **Thorough physical assessment can provide other vital clues** – For example, splenomegaly or hepatomegaly are often noted with regenerative anaemia, but can also indicate neoplasia or masses of other origin (e.g. splenic hematoma). If a splenic mass is suspected, then abdominal palpation should be conducted with care to prevent potential rupture of the mass.

What is the PCV?

Further investigation can be divided into two groups: in-house tests that will direct immediate treatment; and tests by external laboratories that are likely to deliver a diagnosis. Of these, correct evaluation and interpretation of an in-house PCV and blood smear examination are the most important and will direct which further investigative steps are appropriate.

Jugular samples should be avoided in animals with any suspicion of thrombocytopenia or coagulopathy.

In-house evaluation

■ **PCV (Figure 4A)** – If a patient presents with lethargy, pallor and tachycardia, and anaemia is suspected, the most important (and simple) confirmatory test is a *manual packed cell volume measurement*. It is essential that the blood sample is anticoagulated (heparin or EDTA) and adequately mixed prior to measuring the PCV; otherwise the result may be significantly inaccurate (either high or low). This should help to rule out the main differential of hypoperfusion (e.g. resulting from cardiac disease or distributive shock) – in which case the PCV would be normal or only very mildly reduced. **Care is needed in interpretation, as *acute* blood loss will not necessarily**

result in marked changes in the PCV or total solids; this takes time (hours) for the effects to be seen.

At the same time further valuable information is obtained:

■ **Plasma colour** – The plasma in the capillary tube can also be assessed for icterus or haemolysis when the PCV is tested (Figures 4B and C).
■ **Total plasma solids** – Can be measured to help differentiate between haemolysis or decreased red cell production (normal total solids), and blood loss (reduced total solids).

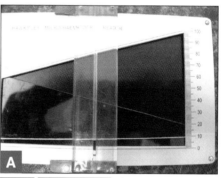

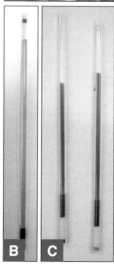

Figure 4: Manual determination of PCV confirms anaemia in patients with (A) clear plasma, (B) icterus and (C) haemolysis

If the **PCV is normal** but the animal is pale, then the following list of differential diagnoses should be considered:

- Cardiogenic shock
- Distributive shock
- Early hypovolaemic/blood loss shock
- High sympathetic tone.

If anaemia is confirmed, it can be graded as **mild, moderate, or severe** (see Figure 1). This is helpful in determining pathogenesis (e.g. severe anaemia is most likely to result from haemolysis or bone marrow disorders, whereas mild anaemia is more likely to result from chronic disease, or acute blood loss), as well as determining what immediate treatment, if any, is required.

Key decision: Is the anaemia regenerative?

In-house haematology and blood smear examination in anaemic patients can help to distinguish signs of a regenerative anaemia (macrocytosis, polychromasia and anisocytosis) from a non-regenerative anaemia.

Regenerative anaemias can be caused by either blood loss or haemolysis.

Non-regenerative anaemias can be caused by disorders of the bone marrow, or by external factors that prevent the bone marrow from responding appropriately to anaemia, such as iron deficiency or a lack of erythropoietin (as seen in CRF).

HELPFUL HINTS

- Automated reticulocyte counts from in-house machines can be very inaccurate and should not be relied upon to decide whether the anaemia is regenerative. ➡️

- Automated, in-house platelet counts can also be unreliable, so it is vital to look at a blood smear for all patients that may be bleeding. Dogs are unlikely to bleed spontaneously if they have an average of more than 2 platelets per high power field (average number of platelets per high power field x20 approximates to platelet count x10^9/l).
- Regeneration can take up to 96 hours to become apparent following acute blood loss or haemolysis.

Key decision: Is there haemolysis?

A key distinction in the investigation of regenerative (or pre-regenerative) anaemia is the differentiation of blood loss from haemolysis. Much of the supporting information for haemolysis will have been gained through the preceding steps, through assessment of mucous membrane colour (icterus) and plasma colour (icteric or haemolysis). Further supporting evidence will come from assessment of the serum biochemistry (bilirubinaemia) and urine analysis (haemoglobinuria, bilirubinuria). Further specific tests that can be performed in house include:

- **An in-saline autoagglutination test (Figure 5)** – Can also be performed to check for IMHA. This is performed by placing 1 drop of anti-coagulated blood in 1 drop of saline on a microscope slide and assessing for agglutination both grossly and microscopically. Care must be taken to differentiate rouleaux from agglutination (Figures 6A and B). If in doubt, another drop of saline can be added. It is worth remembering that in-saline agglutination confirms the presence of anti-erythrocyte antibodies and therefore a Coombs' test is not required for diagnosis.

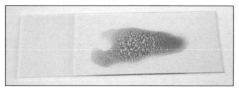

Figure 5: In-saline autoagglutination

KEY POINT: INVESTIGATION OF UNDERLYING CAUSE

The investigation thus far will have allowed the differentiation of anaemia from other causes of pallor, classified the anaemia as regenerative, non-regenerative (or pre-regenerative) and probably distinguished blood loss from haemolysis in the case of regenerative anaemia. Further investigation is centred on differentiation of the cause of the identified anomalies. Not all the diagnostic tests are appropriate in all circumstances and by following the algorithm, only those tests which are appropriate to the patient can be selected.

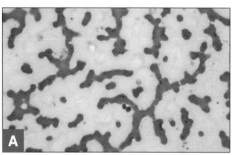

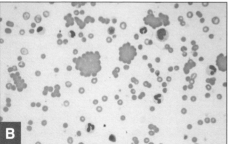

Figure 6: (A) Rouleaux formation. (B) Autoagglutination. Courtesy of Dr Andrew Torrance

It is very important to collect all samples **before** commencing any treatment, as fluids, corticosteroids and antibiotics can all interfere with obtaining an accurate diagnosis and some treatments are contraindicated in certain conditions (e.g. steroids/NSAIDs in GI bleeding; steroids for infectious causes of haemolysis). Depending on the patient's coagulation status, the potential risks associated with sampling should be considered.

- **Biochemistry can:**
  - Help to distinguish blood loss from haemolysis (low albumin and globulin versus raised liver enzymes and raised bilirubin)
  - Give evidence for non-regenerative causes of anaemia such as renal disease or hypothyroidism (high cholesterol)
  - Suggest other causes for blood loss anaemia or haemolytic anaemia, e.g. hypophosphataemia (which can cause haemolysis), hypoadrenocorticism (which can cause blood loss anaemia as well as a reduced regenerative response associated with hypocortisolaemia).

HELPFUL HINTS

- If hypoadrenocorticism is suspected the electrolytes should be checked; however, these may be normal with atypical hypoadrenocorticism in which case an ACTH stimulation test should be performed.
- Primary liver disease causing coagulopathy can be confused with haemolytic anaemia. This is because anaemia, raised liver enzymes and hyperbilirubinaemia can be present in both conditions.

■ **Urinalysis** – Is there evidence for haematuria (red cells in the sediment) or haemoglobinuria/bilirubinuria (Figure 7)?

HELPFUL HINT

■ Myoglobinuria can cause marked discoloration of urine and will give a positive dipstick reaction for haemoglobin.

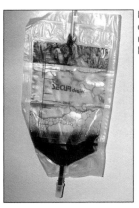

Figure 7: A urine collection bag revealing gross bilirubinuria

■ **Blood typing (Figure 8)** – Prior to transfusion, blood typing is advisable in dogs but not essential if this is the first blood transfusion the patient has received.

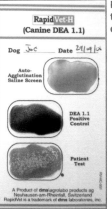

Figure 8: A canine blood typing test reveals this dog is DEA-1.1 positive

■ **Thoracic radiography/ultrasonography** – Can help distinguish between cardiac disease and hypovolaemic shock (is there cardiomegaly or microcardia?). It can also be used to identify pleural or pericardial effusions (Figure 9) (which may be haemorrhagic and causing anaemia, or may be the result of cardiac or neoplastic disease). Imaging can also identify other mass lesions which may be causing anaemia.

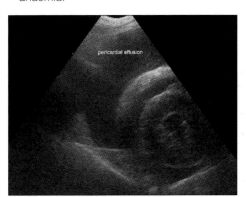

Figure 9: Echocardiogram revealing a pericardial effusion. Courtesy of Irene Schaafsma

■ **Abdominal imaging** – Can be used to look for organomegaly, mass lesions, and the presence of free abdominal fluid (Figure 10). Ultrasonography, if available, is more

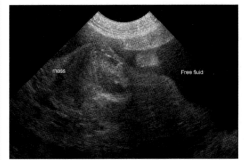

Figure 10: Abdominal ultrasound image revealing the presence of a liver mass with echogenic free abdominal fluid. Courtesy of Irene Schaafsma

sensitive than radiography, does not require sedation, and can be used to guide abdominocentesis if free abdominal fluid is identified (blood is usually echogenic) helping to distinguish haemoabdomen from other forms of ascites. Ultrasonography is much more sensitive for the detection of fluid than is blind abdominocentesis.

External laboratory evaluation

- **Platelet number, white cell count, red cell count and cell morphology** – The presence or absence of other cytopenias can be identified. Abnormal morphology may provide evidence for: microangiopathic conditions (schistocytes); IMHA (spherocytes); or neoplastic conditions (e.g. immature blastic cells in acute lymphoid leukaemia). Reduction in all three cell lines (red, white and platelets) points towards a bone marrow disorder and would help rule out blood loss or haemolysis as a cause for anaemia. Reduction in red blood cells and platelets only can be more difficult to interpret, as it can be seen with immune-mediated disease, blood loss and bone marrow disorders (such as granulocytic leukaemia).
- **A reticulocyte count** – Confirms the presence and magnitude of the regenerative response.
- **Coombs' test** – Ideally, check for IgG, IgM and complement at a range of temperatures. Assess the significance of titre. Note – not all haemolytic anaemias are Coombs'-positive and other diseases such as splenic haemangiosarcoma can cause a weak positive Coombs' test.
- **PCR** – For infectious agents (e.g. *Ehrlichia*, *Leishmania*, *Babesia*, *Mycoplasma*). This requires an EDTA sample.
- **Coagulation tests** – Require a citrated plasma sample.
- **Specific coagulation factor/von Willebrand factor (vWf) assays** – It is

important to distinguish between consumption of factors due to recent bleeding and deficiency states which have caused bleeding.

- **Oestrogen level** – Can be helpful in non-regenerative anaemias.
- **Faecal occult blood** – Useful to help identify gastrointestinal blood loss, but chronic bleeding does not always cause melaena. This needs a meat-free diet to be fed 3 days before testing.
- **Iron and iron-binding proteins** – Can be used to help confirm or exclude gastrointestinal bleeding and iron deficiency as a cause for a non-regenerative anaemia.
- **Erythropoietin** – Can be helpful in non-regenerative cases to exclude renal disease as an underlying cause.
- **Thyroid hormone tests, adrenocortical hormone evaluation** – Endocrine diseases are often associated with mild anaemia. They are very rarely the sole cause of a moderate to severe anaemia, but may contribute to clinical signs and may influence response to treatment.
- **Bone marrow evaluation (Figure 11)** – Non-regenerative anaemias (particularly if other cytopenias are present) will often require cytology of bone marrow aspirates and histopathology of core biopsy specimens, to help distinguish the underlying disease process.

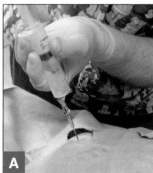

Figure 11:
(A) Obtaining a bone marrow aspirate (continues) ➡

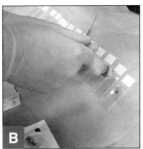

Figure 11:
(continued) (B)
Slide preparation

Conclusion

Using the algorithm (see Figure 1) supported by an in-house PCV and smear examination with appropriate imaging it is usually possible to classify the anaemia into regenerative or non-regenerative, haemorrhagic or haemolytic. This allows appropriate, rational treatment to be initiated (such as a blood transfusion) whilst waiting external laboratory results. ∎

How to...

Provide effective oxygen supplementation

by Karen Humm

Respiratory distress is triggered by hypoxia, hypercapnia or a marked increased in the work of breathing. Hypoxia is by far the most common of these causes and generally patients with hypercapnia or a marked increase in the work of breathing have concurrent hypoxia. Therefore oxygen supplementation is of key importance in managing any patient with respiratory distress. If there is uncertainty as to whether a patient is in respiratory distress, supplemental oxygen should be administered while they are evaluated.

Oxygen supplementation methods

Oxygen makes up approximately 21% of the gaseous component of room air. Various methods of increasing this percentage are available, each with its own advantages and disadvantages. For both short and long term options the percentage inspired oxygen achieved will be affected by the size of the patient, their respiratory rate and the flow rate of oxygen used. Rough guides for flow rates are given below but they only act as a starting point and adjustments may need to be made on a patient by patient basis.

Oxygen source

The source of oxygen for patients in respiratory distress will vary between practices depending on their facilities.

However most practices will use one (or more) of 4 options:

- Direct from a cylinder using oxygen tubing
- Breathing system attached to an anaesthetic machine
- Piped source:
  - Using oxygen tubing
  - Using a breathing system.

Humidification

Irrespective of the method of administration, oxygen is supplied in cylinders or tanks of dry gas or produced as a dry gas from an oxygen generator. Administration of dry oxygen at high rates can lead to increased viscosity of respiratory secretions, impaired mucociliary clearance, mucosal desiccation and an increased risk of respiratory tract infection. Therefore if oxygen is to be administered for longer than an hour or so, it should be humidified. This is particularly important in patients with nasal or tracheal catheters or those undergoing mechanical ventilation as the administered oxygen bypasses the upper airway, the natural site of humidification in an animal. Humidification is achieved simply by allowing oxygen to bubble through sterile water. Bubble humidifiers are cheap (Flexicare Medical Ltd) and will fit on to flow meters designed for piped oxygen (Figure 1). If a humidifier is not available, regular

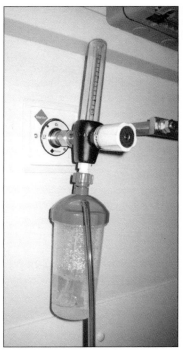

Figure 1: Bubble humidifier

nebulisation can be performed but this requires intensive nursing care and expensive equipment. Alternatively, some commercially available oxygen cages have an integral humidification system.

Short term methods of oxygen supplementation

When a patient in respiratory distress presents to the practice, a quick but thorough physical examination should be performed (focused on the patient's respiratory, cardiovascular and neurological systems) and initial stabilisation performed. During this period oxygen is generally supplemented non-invasively. However, the requirement for a member of staff to stay with the patient constantly means that this is usually a short term option and facilities for administering oxygen on a longer term basis may need to be organised.

Mask supplementation

Using a mask to provide oxygen to a patient is simple and effective. An oxygen flow rate of 1 (for cats and small dogs) to 10 (for giant breeds) litres/minute should be used. Whilst a high percentage of inspired oxygen (80–90%) can be achieved in anaesthetised dogs using a tight fitting mask, the majority of conscious dyspnoeic patients will not tolerate a tight fitting mask and therefore the actual percentage of inspired oxygen in clinical patients is closer to 35–55%. Calmer patients will tolerate a mask gently held over the muzzle allowing free movement, but many patients, particularly cats, will not allow a mask near their head. Struggling with a patient to administer oxygen is counterproductive as their oxygen demand will be increased by the stress and increased muscular activity. Collapsed or weak patients are ideal candidates for mask oxygen supplementation as they do not move (although unconscious patients need intubation to protect their airway from the risk of aspiration) (Figure 2). Care should be taken as a tight fitting mask can easily lead to hyperthermia and inadvertent use of lower oxygen flow rates than the patient's minute volume re-breathing will result in hypercapnia.

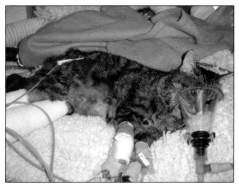

Figure 2: Oxygen delivered by mask is most suitable for weaker patients

Flow-by supplementation

Flow-by supplementation is not an efficient means of oxygen supplementation (Figure 3). The conscious patient is likely to receive an inspired oxygen percentage of considerably less than the maximum, 40%, achievable by this method. However, flow-by is usually ready within seconds, is non-invasive and is less stressful than mask supplementation. Flow rates of 2–10 litres/minute should be used and the oxygen outlet should be held as close to the patient's nose (or mouth if they are panting) as possible without causing distress. Sometimes a patient will tolerate flow-by when tubing is directed to the side of their mouth rather than in front of it.

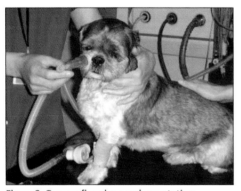

Figure 3: Oxygen flow-by supplementation

Tracheal oxygen supplementation

If a patient is showing signs of severe respiratory distress secondary to upper respiratory tract obstruction (increased inspiratory effort and marked inspiratory noise audible without a stethoscope) a catheter can be placed percutaneously into the trachea. A brief clip and clean of the overlying skin is required and a large bore, 14 or 16 gauge, catheter is inserted into the space between the tracheal rings 4 and 5, or 5 and 6. Once the stylet is within the trachea the catheter is advanced into the tracheal lumen in the

direction of the carina and the stylet removed. Oxygen is then administered in a flow-by fashion directed at the catheter. This technique is only useful in dogs over approximately 10 kg who have a sufficiently large tracheal lumen to allow catheter placement. Invasive tracheal oxygen can be difficult to maintain and so is really only suitable for short term oxygen supplementation.

Longer term oxygen supplementation

Following an initial physical examination and emergency stabilisation (e.g. furosemide administration or thoracocentesis) it is often beneficial to allow a patient to calm in a kennel prior to further manipulation. Oxygen supplementation is continued with flow-by or mask supplementation whilst preparations for delivery of oxygen supplementation in the longer term are made.

Nasal catheters

Oxygen can be supplied direct into the respiratory tract via nasal catheters in both dogs and cats. Feeding tubes are commonly used as catheters with a 5 French catheter being suitable for a cat and an 8 or 10 French for most dogs. Before placement the catheter should be pre-measured against the animal from the nostril to the lateral canthus of the eye. A few drops of 0.5% proxymetacaine or 2% lidocaine should be administered into the nostril 10 minutes prior to placement of the catheter. The patient is gently restrained with their nose pointing dorsally and the catheter is advanced into the ventral meatus. Pushing the nasal planum dorsally while aiming the catheter ventro-medially can aid correct placement. The catheter should be gently but rapidly advanced as patients often move and sneeze during this part of the procedure. If the catheter is not in the ventral meatus it will not advance the pre-measured distance as the dorsal and middle meatuses end at the ethmoid turbinates rather than in the nasopharynx. Once the catheter is in the correct position it should be fixed in place with sutures or tissue glue attached to 'butterfly wings' of tape round the catheter. The catheter should loop round the alar cartilage with fixation close to the nasal orifice to prevent dislodgement (Figure 4). The catheter is then looped dorsally between the eyes (which may decrease the chance of the patient removing it) or on to the lateral aspect of the head to be secured just below the ear.

The procedure should be abandoned if an animal becomes distressed as this may lead to marked worsening of their hypoxia. The procedure is also contraindicated in coagulopathic animals. Once *in situ* catheters can be displaced by determined patients, so a buster collar may be required which again can be stressful. However, if a patient will tolerate placement and maintenance of a nasal oxygen catheter they can provide a consistent inspired oxygen percentage of 40–50% with an oxygen flow rate of 50–100 ml/kg/min. The placement of a second nasal catheter can increase this percentage further to 60–70%. Unfortunately, if a patient consistently pants then the mixing of air in the pharynx leads to a decrease in the percentage inspired oxygen.

Nasal prongs/cannulas

Prongs designed for oxygen supplementation in humans can be used for dogs. They come in 2 sizes (paediatric and adult – Flexicare Medical Ltd). The prongs advance approximately 1 cm into the nostril and will provide a percentage inspired oxygen of around 40%. They are minimally invasive but are therefore easily displaced by an intolerant patient. Administration of proxymetacaine or lidocaine into each nostril approximately 10 minutes before placing the prongs can be useful as can taping the prong tubing together (but not to the dog) over the dorsal aspect of the muzzle (Figure 5). As with a nasal catheter this method is less efficacious in the panting patient.

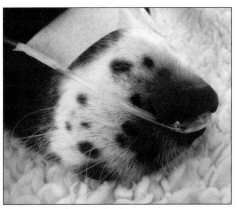

Figure 5: Nasal prongs *in situ*

Tracheal catheters

Some texts describe administering oxygen via a tracheal catheter on a longer term basis, particularly for patients with facial or upper airway injury. A standard intravenous catheter can be used or a long stay catheter of increased length placed as described above. In the author's hands this is not an effective method for longer term supplementation as the catheter is difficult to secure and prevent from kinking.

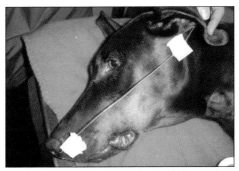

Figure 4: Nasal catheter looped around alar cartilage and fixed in place using bandage butterflys

Buster collar oxygen hoods

Oxygen can be administered into an enclosed buster collar (either practice-made or commercially produced (Kruuse UK Ltd)). Practice-made collars should have a small gap left at the top of the collar to allow venting of humid air and carbon dioxide. Despite this vent hole, many dogs and some cats become hyperthermic, particularly in hot conditions. Placement of the collar may be poorly tolerated, however most dogs and cats do settle if left in a kennel. A high flow rate should be used initially to fill the collar with oxygen and then a rate of approximately 1 litre/min is suitable for a medium-sized dog and should result in a percentage inspired oxygen of approximately 40%.

Oxygen cages

Collapsible (Figure 6) or lightweight oxygen cages are commercially available in various sizes (e.g. J.A.K. Marketing Ltd or Kruuse UK Ltd). They have adaptors for breathing systems and are simple to use. Models vary in presence of means of thermoregulatory or humidity control. Some practices also have permanent fixed oxygen cages although again they are rarely temperature or humidity controlled. As the cages are completely sealed hyperthermia can rapidly develop, particularly in dogs. It is of note that once a

cage is opened the level of oxygen within it rapidly drops to room level. This can mean that if a patient is frequently being handled their inspired oxygen fraction is barely increased.

An oxygen cage can be made in the practice when required by placing cling-film over the front of a cage although the gaps present and the large volume of the cage relative to the patient within it, mean that even with very high flow rates the percentage of oxygen is often barely increased.

Endotracheal intubation and ventilation

It is very rare that an animal in respiratory distress requires anaesthetising and intubation allowing provision of 100% oxygen. This most commonly occurs in patients with upper respiratory tract obstruction when intubation allows by-passing of the obstruction such as in cases of laryngeal paralysis. Judging when intubation is required can be difficult. Less invasive oxygen supplementation techniques in conjunction with stabilisation should be attempted first and the patient's response assessed. If a patient still has marked respiratory distress despite treatment then intubation and ventilation may be required. If the cause of respiratory distress is not upper respiratory tract in origin the prognosis for patients that require intubation and ventilation is unfortunately very poor.

Oxygen toxicity

Exposure of the lungs to an inspired oxygen fraction greater than 60% for greater than approximately 24–72 hours can lead to oxygen toxicity. This causes damage to the alveoli potentially worsening any lung disease present. Ideally therefore oxygen supplementation should be kept below 60% for longer term supplementation. As most methods of oxygen supplementation in the practice situation do not achieve an inspired percentage greater than 60% this is generally a theoretical concern. ∎

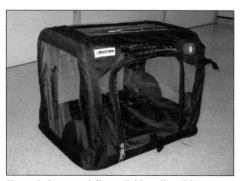

Figure 6: Commercially available collapsible oxygen kennel

How to approach the hypertensive patient

by Rosanne Jepson

Systemic hypertension can be defined as persistently raised blood pressure (BP) and is increasingly recognised in both the canine and feline populations, particularly in older patients. The presence of systemic hypertension can be damaging not only to the cardiovascular system but also to other target organs, such as the eye, kidney and central nervous sy stem. It is therefore extremely important to monitor BP and, when a diagnosis of systemic hypertension is confirmed, to implement appropriate long-term treatment and monitoring strategies in order to prevent ongoing target organ damage (TOD).

Categories of hypertension

Systemic hypertension is usually categorised into one of three classes, depending on underlying aetiology.

- **Secondary hypertension:** This is where systemic hypertension results from an underlying disease process (Figure 1). Secondary hypertension can also be attributable to the administration of certain drugs that can result in increased BP, e.g. phenylpropanolamine, glucocorticoids, mineralocorticoids or erythropoietin.

- **Idiopathic hypertension:** This refers to the presence of systemic hypertension where no underlying disease state can be identified. Idiopathic hypertension has been reported to affect approximately 20% of cats diagnosed with systemic hypertension but is considered rare in dogs.

Disease condition	Reported prevalence of hypertension with underlying disease condition	
	Dogs	Cats
Chronic kidney disease	10–80%	20–65%
Hyperthyroidism	NA	Pre-treatment 10–25% Post-treatment 20%
Hyperadrenocorticism	Pre-treatment 60–85% Post-treatment 40%	NA
Diabetes mellitus	25–50%	No association made
Primary hyperaldosteronism	Unknown	50–100% (Uncommon condition)
Phaeochromocytoma	40–85% (Rare condition)	Unknown (Extremely rare condition)

Figure 1: Clinical conditions associated with the development of secondary hypertension

- **White-coat hypertension:** This is the phenomenon whereby systemic BP is transiently increased due to activation of the sympathetic nervous system with excitement or anxiety during a clinic visit. Distinguishing white-coat hypertension from idiopathic hypertension can be challenging.

How to recognise the hypertensive patient

In human medicine, systemic hypertension is often referred to as 'the silent killer' because there can be very few warning signs – and the same is true for many of our veterinary patients. In some patients suspicion for the presence of systemic hypertension can be raised by evidence of TOD (Figure 2). These changes can be dramatic, such as the cat that presents with sudden-onset blindness as a consequence of retinal detachment or gross hyphaema, or the very rare patient presenting with neurological signs associated with hypertensive encephalopathy (e.g. obtundation or seizures). In most instances, however, clinical signs associated with systemic hypertension are minimal and vague. More often the clinical signs reported will be those related to an underlying disease process. Systemic hypertension is therefore most often diagnosed on the basis of careful and repeated assessment of blood pressure (Figures 3 and 4).

In which patients should we be monitoring blood pressure?

- Regular monitoring should be performed in any patient diagnosed with an underlying condition that has previously been associated with systemic hypertension (see Figure 1), even if initially normotensive. For example: *approximately 20% of cats that are normotensive at diagnosis of hyperthyroidism, will develop systemic hypertension after instituting anti-thyroid medication.*

- Any patient with TOD but especially those presenting with ocular or neurological signs that could be associated with systemic hypertension and which may require immediate anti-hypertensive therapy.
- Any patient started on medication that can cause increase in BP particularly if there is any evidence of underlying TOD.
- Part of a geriatric screening programme for cats and dogs over approximately 9 years.
- Any patient receiving anti-hypertensive medication.

How do I diagnose systemic hypertension?

One of the main difficulties when approaching a patient that you suspect to be hypertensive is deciding exactly 'when to make the diagnosis' and 'when to start treatment'. Recently the tendency has been to move away from a single BP value which defines systemic hypertension. Instead guidelines have been formulated as part of the American College of Veterinary Internal Medicine (ACVIM) Hypertension Consensus Statement, which consider diastolic and systolic BP as continuous variables and categorise them according to the risk of developing TOD.

The risk categories for systolic hypertension are listed in Figure 5. In general, unless there is evidence of hypertensive retinopathy/choroidopathy or hypertensive encephalopathy it is not currently advocated to start anti-hypertensive medication for those patients that fall within the 'minimal' or 'mild' risk categories (systolic BP <160 mmHg).

A flow diagram for a patient in which you have performed a BP measurement and to aid with diagnosis of systemic hypertension is shown in Figure 6. If hypertensive encephalopathy or hypertensive retinopathy/choroidopathy is identified, immediate anti-hypertensive therapy should be started.

Systemic hypertension can cause damage to a number of target organs, for example the eye, kidney, cardiovascular system and central nervous system.

- **Eyes:** Studies suggest that approximately 60–100% of cats with systemic hypertension will have evidence of ocular damage, namely hypertensive retinopathy/choroidopathy. Lesions can be relatively subtle but may include multifocal bullous retinal detachments, retinal detachment, fresh or resolving retinal haemorrhages, retinal vessel tortuosity or perivascular oedema creating the impression of vessel narrowing and hyphaema (Figure 2). Ocular manifestations of systemic hypertension are much less common in the dog, with the prevalence reported to be only 5–20%.
- **Kidney:** In order to maintain glomerular filtration rate and protect the kidney, glomerular capillary pressure is tightly controlled in the afferent arteriole by autoregulation. Systemic hypertension can override this autoregulatory process so that the glomeruli are exposed to elevated pressures resulting in glomerular hypertension, glomerulosclerosis and proteinuria.
- **Cardiovascular system:** Cardiovascular changes that have been associated with systemic hypertension include left ventricular hypertrophy and associated murmurs, arrhythmias and gallop rhythms. Epistaxis can also be a primary clinical sign of vascular damage secondary to systemic hypertension.
- **Central nervous system:** Neurological signs of systemic hypertension have most often been documented in experimental studies and include obtundation and seizures but are rare in clinical patients. However, neurological complications of systemic hypertension may be under-recognised and many owners will report an improvement in demeanour of their pet with successful management of systemic hypertension.

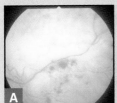 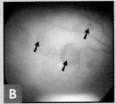 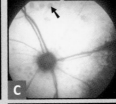 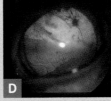

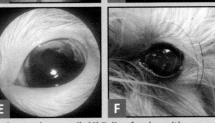

Figure 2: Ocular lesions secondary to systemic hypertension. (A) Feline fundus with evidence of multifocal intraretinal haemorrhages, large bullous retinal detachment and oedema. Marked variation in vessel calibre, with marked apparent loss/attenuation of retinal arterioles, is present (likely due to detachment/oedema). (B) Feline fundus with central focal bullous retinal detachment; peripherally similar smaller circular lesions can also be identified. There is also generalised oedema. Note how the blood vessel is raised by the bullous detachment (arrowed). (C) Feline fundus with multifocal areas of pigmentary disturbance. These represent old/inactive lesions likely to be secondary to small bullous detachment in the past (for example, that indicated by arrow). This cat did not have any detectable visual problem. (D) Feline eye demonstrating an area of total bullous retinal detachment, with large folds of retina displaced anteriorly within the vitreous and therefore now visible directly via the pupil with a focal light source (optic disc more posterior and obscured by retinal folds in this image). Multifocal intraretinal haemorrhages are present. Note also the marked mydriasis. This cat was clinically blind on presentation with similar changes observed bilaterally. (E) Feline eye with evidence of gross hyphaema (blood in anterior chamber). The blood has formed a solid clot. Also note the mydriasis, which is suggestive of concurrent fundic damage. (F) Canine eye with evidence of gross hyphaema. A–E Courtesy of R. Elks. Reproduced from *BSAVA Manual of Canine and Feline Cardiorespiratory Medicine, 2nd edition*

HOW TO MEASURE BLOOD PRESSURE

Techniques available

The gold standard for measuring BP is via direct arterial catheterisation. This technique provides continuous assessment of mean, systolic and diastolic BP. However, it is an invasive procedure which is not applicable to routine monitoring requirements. Direct arterial BP monitoring is therefore most often performed in those emergency patients requiring parenteral anti-hypertensive medication within an intensive care environment or during general anaesthesia.

Most often BP is assessed using an indirect technique, e.g. using an oscillometric device (Figure 3) or Doppler sphygmomanometry (Figure 4). Oscillometric devices rely on the detection of pressure oscillations of air within the cuff when the artery is partially occluded. When using an oscillometric device the mean BP is measured and systolic and diastolic pressures are calculated using inbuilt algorithms.

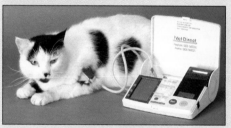

Figure 3: Oscillometric blood pressure measurement in the cat

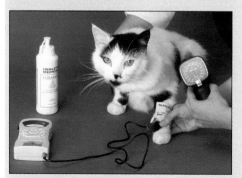

Figure 4: Doppler blood pressure measurement in the cat

The primary advantage of an oscillometric device is that, after cuff placement, the process is automated. This means that the technique requires little training and may make the machine easier to use in a fractious patient. However, oscillometric machines can be slow to take readings and may fail to obtain a measurement in patients with higher heart rates, arrhythmias or if the patient does not remain still throughout measurement.

The Doppler technique utilises a piezoelectric crystal to detect blood flow, converting this signal into an audible sound. The Doppler technique requires some degree of operator experience, but with a small amount of practice is easily mastered. However, it provides only reliable assessment of systolic BP. It is important to realise that in human medicine standards have been set for the validation of indirect BP measuring devices but that no veterinary device currently meets these criteria in conscious dogs and cats.

Tips for performing a BP measurement

- Choose a quiet and relaxed environment away from loud noise, disturbance and other animals.
- Every pet should have the opportunity to explore and acclimatise to their environment for approximately 5–10 minutes prior to BP measurement.
- Allow the owner to be present in order to relax their pet.
- Careful and gentle restraint by the owner or an experienced handler.
- More reliable measurements are usually obtained by allowing the patient to adopt their preferred position.
- BP measurements should always be performed prior to other procedures, e.g. physical examination, blood sampling or obtaining a temperature.
- Avoid performing BP measurements if the patient has received any sedation or undergone general anaesthesia.

For both the Doppler and oscillometric techniques, the BP cuff is most commonly placed on the mid antebrachium, although other sites can be used, e.g. hindleg or tail base. The limb circumference should be measured with a soft tape measure and a cuff width chosen that is 30–40% of limb circumference. Choosing a cuff which is too narrow may lead to falsely elevated BP measurements, whilst a cuff that is too large may underestimate BP. Ideally the patient should be positioned so that the cuff is approximately at the level of the heart.

For the Doppler technique, it is usual to perform an alcohol wipe and apply acoustic jelly in order to obtain adequate contact. In most instances clipping of fur adds additional stress for the patient and is not required. In long-haired patients clipping may be advantageous but the patient should be allowed to reacclimatise afterwards.

It is widely advised that the first measurement obtained is discarded and that subsequently a series of five consecutive and consistent measurements should be recorded and the mean calculated. For readings to be consistent, ideally there should be <20% variability between systolic measurements.

It is often helpful to produce a standard form to allow documentation of BP recordings for each patient. This form could also contain a record of the limb circumference, cuff size, the limb/tail used, the position and temperament of the patient during measurement and other clinical data such as heart rate. A record of this information allows operators to compare BP measurements on consecutive visits knowing that a similar approach and technique has been used.

Risk category	Systolic blood pressure (mmHg)	Recommendation for starting treatment
Minimal	<150	■ Minimal to mild risk of developing target organ damage (TOD) ■ Limited evidence that anti-hypertensive medication required
Mild	150–159	■ May represent cases of 'white-coat' hypertension ■ Treatment should be considered if evidence of ocular or central nervous system TOD ■ Continued monitoring recommended ■ Target categories for patients treated with anti-hypertensive therapies
Moderate	160–179	■ Moderate risk for the development of TOD ■ Anti-hypertensive therapy recommended in patients with evidence of TOD or where concurrent clinical conditions associated with hypertension have been identified ■ Confirmation of hypertensive category status should be made on at least two occasions unless there is evidence of ocular or CNS TOD, when therapy will be required immediately ■ Patients in this category which have no evidence of TOD or clinical conditions associated with systemic hypertension should be monitored carefully to exclude white-coat hypertension before a diagnosis of idiopathic hypertension is made and long-term treatment started
Severe	>180	■ The risk of development and progression of TOD is high ■ White-coat hypertension is uncommon ■ Immediate anti-hypertensive therapy indicated if ocular or CNS TOD present otherwise confirmation of category status should be made on at least two occasions

Figure 5: ACVIM risk categories for systolic hypertension

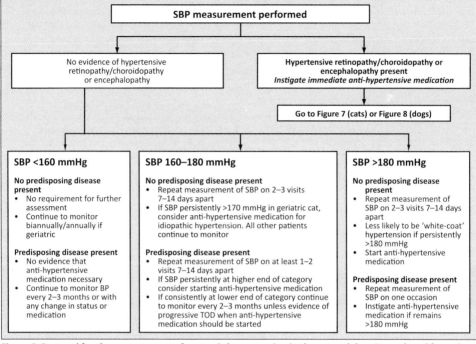

Figure 6: Protocol for the management of systemic hypertension in the cat and dog. Reproduced from the
BSAVA Manual of Canine and Feline Cardiorespiratory Medicine, 2nd edition

In all other patients where an underlying disease process has been identified but there is no evidence of hypertensive retinopathy/choroidopathy, measuring BP on at least two occasions 7–14 days apart is appropriate in order to confirm the diagnosis.

For all patients in which you suspect systemic hypertension it is advisable to obtain a minimum database:

- Complete history
- Full physical examination
- Serum biochemical profile
- Packed cell volume and total solids
- Urinalysis (specific gravity, dipstick, urine protein:creatinine ratio and sediment examination)
- Ophthalmological examination.

If there is clinical suspicion and supportive evidence from your minimum database you may wish to consider:

- Total T4 (cats)
- ACTH stimulation test/low dose dexamethasone suppression test
- Total T4/TSH (dogs)
- Ultrasound assessment of kidneys and adrenal glands
- Evaluation of urinary/plasma metanephrines
- Plasma aldosterone concentrations.

It is also important to consider other clinical factors that could influence BP measurements in your patient:

- Age: Systemic hypertension is more common in older patients (>9 years)

- Breed: Sight hounds are reported to have systemic BP 10–20 mmHg higher than other breeds. The exception to this rule is Irish Wolfhounds, that reportedly have BP lower than other sight hounds. So far no breed associations have been made in the cat
- Medications being administered (e.g. phenylpropanolamine, corticosteroids, mineralocorticoids, erythropoietin)
- Hydration status
- Recent intravenous fluid therapy.

How to diagnose idiopathic hypertension

A diagnosis of idiopathic hypertension should only be made if persistent hypertension is documented, perhaps with evidence of hypertensive ocular changes in combination with a full and unremarkable diagnostic work-up. BP should be assessed on at least two or three occasions 7–14 days apart. Theoretically the diagnostic evaluation should include direct assessment of glomerular filtration rate (GFR) to exclude the possibility of non-azotaemic kidney disease, although in practice this is rarely performed.

Some patients with systemic hypertension but no evidence of increased creatinine concentration demonstrate an inappropriate urine-concentrating ability (urine specific gravity <1.030). In this scenario the reduced urine concentrating ability could reflect hypertensive pressure diuresis and does not automatically imply reduced renal function.

How to diagnose white-coat hypertension

It can be difficult in some patients to distinguish between idiopathic hypertension and white-coat hypertension. A diagnosis of white-coat hypertension should only be made if: high BP readings have been documented on multiple occasions in the absence of other clinical signs; there is no evidence of TOD or underlying disease condition; the individual is at low risk for systemic hypertension; and the clinician is convinced that elevated BP measurements can be attributed to the clinic situation.

How do I treat systemic hypertension?

What are the goals of anti-hypertensive therapy?

- Gradual but persistent decline in BP.
- Avoidance of sudden fluctuations, precipitous drops in BP and periods of hypotension.
- Prevent severe TOD (e.g. ocular or CNS damage).
- Minimise ongoing chronic TOD (e.g. vascular damage within the kidney/ left ventricular hypertrophy).

Current evidence suggests that reducing BP to the 'minimal' or 'mild' ACVIM risk category (systolic blood pressure of <160mmHg) is a suitable target for most patients.

Preliminary considerations

- Any underlying disease process that may be contributing to the development of systemic hypertension or to target organ damage (e.g. chronic kidney disease or cardiac disease) should be identified and treated. *For some conditions, e.g. hyperadrenocorticism, this may lead to the partial or complete resolution of systemic hypertension. However, more often adjunctive anti-hypertensive therapy will be required and in some instances, such as feline hyperthyroidism, systemic hypertension may only be detected after treatment has been started.*
- If possible, any medications that could be contributing to increased BP should be discontinued.
- Some disease conditions will need specific anti-hypertensive therapy. *For example, an aldosterone-secreting tumour would require*

an aldosterone antagonist (e.g. spironolactone) combined with surgical adrenalectomy, whilst treatment of a pheochromocytoma would usually include an alpha-blocker (e.g. phenoxybenzamine), beta-blocker (e.g. atenolol) and surgical management.

Suggested guidelines for instituting and modifying anti-hypertensive treatment are outlined in Figure 7 (cats) and Figure 8 (dogs). Currently there is no indication in veterinary medicine to treat those patients with white-coat hypertension.

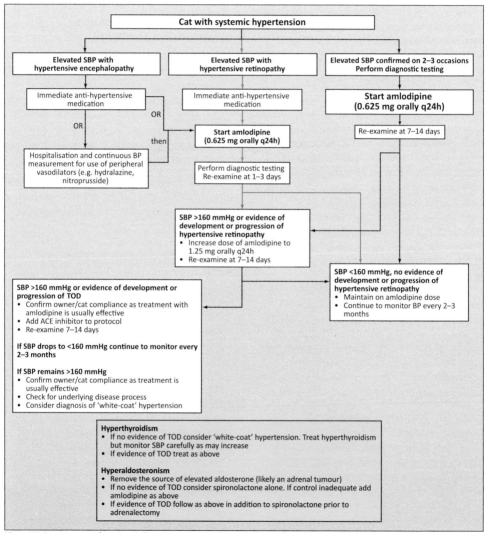

Figure 7: Treatment of systemic hypertension in the cat. Reproduced from *BSAVA Manual of Canine and Feline Cardiorespiratory Medicine, 2nd edition*

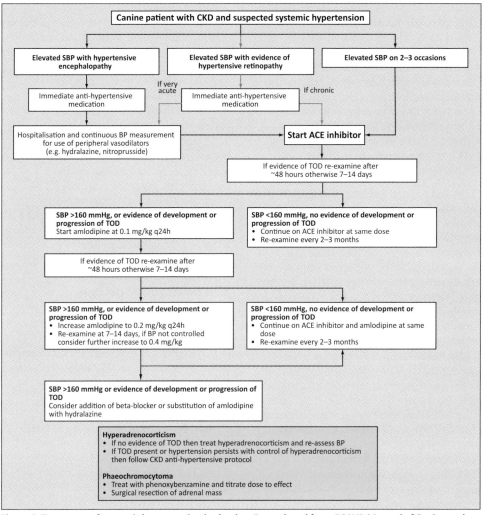

Figure 8: Treatment of systemic hypertension in the dog. Reproduced from *BSAVA Manual of Canine and Feline Cardiorespiratory Medicine, 2nd edition*

When starting anti-hypertensive therapy:

- Always explain and discuss the rationale for anti-hypertensive therapy with owners so that they understand the importance of long-term management and BP monitoring for their pet

- Introduce anti-hypertensive agents at the lowest therapeutic dose
- Monitor BP more frequently, e.g. after approximately 24–48 hours if there is concern regarding TOD (e.g. ocular changes). Monitoring after 7–14 days is appropriate in most other situations

- If a single anti-hypertensive agent fails to adequately control BP consider increasing the dose or adding a second anti-hypertensive agent
- Always confirm owner and patient compliance prior to any dose adjustment
- Always reassess BP approximately 7–14 days after any dose adjustment or sooner if there is TOD (e.g. ocular)
- Aim to achieve BP in the 'minimal' or 'mild' ACVIM risk category (systolic BP <160 mmHg).

The first line anti-hypertensive agent in cats is amlodipine besylate, a calcium channel blocker. Cats appear to have a unique sensitivity to this anti-hypertensive agent and invariably a reduction in blood pressure of 20–30 mmHg can be expected. Angiotensin-converting enzyme inhibitors (ACEis) are the most common second line anti-hypertensive agents but have a relatively limited anti-hypertensive action, reducing BP by approximately 5–10 mmHg.

Care should always be taken when introducing an ACEi, particularly in cats with moderate to severe chronic kidney disease (CKD) or evidence of dehydration, when use of an ACEi may result in a rapid reduction in renal function and worsening azotaemia. Monitoring of renal function is advocated after introduction of this medication.

Systemic hypertension in dogs is much more challenging to manage than in cats. In dogs with CKD and systemic hypertension the first line anti-hypertensive agent is an ACEi, although response to this agent can be variable and disappointing. However, there is evidence that ACEis may have additional benefits in dogs with CKD by reducing proteinuria. Once again care must be taken if introducing this class of medication to dogs with moderate to severe kidney disease or dehydration due to the concerns regarding decline in GFR.

If BP is inadequately controlled with an ACEi alone, then amlodipine besylate is often added to the regime. Hydralazine, beta-blockers and aldosterone antagonists can be considered if the combination of an ACEi and amlodipine are ineffective, but great care must be taken and frequent monitoring performed to ensure against episodes of hypotension (systolic BP <120 mmHg).

Currently the evidence for a salt-restricted diet in dogs and cats with systemic hypertension is controversial and use of a salt-restricted diet alone is unlikely to modulate BP. High-salt diets should be avoided but there is limited evidence that a salt-restricted diet should be used and instead a diet appropriate to any underlying disease condition (e.g. CKD) should be considered.

The emergency patient

Occasionally patients will present as an emergency with evidence of hypertensive encephalopathy and/or severe ocular TOD (e.g. hypertensive retinopathy/choroidopathy, retinal detachment, retinal haemorrhage or hyphaema). Such patients will require immediate hospitalisation and more aggressive anti-hypertensive therapy.

A number of parenteral anti-hypertensive medications are available, e.g. sodium nitroprusside and hydralazine. However, these agents should only be used with continuous BP monitoring, ideally via direct arterial catheterisation, or (at a minimum) an intensive care environment which allows frequent BP assessment.

The exception is those cats which present with ocular TOD, where oral amlodipine besylate therapy is successful in rapidly reducing BP. In these patients hospitalisation is not an absolute requirement but more frequent follow-up, for example within 24–48 hours, would be recommended in order to ensure reduction in BP and prevent further TOD.

Management and monitoring of the treated patient

- Once BP has been stabilised, routine monitoring approximately every 2–3 months is recommended.
- Aim to maintain BP in the 'mild' or 'minimal' ACVIM risk category (systolic BP <160 mmHg).
- Continue routine monitoring to achieve optimal management of any underlying disease condition.
- Adjust anti-hypertensive medication carefully to maintain BP control.
- Monitor BP more frequently if there is a change in:
  - The patient's clinical status
  - The underlying disease condition
  - The patient's medication. ∎

How to…

Microchip chelonians

by Mike Jessop

mplantation of a microchip into tortoises is a safe and effective technique, provided extra precautions are taken to minimise the risk of sepsis.

It is not uncommon to see an abscess following injections in chelonians (Figure 1). The problem arises due to the nature of the reptile integument. The scaled skin, with low surface shedding, leads to high levels of surface microorganisms. Reptiles are non-groomers and if housing conditions are not optimal skin contaminants can be present in high levels. The skin is inelastic, hence the injection site stays open after withdrawal of the needle. This increases the risk of chip loss and infection.

Thus, attention to sterility prior to implantation is paramount. Wound closure is necessary and implant site analgesia is required. For these reasons, the procedure is deemed to be an act of veterinary surgery and so should only be carried out by a veterinary surgeon as an in-patient procedure.

The animal should be admitted with informed consent, for the procedure and secondly for the use of non-licensed medications.

As with all microchipping procedures, remember first to check thoroughly for prior implanted chips. Make sure a check is made for non-standard sites, especially the forelimbs.

Equipment (Figure 2)
- Toothbrush.
- Skin scrub.
- Local anaesthetic.
- Sedative/general anaesthetic (if required).
- Chip and implanter.
- Scanner.
- Sterile cotton buds.
- Tissue glue or suture kit.

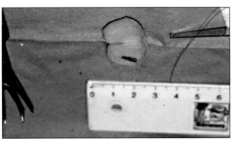

Figure 1: Sectioned abscess to reveal microchip as the nidus. Note reptile 'pus' is a fibrinous material that solidifies around the infection

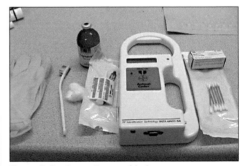

Figure 2: Equipment assembled

The site

The internationally agreed site is the left hindleg and the preferred position is over the quadriceps muscle mass. The chip can be placed subcutaneously if the animal is large enough, or intramuscularly in smaller animals.

Access is straightforward in most species of tortoise. Certain species and some individuals can be more difficult. Nervous individuals, especially recently wild-caught animals, may retract the limb. Box turtles and hingeback species are able to close the femoral fossa completely. Some species become so large and powerful that sustained extension of the hindlimb is impossible. In some situations sedation is required. Refer to specific texts for advice on drugs and dosages.

For the above reasons, there have been some calls to change the site to a subcarapacial position, caudally on the left side. This has the advantage of easier access and a more superficial position in large tortoises. However, until there is international agreement, it is advised to maintain the left hindleg site.

Site preparation

The limb is gently extended. A surgical scrub of the site is essential (Figure 3). Abscessation following implantation is occasionally seen and entirely preventable. The scaled skin of tortoises requires meticulous cleaning. The preferred technique is gentle scrubbing with a toothbrush and iodine scrub. This may need to be extensive if the skin is heavily soiled. The soap is then rinsed off with surgical spirit.

Analgesia

The implant site is infiltrated with local anaesthetic (Figure 4). In adults the skin is thick; therefore intradermal and subcutaneous infiltration is needed to ensure effective analgesia. Standard veterinary formulations of local anaesthetics appear to

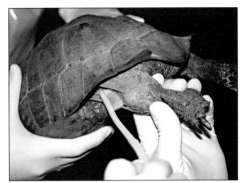

Figure 3: Scrubbing the site

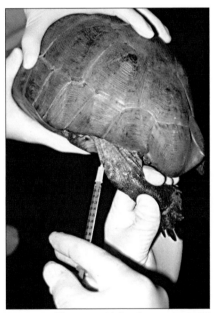

Figure 4: Infiltration with local anaesthesia (30 G needles are ideal)

be well tolerated in chelonians but take care to keep volumes to a minimum, especially in small individuals. Use of insulin syringes with 30 G needles is recommended.

If the chip is to be placed intramuscularly some infiltration into the muscle is required.

It is important to advise the owner that a functional lameness is possible due to the slow clearance of the local anaesthetic. Otherwise this will be blamed on the microchip.

The incision

In older animals it is recommended to incise the skin with a scalpel. In younger animals one can use the implant needle alone. Position the needle either subcutaneously or intramuscularly and insert the chip.

The insertion point for the implant needle is just above the stifle. The needle is inserted in a proximal direction away from the stifle and toward the hip along the anterior (dorsal) thigh. Length of insertion will vary with size of the animal, aiming to achieve a final chip site in the upper half of the upper limb.

The chip

All standard microchips are acceptable for implantation into tortoises (Figure 5). The newer smaller gauge mini-microchips are available for smaller animals and can be implanted in animals <100 mm in length.

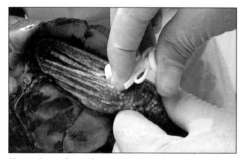

Figure 5: Implantation

Closure

Very occasionally haemorrhage occurs on needle withdrawal. This is more commonly seen on intramuscular implantation. In some individuals this can be marked and risks flushing the chip back to the skin incision. Use sterile cotton buds to apply local pressure.

Cotton bud swabbing is important to dry the site prior to closure. Suturing is acceptable with a single mattress suture to ensure eversion of skin edges. Skin staples are effective. The reptile skin heals more quickly if closed in an everted position.

The preferred technique is to use tissue glue (Figure 6A). The skin is bonded in an everted pattern. The use of liquid skin (Figure 6B) or liquid bandage adds additional wound protection.

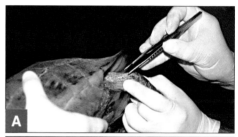

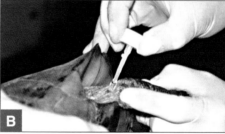

Figure 6: (A) Apposing the skin edges after applying the tissue glue. (B) Applying 'liquid skin' as a dressing

Post-procedural care

Keep the animal hospitalised for at least 2 hours after the procedure. Check the wound and microchip placement (Figure 7) just prior to returning to the owner.

It is recommended to maintain the tortoise in a clean environment for a few days, especially for digging species or those allowed free roam in a garden.

If sutures or staples are used, they should be left in place for a minimum of 4 weeks.

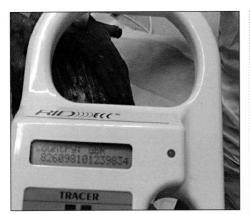

Figure 7: Post procedure confirmation

Aquatic species

Terrapins require extra care following the procedure. It is advised that water quality and hygiene is stressed to the owner prior to implantation. If possible, maintain in a dry environment for 2 days after the procedure. Daily wound cleansing with iodine, drying, then application of a waterproof dressing such as Orabase will reduce any problems. Terrapins will generally heal more quickly and 2 weeks post-procedural care should be all that is required. Most risk of infection is from contamination via poor water quality.

Timing

In non-hibernating species timing is not an issue. In hibernating species, do not implant less than 6 weeks prior to hibernation. If licensing regulations force implantation close to hibernation it is important to keep the animal awake for at least 6 weeks after the technique. This is easily achieved with an indoor heated vivarium.

Regulations

Under the Convention on International Trade in Endangered Species of Wild Fauna and Flora (CITES) certain species are required by law to be microchipped for trading. This legislation comes under the jurisdiction of the Animal Health and Veterinary Laboratories Agency (AHVLA).

> Wildlife Licensing and Registration Service
> Zone I/17, Temple Quay House, Temple Quay, Bristol BS1 6EB
> Phone: 0117 372 8691 or 0117 372 8168
> Email: wildlife.licensing@ahvla.gsi.gov.uk

This requirement for action under the legislation only arises on sale of these animals.

Many species are affected, including

- *Testudo graeca* (spur-thighed complex; several different species represented under this name)
- *Testudo marginata* (marginated tortoise)
- *Testudo hermanni* (Hermann's tortoise).

For a complete list of species covered refer to the AHVLA.

The more recently traded species are not covered, e.g. *Testudo horsefieldi* (Horsfield's, Russian, Afghan or Steppe tortoise) and *Geochelone pardalis* (leopard tortoise). Legislation is subject to change and it should be noted that some countries will impose export bans on their native species.

Prior to sale the animal must be microchipped and a licence obtained from AHVLA.

A special exemption exists for tortoises of less than 100 mm straight carapace length.

In the case of captive-bred tortoises covered by CITES the sire and dam need to be microchipped. A breeder's licence is then obtained for the sale of the hatchlings. These can than then be sold along with an Article 10 Certificate. Once they reach 100 mm a chip must be implanted prior to any subsequent sale.

Therefore, when presented with a newly acquired tortoise, it is important to check for certification. If the animal is over 100 mm in length there should already be a microchip implanted and the number should be logged on the certificate. The certificate will have been returned to the AHVLA by the seller but, ideally, a copy should be handed to the new owner. Long-owned animals do not need certification and the CITES regulation is not a registration scheme. Clients with animals that have been in their possession for many years are encouraged to write down the provenance of their animals as far as they can remember. Newly implanted microchips should be registered on the manufacturer's national database. ■

FURTHER READING

Girling SJ and Raiti P (2004) *BSAVA Manual of Reptiles, 2nd edition*. BSAVA Publications, Gloucester
Mader DR (2005) *Reptile Medicine and Surgery, 2nd edition*. Elsevier, Philadelphia
McArthur S, Wilkinson R and Meyer J (2004) *Medicine and Surgery of Tortoises and Turtles*. Blackwell, Oxford

Microchip information and details of companies signed up to the BSAVA Microchip Advisory Group Codes of Practice are available at **www.bsava.com**

Microchip Adverse Reaction forms are available from **www.bsava.com**. It is important that any post-implantation complications are reported as an adverse reaction.

Details of implantation sites for chelonians and other species are available from the WSAVA website via **www.bsava.com**

How to...

Decide whether **CT** or **MRI** is best for your patient

by Victoria Johnson

There has been a rapid increase in the availability of cross-sectional imaging techniques in recent years. CT and MRI are now readily accessible in many referral institutions. In addition, mobile MRI and CT units make frequent visits to veterinary practices all over the UK and some first opinion practices are investing in low field MRI systems and CT scanners. This means that vets are now faced with a situation where they have the choice between these two advanced imaging modalities and a need to understand their respective strengths and weaknesses.

This article aims to simplify that choice and guide you in selection of an appropriate imaging modality. In some situations this is easy and there is a clear clinical benefit to using one modality over the other. There are, however, some circumstances where other factors such as cost, time, accessibility or personal preference become more important in selection.

What is CT?

Computed tomography (CT) (Figure 1) is a cross-sectional imaging modality based on X-ray technology. X-rays are produced from a high-powered X-ray tube and pass through the patient to be received by a panel of detectors. The X-ray beam is attenuated as it passes through the patient and this allows an image to be created based on the relative density of the different body parts. In most modern X-ray machines the tube rotates around the patient as the CT bed moves forwards or backwards. The bed can either move in small steps, creating a single 'slice' of the patient, or can move constantly as the tube rotates. The latter creates a helix of imaging data from the patient (so-called helical CT) that can then be reconstructed by a computer into different formats.

Usually the data are reconstructed into transverse slices of varying thickness, but sagittal, dorsal and three-dimensional reconstructions can also be created and are extremely useful. The most up-to-date CT scanners have multiple panels of detectors to

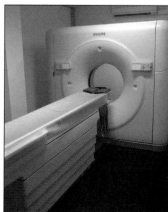

Figure 1: External appearance of a CT scanner

receive the X-ray beam after it has passed through the patient. This multidetector CT (MDCT) technology allows extremely rapid imaging (as little as 10 seconds to image an entire dog from nose to tail) and generates a volume of attenuation information, thus enabling exquisite multiplanar and 3D reconstructions. MDCT also facilitates highly detailed CT angiography to be performed using iodinated contrast media.

CT – KEY FEATURES

- Ionising radiation
- Equipment, setup and maintenance usually cost less than MRI
- Images acquired in transverse plane, but with MDCT additional planes can be reconstructed with equivalent resolution
- Extremely quick, especially MDCT
- Intravenous iodinated contrast media used for most examinations*
- Can easily perform angiography with helical CT scanners

* In general contrast medium is advised for most CT examinations with the exception of cases where its administration could compromise the health of the patient, or in cases where bone imaging alone is required.

What is MRI?

Magnetic resonance imaging (MRI) is based on the use of strong magnetic fields and radiofrequency pulses to generate cross-sectional images. The patient is placed into a large magnet and the powerful magnetic field results in the alignment of hydrogen atoms within the body. Different radiofrequency pulses and additional gradient magnetic fields are then turned on and off to create a complex set of frequency information that can be transformed into an image. Unlike CT, images of the patient can be acquired in any plane (sagittal, dorsal, transverse, or oblique).

Magnetism is measured by means of a unit, the Tesla (T). Two main types of MR scanner

are available: low field and high field (Figure 2). The low field magnets have a smaller magnetic field (0.2–0.5 T usually) and are open devices. These are considerably cheaper than high field magnets and have a smaller field of view. The image quality – especially of the brain and head – is usually good, though sequences generally take longer to acquire than with high field magnets.

High field magnets are supercooled with liquid helium. They are larger, more expensive structures with a closed gantry. The images are quicker to acquire and of high quality due

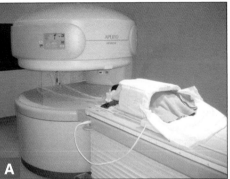

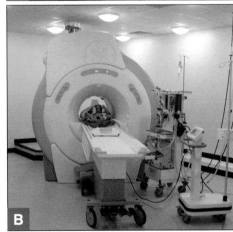

Figure 2: (A) External appearance of a low field MRI scanner. (B) External appearance of a high field MRI scanner. Courtesy of the Animal Health Trust

to the higher signal-to-noise ratio compared to low field systems. High field MR scanners are much more suited to angiography and other advanced imaging techniques than the low field scanners.

In MR imaging different combinations of radiofrequency pulses and gradient magnetic fields are used to create sequences of images with different contrast. Many different MRI sequences are available. By utilising different sequences and techniques and also by the administration of intravenous contrast medium (gadolinium) it is possible to be very precise about the nature of a lesion. For example, haemorrhage (Figure 3), fat, proteinaceous fluid and pure water are amongst substances that have very specific imaging characteristics on MRI.

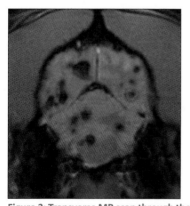

Figure 3: Transverse MR scan through the caudal fossa of a 13-year-old dog. This is a particular sequence called a gradient echo (or T2*) scan, which aids in the detection of haemorrhage. The multiple lesions present are haemangiosarcoma metastases

More advanced imaging techniques are also available. These include: diffusion weighted imaging (used in ischaemic strokes); diffusion tensor imaging (used in fibre mapping and demyelinating disease); and functional MRI (identifies areas of neural activity by evaluation of blood oxygen levels).

MRI – KEY FEATURES

- No ionising radiation
- Relies on magnetic fields and radiofrequency pulses to generate an image
- Creates a map of hydrogen atoms within the body
- Equipment, setup and maintenance usually more expensive than CT
- Two main types of scanner: low and high field strength
- Can acquire images in any plane
- Usually takes longer than CT
- Much greater contrast between the soft tissues than in CT
- Intravenous contrast medium (gadolinium) used in many examinations
- Numerous advanced techniques can be performed (generally with a high field scanner)

Selecting an imaging modality depending on the anatomical region

Often a patient is sent for cross-sectional imaging for evaluation of a particular body part. This usually facilitates the choice of CT or MRI, as there are some clearly defined differences between the modalities when considering specific anatomical regions.

Central nervous system (CNS)

MRI is the imaging modality of choice for the central nervous system due to its superior contrast resolution. There are many subtle changes that are seen on MRI of the brain and spinal cord that simply cannot be detected on CT. Also, CT has limitations in evaluation of the brain and spinal cord due to artefacts created by the surrounding bone of the skull and vertebrae. These artefacts create more of a problem in canine and feline patients (due to their smaller brain size and thicker skull and overlying musculature) than they do in human patients.

Specific MRI sequences can also be used in the CNS and present additional advantages over CT. These include: gradient echo sequences for the diagnosis of haemorrhage (see Figure 3); diffusion weighted imaging in the evaluation of ischaemic disease; FLAIR sequences to assist in diagnosis of perilesional oedema and identification of pure fluid; and STIR sequences to evaluate muscle, bone and nerve root changes.

The use of CT alone to diagnose spinal cord disease in the acutely paretic or plegic patient is controversial. Extruded mineralised disc material in chondrodystrophoid patients is easily visualised in non-contrast CT scans, but CT myelography is necessary to identify significant sites of spinal cord compression or expansion. CT myelography does not, however, allow detailed assessment of the parenchyma of the spinal cord. The presence of related, or unrelated, intramedullary lesions is better recognised on MRI without the inherent risks of myelography (Figure 4).

The use of CT alone to diagnose brain disease should be limited to situations where MRI is not available. CT can be used to identify an intracranial mass effect, areas of severe oedema or acute haemorrhage and contrast-enhancing brain (Figure 5) or meningeal lesions. Brain CT may overlook many subtle, but significant brain lesions that would be easily detected on MRI. Note that CT is not generally suitable for assessment of foramen magnum herniation.

There are many instances where CT is complementary to MRI in evaluation of the CNS – these include skull and vertebral malformations (Figure 4B), trauma cases and lumbosacral stenosis. In some trauma situations CT can be suitable for first line imaging of the CNS to assess for fractures and overt oedema/haemorrhage. This can even be performed in non-anaesthetised comatose patients due to the rapid image acquisition of CT.

CNS – KEY FEATURES

- MRI preferable in almost every situation for brain and spine imaging
- MRI offers many significant advantages in terms of tissue contrast and special sequences to identify particular pathology
- CT can be used if MRI is not available:
  - To identify a mass effect, severe oedema, acute haemorrhage or contrast-enhancing lesions in the brain or spinal cord
  - With myelography for the assessment of extradural compressive lesions in acutely presenting paretic or plegic patients
- CT is often useful in addition to MRI in:
  - Trauma
  - Skull and vertebral malformations
  - Degenerative lumbosacral stenosis

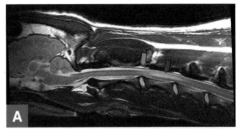

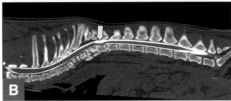

Figure 4: (A) Sagittal T2W MR scan through the cervical spine of a 3-year-old Rottweiler. The patient has a subarachnoid cyst (red arrow). MRI not only demonstrates the presence of the cyst, but also shows the associated parenchymal hyperintensity within the spinal cord at C3 (blue arrow). (B) Sagittal reconstruction from a MDCT scanner of the thoracic and lumbar spine after lumbar myelography. This patient is a 3-year-old French Bulldog and also has a subarachnoid cyst. CT myelography demonstrates the presence and location of the cyst (yellow arrow), but it is not possible to evaluate the spinal cord parenchyma. This patient also has multiple vertebral abnormalities and a kyphosis. Osseous vertebral changes are clearly demonstrated by CT

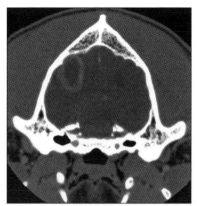

Figure 5: Transverse CT scan of the brain after intravenous contrast medium. A ring enhancing mass is present in the right parietal lobe. CT can demonstrate large contrast-enhancing mass lesions within the brain, but subtle parenchymal lesions will be missed. Note the lack of detail seen within the remainder of the brain parenchyma on a typical brain CT scan

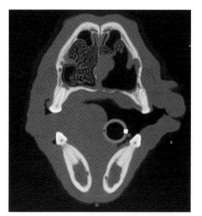

Figure 6: Transverse CT scan through the nose of a 6-year-old dog with aspergillosis. CT provides exquisite detail of the nasal chambers and demonstrates severe left-sided turbinate destruction

Nasal cavities and sinuses

Both CT and MRI are extremely useful in assessment of the nasal cavities and frontal sinuses. CT and MRI are effective in the assessment of turbinate, maxillary and palatine destruction (Figure 6), mass lesions, presence of fluid, osteomyelitis, and contrast-enhancing lesions. Whilst CT and MRI are both able to detect cribriform plate destruction, rostral meningeal/brain enhancement or mass lesion, MRI has the advantage that it may also demonstrate T2W meningeal hyperintensity surrounding the olfactory lobes in cases of nasal neoplasia. The cause of this finding is, as yet, unknown but it may represent micrometastases, secondary meningitis or an accumulation of fluid. It has not been shown to have an effect on neurological deficits or survival time.

CT can be used to guide fine needle aspiration (FNA) and biopsy if required. CT of the thorax can easily be performed at the same time as nasal CT in order to evaluate for metastatic disease.

> **NASAL CAVITIES AND SINUSES – KEY FEATURES**
>
> ■ Both CT and MRI are very useful
> ■ Both can demonstrate cribriform plate invasion and rostral brain involvement in nasal neoplasia
> ■ MRI may show additional meningeal changes surrounding the olfactory bulbs in nasal neoplasia
> ■ CT can be used to guide FNA or biopsy
> ■ CT can be used for thoracic metastatic screening

External, middle and inner ears

CT and MRI are both able to detect the presence of fluid or mass lesions within the tympanic bulla and external ear canal, sclerosis or erosion of the bulla wall, associated retropharyngeal or para-aural lesions and regional lymphadenopathy (Figure 7A). MRI has an additional advantage in enabling evaluation of the facial and vestibulocochlear nerves for thickening and enhancement (Figure 7B) and also allows visualisation of the fluid signal within the cochlea and semicircular canals.

Associated brain disease is also best assessed by MRI, but may be recognised on CT.

CT can be used for thoracic metastatic screening if aural/para-aural neoplasia is suspected.

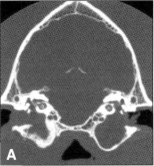

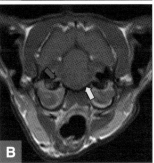

Figure 7: (A) Transverse CT scan (bone algorithm) at the level of the tympanic bullae in a 7-year-old Weimaraner with chronic otitis media. The right tympanic bulla wall is thickened and irregular, and both bullae contain abnormal material.
(B) Transverse T1W/C transverse MR scan through the tympanic bullae of a cat with severe chronic ear disease and clinical signs of otitis interna. In addition to the abnormal material within the bullae, MR also demonstrates contrast enhancement of the right vestibulocochlear nerve (purple arrow) and suspected meningeal enhancement around the brainstem (yellow arrow)

EXTERNAL, MIDDLE AND INNER EARS – KEY FEATURES

- CT or MRI can be used
- MRI can also assess cranial nerves VII and VIII, the cochlea and semicircular canals and the adjacent brainstem
- CT can be used for thoracic metastatic screening

Thorax

The inherent variation in densities within the thorax makes the chest ideally suited to CT evaluation (Figures 8 and 9). Conversely, the low signal from the air-filled lungs and the presence of artefacts means that MRI is far less suited to assessment of the thorax. Overall, CT is the preferred modality for assessment of the thorax, though MRI can be useful in the

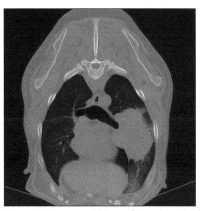

Figure 8: Transverse CT scan (lung algorithm) through the mid thorax of an 11-year-old mix breed dog. A large left-sided lung mass is present. Thoracic CT provides excellent pulmonary detail and also enables assessment of regional lymph nodes and a search for pulmonary metastases. Post-contrast images were also acquired (soft tissue algorithm)

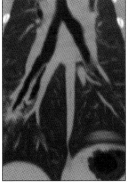

Figure 9: Dorsal MDCT reconstruction of the thorax (at the level of the tracheal bifurcation) in a young dog. The right caudal mainstem bronchus is dilated and contains an abnormal structure. This was found to be a holly leaf at bronchoscopy and surgery was required for removal

assessment of the thoracic wall, mediastinal masses, the pleural space (Figure 10) and, with a suitable scanner and compatible equipment, the heart. Images using either modality should be obtained during periods of apnoea. With rapid CT machines this can usually be achieved by hyperventilating to an apnoeic state or by the use of remote ventilation and breath-hold techniques. Respiratory and cardiac gating techniques are usually required for MRI of the thorax.

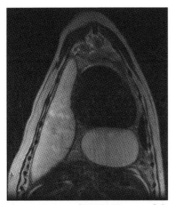

Figure 10: Dorsal T2W MR scan of the ventral part of the thorax of a 3-year-old dog with chronic pyothorax. The scans were obtained prior to surgery (CT was not available) to locate loculated fluid and to assess for possible foreign material. The areas of high signal represent fluid pockets. The low signal structure is the apex of the heart

THORAX – KEY FEATURES

- CT is definitely the modality of choice
  - Extremely useful in the evaluation of pleural, mediastinal, bronchial, pulmonary parenchymal and thoracic wall lesions
  - Superior metastatic screening when compared to radiographs
- MRI can be used for thoracic imaging in some situations
  - Useful for mediastinal masses, thoracic wall masses and the pleural space
  - Respiratory and cardiac gating techniques are usually required
  - Cardiac MRI can be performed with extremely advanced MR scanners

Abdomen

CT provides excellent images of the abdominal organs and peritoneum (Figure 11). Contrast should always be administered (see CT – Key features, earlier) and with helical CT (particularly MDCT) it is also possible to obtain exquisite angiographic studies. Contrast CT is extremely useful for CT excretory urograms, portosystemic shunt diagnosis, presurgical assessment of abdominal masses, and many other indications. It may even be preferable to abdominal ultrasonography in large obese patients.

MRI of the abdomen allows excellent evaluation of the parenchyma of the organs due to the good soft tissue contrast. Body

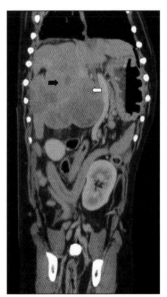

Figure 11: Dorsal MDCT reconstruction of the abdomen after intravenous contrast medium administration. This 11-year-old dog has a large heterogenous right-sided liver mass (black arrow), which can be seen displacing the portal vein (white arrow) to the left. CT was used to perform a full assessment of the mass, regional lymph nodes, other abdominal organs and the thorax

MRI is used widely in people for the assessment of hepatic, splenic and renal nodules and masses and also for prostatic disease. Once again, rapid sequences and/or gating are usually required. Expertise and experience are essential to obtain the most relevant information from abdominal MRI.

ABDOMEN – KEY FEATURES

- CT is the current modality of choice, providing good quality images and being much easier to perform
- MRI can be used but requires special sequences and expertise
- In the future MRI may be used more for the characterisation of abdominal masses and nodules in veterinary patients

Pelvic region

Both CT and MRI are suited to evaluation of the pelvic region. This area is not prone to movement artefact, and therefore MRI may hold the advantage over CT given its superior soft tissue contrast and the ability to assess the adjacent CNS structures more readily.

PELVIC REGION – KEY FEATURES

- Either CT or MRI may be used
- MRI may hold a slight advantage with its benefits of additional soft tissue contrast

Elbow

CT has been the most widely reported cross-sectional imaging technique in the assessment of canine elbow disease. CT is ideally suited to the osseous changes of medial compartment disease, osteochondrosis (OC) lesions and incomplete ossification of the humeral condyle (IOHC). CT and arthroscopy have been shown to be complementary techniques, with CT identifying some lesions not seen on arthroscopy and *vice versa*. CT has also been used quantitatively in the assessment of elbow incongruity.

More recently MRI has been advocated in the detection of subtle intramedullary abnormalities such as bone oedema. MRI also theoretically holds the potential for cartilage imaging, but powerful scanners are required for this level of detail.

ELBOW – KEY FEATURES

- CT usually recommended
- Quick and provides excellent osseous detail
- Ideal for the diagnosis of common elbow conditions (medial compartment disease, IOHC, OC, elbow incongruity)
- Complementary to arthroscopy
- MRI may also be used and could provide additional information concerning bone oedema and cartilage

Shoulder

MRI offers significant potential for the evaluation of muscular, ligamentous and tendinous shoulder injuries in adult dogs. Some of these conditions are not seen arthroscopically and hence may be underdiagnosed. MRI is also well suited to the diagnosis of brachial plexus disease.

CT of the shoulders is generally much less useful. Osteochrondrosis lesions in young patients are usually seen radiographically and assessed and treated arthroscopically. CT may be helpful in fracture assessment and can also be used for assessment of suspected neoplasia with the addition of a thoracic metastatic scan.

SHOULDER – KEY FEATURES

- MRI has great potential for the assessment of muscular, tendinous and ligamentous shoulder injury
- CT is much less useful overall and is reserved for osseous disease

General skeleton

CT offers the advantage of superior multiplanar and volume rendered 3D reconstructions which are extremely beneficial in the planning of fracture repair and other orthopaedic surgeries such as angular limb deformity correction (Figure 12). MRI is more advantageous where neoplastic invasion into bone is suspected. In this scenario the altered intramedullary bone signal may be seen long before lytic changes are recognised on a CT examination.

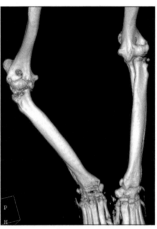

Figure 12: 3D CT reconstructions can be useful to assess the overall alignment of osseous elements of the axial and appendicular skeleton for surgical planning

GENERAL SKELETON – KEY FEATURES

- CT useful for angular limb deformities, fracture repair planning
- MRI advantageous in neoplastic disease (such as mandibular or maxillary tumours)

Whole body MRI and CT for metastatic disease?

Recently protocols for whole body MRI screening for the diagnosis and staging of neoplastic disease have been reported. Some institutions are also routinely performing whole body CT examinations for the same purpose. The CT studies are quick to acquire if MDCT is used, whereas special protocols are required for fast MRI screening techniques. All of these types of studies take a long time to read, but certainly are useful in detecting previously unrecognised metastatic disease. In these whole body techniques the emphasis is generally on contrast rather than spatial resolution and MRI holds the advantage in the detection of bone marrow changes, lymphadenopathy, soft tissue lesions and CNS lesions. CT remains beneficial in metastatic lung and bone imaging, but the latter is probably better assessed using bone scintigraphy.

In the future, positron emission tomography (PET) may become increasingly important in cancer staging. PET/CT or PET/MRI may eventually become the gold standard of cancer imaging in our canine and feline patients.

Patients with metallic implants – CT or MRI?

Metallic implants create problems for both CT and MR examinations.

In MRI *non-ferrous* implants may be placed into the magnet, but can create serious artefacts and hence non-diagnostic studies. The magnitude of these artefacts differs depending on the MR sequence used.

The artefacts identified on CT examinations in patients with metallic implants can also prevent interpretation, but on occasion the gantry can be angled to avoid the metallic region and certain slices and reconstructions can limit their effect on the final image.

CT and MR angiography

Both CT and MR have a role in angiography in our small animal patients. Current applications include evaluation of portosystemic shunts, assessment for pulmonary thromboembolic disease, planning of vascular mass resection and many others. For CT angiography a helical scanner is required and a rapid injection pump is preferable (Figure 13). For MR angiography the best results are achieved with high field scanners and special techniques such as parallel imaging.

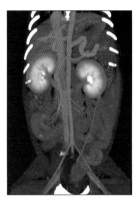

Figure 13: CT angiogram performed with an MDCT unit and a rapid injection pump. The image is displayed as a Maximum Intensity Projection (MIP) which is a useful way to view contrast-enhanced vessels or mineralised lesions

Conclusion

Veterinary practices now have unprecedented access to cross-sectional imaging modalities. In many situations CT and MRI can be used interchangeably and the decision on which to choose may be mostly affected by cost and availability. There are, however, some important situations where the correct choice is extremely important and the wrong modality may make the study non-diagnostic for the disease process in question. ■

How to...
Pick your way through the jungle of **ectoparasite treatments for dogs and cats**

by Peri Lau-Gillard

This article provides a brief summary of the various active ingredients and formulations of insecticides and acaricides currently authorised for use in dogs and cats in the United Kingdom, in order to help the busy practitioner to find his/her way through the jungle of products available. For further reading refer to the datasheets in the NOAH compendium and the guidelines of the European Scientific Counsel on Companion Animal Parasites (ESCCAP).

Insecticides

Insects of veterinary importance in small animals include fleas, chewing and sucking lice, mosquitoes and certain flies (e.g. phlebotomine sandflies).

Imidacloprid (Advantage spot on®, Bayer plc)

- Advantages: Adulticidal activity against fleas on contact within 24 hours; larvicidal in environment; authorised for flea control in rabbits; will control biting lice in dogs.
- Disadvantages: No repellent (anti-feeding) action; reduced efficacy after bathing/swimming; occasional application site reactions.
- Comments: The only flea product authorised for use in rabbits.

Imidacloprid + permethrin (Advantix spot on for dogs®, Bayer plc)

- Advantages: Adulticidal activity against fleas on contact within 24 hours; larvicidal in environment; acaricidal and repellent efficacy against ticks for 3 weeks; repellent activity against sandflies for 2–3 weeks; repellant activity against mosquitoes for 2–4 weeks; repellant activity against stable flies for 4 weeks.
- Disadvantages: Reduced efficacy after bathing/swimming; occasional application site reactions.
- Comments: Do not use on cats (toxic). Has repellent activities.

Imidacloprid + moxidectin (Advocate spot on®, Bayer plc)

- Advantages: Control of canine *Sarcoptes* and *Demodex* mites, feline and canine *Otodectes* mites, feline and canine roundworm and hookworm, canine whipworm, and canine biting lice. Authorised for the prevention of heartworm (active against L3 and L4 larvae of *Dirofilaria immitis*) in dogs, cats and ferrets. Prevention and treatment of canine angiostrongylosis and treatment of canine lungworm (*Crenosoma vulpis*). For the treatment and prevention of flea infestation (*Ctenocephalides felis*) in dogs, cats and ferrets.

- Disadvantages: No repellent action; reduced efficacy after bathing/swimming; occasional application site reactions.
- Comments: The only anti-flea and heartworm prevention product authorised for use in ferrets.

Fipronil (Frontline Spray® or Frontline spot on®, Mérial Animal Health Ltd; Fiprodog® or Fiprocat®, Dechra Veterinary Products Ltd; Fiprospot®, Ceva Animal Health Ltd; Effipro spray® or Effipro spot on®, Virbac Ltd)

- Advantages: All products kill adult fleas. Effipro spot on® also effective for tick infestation in dogs and cats, whereas Frontline spray®, Frontline spot on® and Effipro spray® will additionally treat canine and feline biting lice infestations. Sprays can be used on puppies and kittens older than two days.
- Disadvantages: No repellent action; no larvicidal/ovaricidal activities; reduced efficacy after bathing/swimming; occasional application site reactions; spray is labour-intensive.
- Comments: Do not use on rabbits (toxic).

Fipronil + (S)-methoprene (Frontline Combo spot on for dogs and cats, Mérial Animal Health Ltd)

- Advantages: Adulticidal, larvicidal and ovaricidal activities against fleas; effective against ticks and/or biting lice in dogs and cats.
- Disadvantages: No repellent action; reduced efficacy after bathing/swimming; occasional application site reactions.
- Comments: Do not use on rabbits (toxic).

Fipronil + (S)-methoprene + amitraz (Certifect spot on solution for dogs, Mérial Animal Health Ltd)

- Advantages: Adulticidal, larvicidal and ovaricidal activities against fleas; effective against ticks and/or biting lice in dogs. Affects a wider range of tick species than

Frontline Combo, increased speed of kill (starting at 2 hours and >90% at 24 hours) and a longer duration of activity.
- Disadvantages: Reduced efficacy after bathing/swimming; occasional application site reactions.
- Comments: Do not use on rabbits or cats (toxic). People with diabetes mellitus or taking monoamine oxidase inhibitors (MAOIs) should take particular care when handling the product.

Selamectin (Stronghold spot on®, Pfizer Ltd)

- Advantages: Effective against canine *Sarcoptes* mites, feline/canine *Otodectes* mites, canine/feline adult intestinal roundworms, feline adult intestinal hookworms, canine/feline biting lice. Adulticidal, larvicidal and ovicidal against fleas. Authorised for the prevention of heartworm disease (*Dirofilaria immitis*) in dogs/cats. Usable for pregnant and lactating queens/bitches.
- Disadvantages: No repellent action; reduced efficacy after bathing/swimming; occasional application site reactions reported.
- Comment: Very wide spectrum product.

Metaflumizone (ProMeris spot on for cats®, Pfizer Ltd)

- Advantages: Kills adult fleas on contact.
- Disadvantages: No repellent action; reduced efficacy after bathing/swimming; occasional application site reactions (temporary oily appearance, clumping/spiking of the coat, colour change of fur). Slow acting (2–4 days).
- Comment: Clients may not be happy with oily coat appearance and possible coat colour changes.

Metaflumizone + amitraz (ProMeris spot on for dogs®, Pfizer Ltd)

- Advantages: Kills adult fleas on contact. Authorised for the treatment and prevention of infestations by ticks, treatment of canine demodicosis and canine biting lice.

- Disadvantages: No repellent action; reduced efficacy after bathing/swimming; side effects (sedation, lethargy, CNS depression, hyperglycaemia, bradycardia) can be seen; strong odour of product (author's own experience).
- Comments: People taking MAOI-containing medication or who have diabetes should take particular care when handling the product. Potential risk of dogs developing drug-induced pemphigus foliaceus (Oberkirchner *et al.*, 2011).

Pyriprole (Prac-Tic spot on solution for dogs®, Novartis Animal Health UK Ltd)

- Advantages: Kills adult fleas within 24 hours; kills ticks within 48 hours.
- Disadvantages: Not suitable for cats; no repellent action; fur discoloration, greasy appearance/clumping of the fur, alopecia or pruritus may be observed at the application site.
- Comments: Do not use in rabbits. Weekly immersion in water does not affect efficacy against fleas/ticks, but dogs should not be bathed/shampooed from 48 hours before treatment and/or within 24 hours after treatment.

Indoxacarb (Activyl spot on solution for dogs and cats®, MSD Animal Health)

- Advantages: Active against adult, larval and egg stages of fleas; larvae in the animal's immediate environment are killed following contact with indoxacarb-treated pets; fleas will stop feeding 0–4 hours after treatment, with cessation of egg-laying, paralysis and death then occurring within 4–48 hours.
- Disadvantages: Oily appearance of fur and/or clumping on application side; a dry white residue may also be observed; transient alopecia or pruritus may occur at the application site.

- Comments: Animals should not swim or be bathed for 48 hours after treatment.

Indoxacarb and permethrin (Activyl Tick plus spot on solution for dogs®, MSD Animal Health)

- Advantages: Adulticidal activity against fleas on contact within 4–48 hours; larvicidal in immediate environment after contact with treated pet; acaricidal efficacy against against *Ixodes ricinus* and for up to 3 weeks against *Rhipicephalus sanguineus*.
- Disadvantages: All ticks may not be killed within the first 48 hours but may be killed within a week; oily appearance of fur and/or clumping on application side; a dry white residue may also be observed; transient alopecia or pruritus may occur at the application site.
- Comments: Do not use on cats (use can be fatal); dogs should not swim or be bathed for 48 hours after treatment.

Nitenpyram (Capstar tablet®, Novartis Animal Health UK Ltd)

- Advantages: Kills 95–100% of adult fleas within 6 hours; can be given to animals at all stages of pregnancy or lactation.
- Disadvantages: No repellent action; no larvicidal/ovaricidal activities against fleas.
- Comments: Not for use as sole anti-flea therapy.

Spinosad (Comfortis chewable tablet for dogs®, Elanco Companion Animal Health)

- Advantages: Rapid onset of action and long duration (one month); therefore almost complete prevention of appearance of flea eggs in the environment.
- Disadvantages: Cannot be used in cats. Cannot be used in dogs weighing <3.9 kg as accurate dosing not possible. Do not use in dogs with pre-existing epilepsy. Product may interact with other P-glycoprotein substrates (e.g. digoxin, doxorubicin,

ciclosporin). Vomiting commonly occurs in the first 48 hours after dosing, but is transient, mild and does not require symptomatic treatment.

- Comments: Comfortis is authorised for use in cats in the USA – so watch this space!

Deltamethrin (Scalibor Protectorband for dogs®, MSD Animal Health)

- Advantage: Control of infestations with ticks and sandflies (*Phlebotomus perniciosus*) for 5–6 months; anti-feeding effect on adult mosquitoes (*Culex pipiens*) for 6 months; can be used during pregnancy and lactation. Long acting!
- Disadvantage: Collar may not be convenient for owner; strong smell; local reactions may occur.
- Comments: Remove collar before swimming/bathing the dog because deltamethrin is harmful to aquatic organisms. Prevent dog from swimming in water for the first 5 days of wearing the collar.

Insect growth regulator inhibitors

Lufenuron (Program tablet for dogs®, Program suspension for cats®, Program suspension for injection for cats, Novartis Animal Health UK Ltd)

- Advantages: Can be given to pregnant bitches and queens, lactating queens and puppies/kittens taking solid food; injection for cats lasts 6 months.
- Disadvantages: No effect against adult fleas; time lag of 60–90 days required to disrupt flea life cycle; no repellent activity.
- Comments: Adulticide flea treatment needed concurrently.

Lufenuron + milbemycin (Program Plus tablet for dogs®, Novartis Animal Health UK Ltd)

- Advantages: Prevention of fleas; prevention of heartworm disease (L3 and L4 stages of *Dirofilaria immitis*); treatment of adult stages of gastrointestinal nematodes (hookworms,

roundworms and whipworms) in dogs. It can be used from 2 weeks of age.

- Disadvantages: Not suitable for cats; no effect against adult fleas; time lag of 60–90 days required to disrupt flea life cycle; no repellent activity.
- Comments: For heartworm-positive dogs, adulticidal therapy is indicated before administering Program Plus.

Acaricides
Products for tick control

- **Deltamethrin** (Scalibor Protectorband for dogs®, MSD Animal Health)
- **Fipronil** (Frontline Spray® or Frontline spot on®, Mérial Animal Health Ltd; Effipro spray® or Effipro spot on®, Virbac Ltd)
- **Fipronil + (*S*)-methoprene** (Frontline Combo spot on for dogs and cats, Mérial Animal Health Ltd)
- **Fipronil + (*S*)-methoprene + amitraz** (Certifect spot on solution for dogs, Mérial Animal Health Ltd)
- **Imidacloprid + permethrin** (Advantix spot on for dogs®, Bayer plc)
- **Imidacloprid + moxidectin** (Advocate spot on®, Bayer plc)
- **Indoxacarb + permethrin** (Activyl Tick plus spot on solution for dogs®, MSD Animal Health)
- **Metaflumizone + amitraz** (ProMeris spot on for dogs®, Pfizer Ltd)
- **Pyriprole** (Prac-tic spot on solution for dogs®, Novartis Animal Health UK Ltd)
- **Selamectin** (Stronghold spot on®, Pfizer Ltd)

Products to treat sarcoptic mange

- **Amitraz** (Aludex cutaneous solution for dogs®, MSD Animal Health)
  - Advantages: Very effective.
  - Disadvantages: Not user-friendly (see product insert for handling and application directions); cannot be used on Chihuahuas, pregnant or lactating bitches

or puppies <3 months old; concurrent use with other alpha-2 adrenoceptor agonists not recommended.
- Comments: Amitraz is an MAOI and should not be used on dogs or applied by anyone taking other MAO inhibiting drugs. Care is needed if the drug is being handled by a diabetic owner or applied to a diabetic patient, as they may develop transient hyperglycaemia. Do not use on cats or horses.
- **Selamectin** (Stronghold spot on®, Pfizer Ltd)
- **Imidacloprid + moxidectin** (Advocate spot on®, Bayer plc).

In-contact animals and the environment should be treated concurrently.

Products to treat canine demodicosis
- **Amitraz** (Aludex cutaneous solution for dogs®, MSD Animal Health)
  - Advantages, disadvantages and comments as above for Amitraz in treating sarcoptic mange.
- **Imidacloprid + moxidectin** (Advocate spot on®, Bayer plc)
- **Metaflumizone + amitraz** (ProMeris spot on for dogs®, Pfizer Ltd).

Products to treat cheyletiellosis
Currently there are no products authorised for this use, although reports have shown that fipronil- and selamectin-containing products are effective. Alternative treatments include weekly lime sulphur dips, or weekly bathing with 1% selenium sulphide shampoo over 3 consecutive weeks. In-contact animals and the environment should be treated concurrently.

Products to treat trombiculidiasis
To the author's knowledge there is currently no authorised product available, but there is evidence in the literature that fipronil- and selamectin-containing products may be effective.

Products to treat otocariosis
- **Imidacloprid + moxidectin** (Advocate spot on®, Bayer plc)
- **Selamectin** (Stronghold spot on®, Pfizer Ltd)
- **Tiabendazole** (Auroto ear drop solution®, Dechra Veterinary Products Ltd).

In-contact animals and the environment should be treated concurrently. ■

C = cat, D = dog, F = ferret, R = rabbit; A = adulticidal, L = larvicidal, O = ovaricidal. Endoparsites: *At = Ancylostoma tubaeforme*, *Av = Angiostongylus vasorum*, *Cv = Crenosoma vulpis*, *Di = Dirofilaria immitis*, *Tc = Toxocara cati/canis*, *Tl = Toxascaris leonine*, *Tv = Trichuris vulpis*, *Us = Uncinaria stenocephala*

* Can be used in pregnant bitches/queens
** Can be used during pregnancy and lactation
*** Can be used in nursing bitches/queens

Activyl	
Active ingredient	Indoxacarb
Presentation	Spot on
Species	C, D
Minimum age for first use	8 weeks (bodyweight >1.2 kg)
Spectrum of activity	Fleas
Affected by weekly bath/swim	✓
Frequency of use	4 weeks

Activyl Tick plus	
Active ingredients	■ Indoxacarb ■ Permethrin
Presentation	Spot on
Species	D
Minimum age for first use	8 weeks (bodyweight >1.2 kg)
Spectrum of activity	■ Fleas ■ Ticks
Affected by weekly bath/swim	✓
Frequency of use	4 weeks ➡

Advantage

Active ingredient	Imidacloprid
Presentation	Spot on
Species	C,D,R
Minimum age for first use	■ 8 weeks: C,D ■ 10 weeks: R ***
Spectrum of activity	■ Fleas (A,L,C,D,R) ■ Biting lice (D only)
Affected by weekly bath/swim	✓
Frequency of use	4 weeks

Advantix

Active ingredients	■ Imidacloprid ■ Permethrin
Presentation	Spot on
Species	D
Minimum age for first use	7 weeks **

Spectrum of activity	■ Fleas (A)
	■ Flies
	  – Mosquito
	  – Sandfly
	  – Stablefly
	■ Ticks

Affected by weekly bath/swim	✓
Frequency of use	4 weeks

Advocate

Active ingredients	■ Imidacloprid ■ Moxidectin
Presentation	Spot on
Species	C,D,F
Minimum age for first use	■ 9 weeks: C ■ 7 weeks: D
Spectrum of activity	■ Fleas (A) ■ Biting lice (D only) ■ Demodex (D only) ■ Sarcoptes (D only) ■ Ear mites (C,D)

Spectrum of activity (contd)	■ Endoparasites
	  – *Di*: C,D,F
	  – *Av, Cv*: D
	  – *Tc, At*: C,D
	  – *Tv, Tl, Us*: D

Affected by weekly bath/swim	✓
Frequency of use	4 weeks

Aludex

Active ingredient	Amitraz
Presentation	Emulsion for external use only
Species	D
Minimum age for first use	12 weeks
Spectrum of activity	■ Demodex ■ Sarcoptes
Affected by weekly bath/swim	✓
Frequency of use	Weekly

Capstar

Active ingredient	Nitenpyram
Presentation	Tablet
Species	C,D
Minimum age for first use	4 weeks **
Spectrum of activity	Fleas (A)
Affected by weekly bath/swim	✗
Frequency of use	Use with other

Certifect

Active ingredients	■ Fipronil ■ Amitraz ■ (S)-methoprene
Presentation	Spot on
Species	D
Minimum age for first use	8 weeks **

Spectrum of activity	■ Fleas (A,L,O) ■ Biting lice ■ Ticks
Affected by weekly bath/swim	✓
Frequency of use	Every 2 weeks max.

Comfortis

Active ingredient	Spinosad
Presentation	Tablet
Species	D
Minimum age for first use	14 weeks
Spectrum of activity	Fleas (A,O)
Affected by weekly bath/swim	✗
Frequency of use	4 weeks

Effipro

Spot on

Active ingredient	Fipronil
Presentation	Spot on
Species	C,D
Minimum age for first use	8 weeks
Spectrum of activity	■ Fleas (A) ■ Ticks
Affected by weekly bath/swim	✗
Frequency of use	4 weeks

Spray

Active ingredient	Fipronil
Presentation	Spray
Species	C,D
Minimum age for first use	2 days
Spectrum of activity	■ Fleas (A) ■ Biting lice ■ Ticks

Affected by weekly bath/swim	✗
Frequency of use	4 weeks

Frontline combo

Active ingredients	■ Fipronil ■ (S)-methoprene
Presentation	Spot on
Species	C,D
Minimum age for first use	8 weeks **
Spectrum of activity	■ Fleas (A,L,O) ■ Biting lice ■ Ticks
Affected by weekly bath/swim	✗
Frequency of use	4 weeks

Frontline

Spot on

Active ingredient	Fipronil
Presentation	Spot on
Species	C,D
Minimum age for first use	8 weeks **
Spectrum of activity	■ Fleas (A) ■ Biting lice ■ Ticks
Affected by weekly bath/swim	✗
Frequency of use	4 weeks

Spray

Active ingredient	Fipronil
Presentation	Spray
Species	C,D
Minimum age for first use	2 days
Spectrum of activity	■ Fleas ■ Biting lice ■ Ticks

Affected by weekly bath/swim	✗
Frequency of use	4 weeks

Fiprocat	
Active ingredient	Fipronil
Presentation	Spot on
Species	C
Minimum age for first use	8 weeks
Spectrum of activity	Fleas (A)
Affected by weekly bath/swim	✗
Frequency of use	4 weeks

Fiprodog	
Active ingredient	Fipronil
Presentation	Spot on
Species	D
Minimum age for first use	8 weeks
Spectrum of activity	■ Fleas (A) ■ (Ticks)
Affected by weekly bath/swim	✗
Frequency of use	4 weeks

Fiprospot	
Active ingredient	Fipronil
Presentation	Spot on
Species	C,D
Minimum age for first use	8 weeks
Spectrum of activity	■ Fleas (A) ■ (Ticks) (D)
Affected by weekly bath/swim	✗
Frequency of use	4 weeks

Prac-Tic	
Active ingredient	Pyriprole
Presentation	Spot on
Species	D
Minimum age for first use	8 weeks
Spectrum of activity	■ Fleas (A,O) ■ Ticks
Affected by weekly bath/swim	✗
Frequency of use	4 weeks

Program	
Active ingredient	Lufenuron
Presentation	Tablet; suspension; injectable
Species	D, C
Minimum age for first use	Puppies/kittens taking solid food *
Spectrum of activity	Fleas (L,O)
Affected by weekly bath/swim	✗
Frequency of use	4 weeks

Program Plus	
Active ingredients	■ Lufenuron ■ Milbemycin oxime
Presentation	Tablet
Species	D
Minimum age for first use	
Spectrum of activity	■ Fleas (L,O) ■ Endoparasites (*Di, Ac, Tc, Tv*)
Affected by weekly bath/swim	✗
Frequency of use	4 weeks

ProMeris	
Active ingredient	Metaflumizone
Presentation	Spot on
Species	C
Minimum age for first use	8 weeks**
Spectrum of activity	Fleas (A)
Affected by weekly bath/swim	✓
Frequency of use	4 weeks

ProMeris Duo	
Active ingredients	■ Metaflumizone ■ Amitraz
Presentation	Spot on
Species	D
Minimum age for first use	8 weeks**
Spectrum of activity	■ Fleas (A) ■ Biting lice ■ Flies ■ Ticks ■ Demodex
Affected by weekly bath/swim	✓
Frequency of use	4 weeks

Scalibor	
Active ingredient	Deltamethrin
Presentation	Collar
Species	D
Minimum age for first use	7 weeks**

Spectrum of activity	■ Flies
	  – Mosquito
	  – Sandfly
	■ Ticks

Affected by weekly bath/swim	✓
Frequency of use	5–6 months

Stronghold	
Active ingredient	Selamectin
Presentation	Spot on
Species	C,D
Minimum age for first use	6 weeks**
Spectrum of activity	■ Fleas (A,L,O) ■ Biting lice ■ Sarcoptes (D only) ■ Ear mites ■ Endoparasites (At C only, Tc)
Affected by weekly bath/swim	✗
Frequency of use	4 weeks

FURTHER READING

Oberkirchner U, Linder KE, Dunston S, Bizikova P and Olivry T (2011) Metaflumizone–amitraz (Promeris)-associated pustular acantholytic dermatitis in 22 dogs: evidence suggests contact drug-triggered pemphigus foliaceus. *Veterinary Dermatology* **22**, 436–448

How to...

Perform rhinoscopy
in the dog and cat

by Philip Lhermette

The nose is a difficult site both to
image effectively and to access.
Surgical rhinotomy is an extremely
invasive and painful procedure and is
rarely necessary except for extensive
debulking of tumours prior to radiotherapy.
CT and MRI provide the best means for
delineating the margins of nasal masses but
rhinoscopy is the gold standard for visualising
nasal lesions, taking biopsy samples and
removing foreign bodies. Treatment of various
nasal conditions can also be carried out
rhinoscopically, including treatment for nasal
aspergillosis, removal of polyps, and laser
debulking of tumours.

Instrumentation

A 2.7 mm 30 degrees rigid endoscope with a
working length of 18 cm is used for the
majority of rhinoscopic examinations in both
the dog and cat. The endoscope is most
commonly used with a matching cystoscope
sheath, which provides an instrument channel
through which grasping or biopsy forceps can
be introduced (Figure 1). In some cats a
smaller arthroscope sheath is required but this
lacks an instrument channel, requiring
instruments to be placed alongside the
endoscope in order to take biopsy samples. A
9.5 Fr operating telescope is also available
from Karl Storz, which is essentially a 1.9 mm
telescope and cystoscope sheath combined.

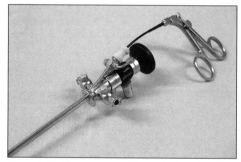

Figure 1: Rigid endoscope with protective sheath

It has a 3 Fr instrument channel and is ideal
for rhinoscopy in cats but is not as versatile or
robust as the 2.7 mm endoscope and costs
around the same amount. Rigid endoscopes
smaller than 4 mm should *never* be used
without a protective sheath of some kind as
they are very easily damaged.

A protective sheath also provides an
irrigation port, and effective saline irrigation
is the key to performing an effective
rhinoscopic examination.

A second pair of 3 mm rigid biopsy forceps
is invaluable. Nasal mucosa swells rapidly
when inflamed and can easily obscure
underlying pathology. Small superficial pinch
biopsy may not be diagnostic so getting a
sufficiently large and deep sample is
imperative if a diagnosis is to be obtained.

A flexible bronchoscope of around 3.5–
4 mm diameter is also useful to obtain a

retroflexed view of the choanae over the free edge of the soft palate. In large dogs a small gastroscope can be used.

Finally, a good light source, preferably xenon, and a camera system are essential.

Patient preparation

Radiographs should always be taken prior to rhinoscopy as the procedure will inevitably result in changes that will make subsequent radiography impossible to interpret. Intra-oral, lateral and skyline views should be taken to examine the turbinates, tympanic bullae and frontal sinuses in detail. If dental disease is suspected, additional dental radiographs may also be taken. In any case a complete oral and dental examination should be undertaken under anaesthesia prior to rhinoscopy.

Blood samples for *Aspergillus* serology and routine biochemistry and haematology can also be useful, and a basic clotting profile is advised. Nasal mucosa is extremely well vascularised and haemorrhage can be a problem, especially when the mucosa is inflamed. Adequate clotting ability is a prerequisite to a successful procedure. Culture of nasal bacterial swabs is rarely helpful and usually only returns commensal organisms. Similarly, examination of discharge for *Aspergillus* may be attempted but is often unrewarding. True primary bacterial rhinitis is extremely rare if it occurs at all.

Caudal (flexible) retroflexed rhinoscopy

The anaesthetised patient is placed in sternal recumbency with the head positioned over a wet table or gridded tray. It may be helpful to place a rolled up towel under the lower jaw to raise the nose a little. A mouth gag is inserted and the flexible endoscope is inserted to the free edge of the soft palate and then retroflexed up and around into the nasopharynx in a 'J' manoeuvre. Alternatively,

where there is space, the tip may be preflexed and pushed past the free edge of the soft palate, then hooked over the dorsal edge. This gives an inverted view of the choanae on the monitor so up is down and left is right (Figure 2). This is a common site for foreign bodies and nasal masses including nasopharyngeal polyps in cats, but strictures and *Aspergillus* colonies may also be seen here.

Tissue samples may be taken but it is important to remove the endoscope from the mouth first and straighten the end before inserting the biopsy forceps right to the tip. The endoscope is then replaced and the sample taken before removing and straightening the endoscope prior to withdrawing the forceps. Forcing instruments through a flexed endoscope will damage the lining of the instrument channel, resulting in expensive repairs or a worthless endoscope.

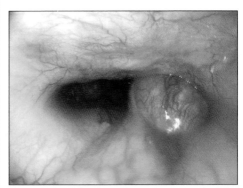

Figure 2: The right choanal mass is seen on the left

Anterior (rigid) rhinoscopy

Following examination of the nasopharynx the cuff of the endotracheal tube is checked to ensure a good seal and a swab is placed over the larynx. Anterior rhinoscopy is invariably carried out with a rigid endoscope under vigorous saline irrigation. Flexible endoscopes do not have a large enough channel to permit irrigation and any haemorrhage will make further examination impossible. Rigid endoscopes have superior optics, magnification and illumination and are used within a sheath that can provide copious irrigation to wash away mucus debris and haemorrhage.

The endoscope is placed into the cystoscopy sheath and attached to the light guide cable and camera system. The system is then white balanced to ensure accurate representation of the image. A litre bag of normal saline is attached to one of the irrigation ports via a standard giving set and the valves opened to allow flow to be controlled via the tap on the cystoscopy sheath. Saline should be at room temperature; cold saline can result in hypothermia during a prolonged procedure due to the highly vascularised nasal mucosa acting as a heat sink. Raising the drip stand should give sufficient gravity flow for most cases, but a pressure bag can be useful where increased irrigation is required to dislodge mucus or where there is extensive haemorrhage. When visualisation is poor, the depth to which the scope can be inserted without passing the medial canthus of the eye should be marked with tape to prevent iatrogenic damage to the cribriform plate.

Visualisation

The 'normal' side is usually examined first. A small amount of sterile water-soluble lubricant is applied to the outside of the sheath. Then the alar cartilage is elevated to allow insertion of the tip of the endoscope into the anterior nares and saline flow is started. Extreme care must be taken to prevent unnecessary trauma to the delicate nasal mucosa. It is helpful for the surgeon to be sitting down with one hand placed on the top of the animal's nose with the index finger and thumb controlling and stabilising the tip of the endoscope.

The other hand holds the camera and provides directional control. It is vital to remember that the angle of view is at 30 degrees to the long axis of the endoscope and is directed diagonally opposite to the light guide post. This means that when the endoscope is placed in a tubular structure with the light guide post in the ventral position, the lumen should appear at the bottom of the picture on the monitor. This can be appreciated more fully by attaching a camera to a bare endoscope and then inserting it into a sheath and watching the position of the lumen on the monitor. If the surgeon attempts to keep the lumen in the centre of the picture on the monitor then the tip of the endoscope will actually be gouging a neat trough in the ventral nasal mucosa! If the endoscope is turned on its side during the procedure, as it often is, compensation must be made for the direction of insertion relative to the position of the lumen on the monitor.

Following a set routine will help prevent mistakes and ensure nothing is missed

1. The nasal cavity (Figure 3) is divided into the dorsal, middle, common and ventral meati by the dorsal, ventral and ethmoidal nasal conchae or turbinates. Following insertion into the rostral nares, the endoscope is aligned with the nasal septum and the rostral nares examined first. The dorsal and ventral meati are identified and examined separately.

2. The dorsal meatus is examined first by directing the tip of the endoscope dorsally and medially towards the septum. The dorsal meatus is a single domed area delineated by the dorsal turbinate and is easily identified (Figure 4) and followed back towards the cribriform plate until it gets too narrow to proceed further. Nasal mucosa should be uniformly pink and smooth and should not bleed excessively on touch. There should be no visible mucus or discharge. Any discharge is abnormal and indicates underlying

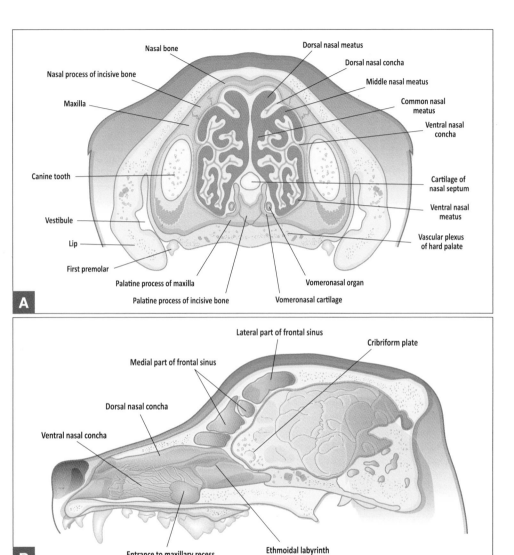

A

Dorsal nasal meatus
Nasal bone
Dorsal nasal concha
Nasal process of incisive bone
Middle nasal meatus
Maxilla
Common nasal meatus
Ventral nasal concha
Canine tooth
Cartilage of nasal septum
Ventral nasal meatus
Vestibule
Lip
Vascular plexus of hard palate
First premolar
Palatine process of maxilla
Vomeronasal organ
Palatine process of incisive bone
Vomeronasal cartilage

B

Lateral part of frontal sinus
Cribriform plate
Medial part of frontal sinus
Dorsal nasal concha
Ventral nasal concha
Entrance to maxillary recess
Ethmoidal labyrinth

Figure 3: (A) Transverse and (B) longitudinal sections to show the anatomy of the canine/feline nose

pathology. Mucus can be quite tenacious and it may be necessary to attach a syringe of saline to the other accessory port and direct a forceful jet directly at the mucus to dislodge it.

3. The endoscope is withdrawn and the middle meatus is then examined as far back as the ethmoid turbinates which appear as a corrugated area (Figure 5).

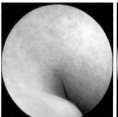
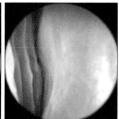
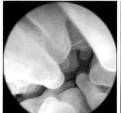
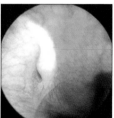

Figure 4: Normal dorsal meatus

Figure 5: Normal ethmoid turbinates (left)

Figure 6: Normal ventral turbinates

Figure 7: Normal Eustachian tube opening

4. The common meatus can then be examined before pointing the tip of the endoscope ventrally to enter the ventral meatus. Here the ventral turbinates appear as folds which should almost interdigitate (Figure 6).
5. The ventral meatus can be followed back to the nasopharynx. Great care should be taken especially in small dogs and cats. As the cystoscope has an oval cross section, gently rotating the endoscope to move the turbinates out of the way allows passage of the endoscope, always being aware of the 30 degree angle of view. The curve of the caudal septum becomes visible as the nasopharynx is entered and the openings of the Eustachian (auditory) tubes can be clearly seen (Figure 7).
6. As the nasopharynx is entered the wide space often leads to turbulence in the saline irrigant, obscuring the view. Turning off the saline flow will improve the view and allow examination of the nasopharynx in air. If visualisation is poor, for instance in the presence of severe haemorrhage, inserting the scope to a depth necessary to enter the nasopharynx is not advised.

With care the 2.7 mm 30 degrees endoscope and cystoscopy sheath will get back as far as the nasopharynx in most adult cats. However, in smaller cats it may be necessary to use an arthroscopy sheath with this endoscope as it has a smaller cross-sectional area. In kittens a 9.5 Fr operating telescope is used or alternatively a 1.9 or 2.4 mm endoscope may be used with an appropriate sheath. Sometimes nasal pathology or severe haemorrhage can seriously hamper visualisation and where this occurs a rigid endoscope should never be inserted beyond the level of the medial canthus of the eye to prevent damage to the delicate cribriform plate.

Obtaining good biopsy samples

Lesions should always be noted on the way in, as iatrogenic damage may otherwise be mistaken for pathology. Multiple biopsy samples should always be taken. Nasal mucosa is very reactive and it is not possible to make a diagnosis on gross appearance alone as many different conditions may appear very similar. Specimens taken with flexible forceps through the instrument channel are necessarily small and may only be quite superficial. Taking several samples at the same site can obtain specimens of deeper tissues that may be more diagnostic. A pair of 3 mm oval cupped biopsy forceps is used to obtain larger samples once the initial ones have been taken. These forceps must be inserted alongside the endoscope until the tips come into view. Placing them alongside the sheath before inserting the endoscope into the patient will enable the surgeon to match landmarks on the sheath with points on the forceps when the tips are aligned. In this way the depth of insertion can be judged accurately and the surgeon knows when the forceps should come into view.

With the endoscope in position in the nose the tip of the forceps is walked along the top edge of the endoscope sheath. This is essential since the angled view of the endoscope looks up, so insertion of the forceps at the side or beneath the endoscope will prevent the forceps being seen at all. If the forceps do not appear when inserted to the correct depth, they may have passed to one side of a turbinate with the endoscope on the other. Withdraw the forceps and try again. With practice the forceps can be visualised and large biopsy samples taken under direct guidance.

Monitoring recovery

At the end of the procedure the endoscope is removed and the nose flushed with saline via a 50 ml syringe. The pharynx is cleaned, preferably with suction, the swab removed and the nose lowered to allow drainage forward to the anterior nares. Anaesthesia is maintained until any haemorrhage is controlled. Postoperative acepromazine may be considered to ensure a smooth recovery and to lower blood pressure to reduce haemorrhage. Extubation is left until pharyngeal gag reflexes return. Analgesia and antibiotic therapy may be required depending on the procedure performed and the underlying condition.

Sinusoscopy

Examination of the frontal sinuses is not normally possible during anterior rhinoscopy unless there is extensive turbinate destruction such as occurs in some cases of aspergillosis. Access to the frontal sinuses for sinusoscopy is obtained by making a small incision and drilling a 5–6 mm hole directly into the frontal sinus, halfway between the midline of the skull and the zygomatic process of the frontal bone, with a sterile surgical drill. The endoscope can then be inserted and the sinus examined under saline irrigation. Samples for cytology or culture can be obtained in the normal way and skin closure is routine.

Acknowledgements

The line diagrams in this article have been reproduced from the *BSAVA Manual of Canine and Feline Endoscopy and Endosurgery*, edited by Philip Lhermette and David Sobel. These diagrams were drawn by Samantha Elmhurst BA Hons (www.livingart.org.uk) and are printed with her permission.

GALLERY OF NASAL PATHOLOGY

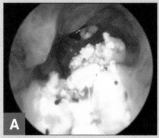 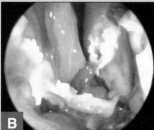 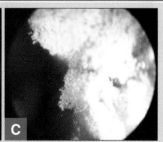

Nasal aspergillosis. (A,B) Colonies in the noses of two dogs: (A) demonstrating the classic white plaques; and (B) showing a greenish tinge due to secondary infection. Note the extensive turbinate damage, leading to an abnormally large airspace. In (A) turbinate destruction has exposed the frontal sinus and *Aspergillus* plaques can be seen within the sinus cavity (rear of the image). (C) Close-up view of the *Aspergillus* colony showing the 'cotton wool' appearance of the fungal hyphae ➡️

GALLERY OF NASAL PATHOLOGY

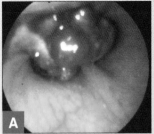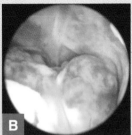

Nasal adenocarcinoma at the choanae viewed by (A) posterior rhinoscopy and (B) anterior rhinoscopy. Note the difference in appearance when viewed under saline irrigation

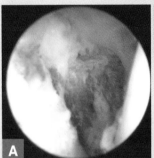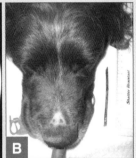

A piece of stick (A) embedded in the nose of a spaniel (middle of the image). (B) A piece of stick following removal from the nose of a spaniel

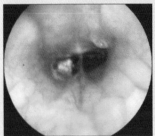

Aspergillus colonies at the choanae, viewed by posterior rhinoscopy. The endoscope is retroflexed through 180 degrees, giving an inverted image, so this colony is in the right nostril

BSAVA members can see Phil Lhermette's video accompanying this article online on the **companion** extra page of the BSAVA website – **www.bsava.com**

How to...
Approach the **smelly ear**
by Janet Littlewood

Ear disease is a common reason for the presentation of small animals in general veterinary practice. After preventive health care, dermatological conditions are the most common reason for pet owners seeking veterinary attention. Otitis is the third most common dermatological presentation for dogs, and second commonest for cats, accounting for 22% and 19% of dermatological cases, respectively (Hill *et al.*, 2006).

Otitis is a variably painful condition, usually accompanied by an aural exudate, which is often malodorous. Ear and head carriage are often affected due to discomfort, but cranial nerve and central neurological deficits may also be present. Head shaking and scratching at the ear are common signs. With increasing chronicity and pain this may reduce, but animals will resent being handled or touched around the head and may be depressed, appear systemically unwell and even become aggressive towards owners.

When presented with an animal with ear disease the practitioner has to consider both the need to initiate appropriate therapy to relieve the discomfort of the otitis and the need to identify the underlying cause of the inflammatory condition. The ear is a specialised skin structure and is subject to a range of primary dermatological conditions which may initiate pathology (Figure 1),

allowing secondary infections to develop (Figure 2). Of all the potential primary causes of otitis externa, the most common underlying problem in chronic or recurrent cases is an allergic dermatosis, principally atopic dermatitis (Figures 3 and 4).

- Foreign bodies
  Grass awns
- Parasites
  Otodectes cynotis
  Demodex canis/felis
  Sarcoptes scabiei (pinnal)
- Hypersensitivity disorders
  Atopic dermatitis
  Adverse cutaneous food reactions
  Contact, particularly drugs
- Keratinisation defects
  Endocrinopathies
  – Hypothyroidism
  – Sex hormone imbalance
  – Primary idiopathic seborrhoea
- Neoplasia
  Ceruminal gland adenocarcinoma
  Other skin tumours
- Inflammatory masses
  Feline nasopharyngeal polyps
  Proliferative otitis
  – Eosinophilic
  – Necrotising
- Immune-mediated
  Erythema multiforme
  Other autoimmune conditions, usually pinnal
  Juvenile cellulitis

Figure 1: Primary causes of otitis externa

- Yeast infection
  Malassezia spp., predominantly
  M. pachydermatis
- Bacterial infection
  Staphylococcus pseudintermedius
  β-haemolytic streptococci
  Gram-negative bacteria
  - *Escherichia coli*
  - *Proteus* spp.
  - *Klebsiella* spp.
  - *Pseudomonas aeruginosa*
  Anaerobes
  - *Bacteroides* spp.
- Otitis media
  Descending
  Ascending
- Chronic progressive pathology

Figure 2: Secondary causes and perpetuating factors in otitis externa

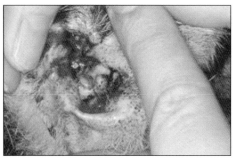

Figure 3: Ceruminous otitis externa in a cat with atopic dermatitis and flea bite hypersensitivity

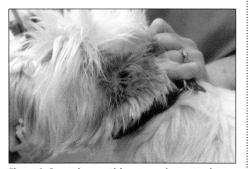

Figure 4: Ceruminous otitis externa in an atopic West Highland White Terrier; the condition was unilateral in this case

Aetiology and pathogenesis

The normal healthy ear canal produces minimal secretions from the sebaceous and modified apocrine (ceruminous) glands. The secretions are carried upwards and distally, with the upward migration of the epithelial cells of the stratum corneum, and out of the external auditory meatus. Inflammation results in an increase and alterations in glandular secretions, overcoming the normal upward escalatory cleaning mechanism, which in turn enhances the growth of microbes.

Malassezia organisms are part of the normal flora of the canine and feline ear and are found in small numbers in up to 36% of normal dogs (Baxter, 1976). Increased humidity, from both secretions and water in the ear canals, enhances the growth of yeast organisms (Mansfield *et al.*, 1990) and *Malassezia* organisms are present in up to 76% of cases of otitis externa (Crespo *et al.*, 2002), often in combination with *Staphylococcus pseudintermedius*.

With increasing chronicity bacterial infection tends to supersede yeast infection. A range of opportunistic organisms may be implicated. This picture may then be further modified by the use of antimicrobial preparations which may select for resistant organisms, resulting in the therapeutically challenging clinical presentation of *Pseudomonas* otitis. This progression of disease is accompanied by a change in the gross nature of the aural exudate, initially ceruminous brownish and waxy or more yellow-orange in colour, to a purulent off-white to greenish exudate which may be obviously slimy or mucoid and often with an offensive odour (Figure 5).

Inflammation of the external ear canal results in hyperplasia of the integument lining the canal and of the glands. The resulting narrowing of the lumen of the canal further impairs the normal drainage function of the ear and enhances the microenvironment for microbial multiplication (Figure 6). Chronic

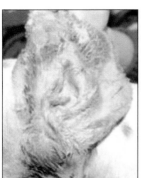

Figure 5: Purulent otitis externa due to *Pseudomonas aeruginosa* infection in an atopic Basset Hound

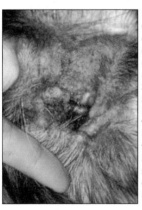

Figure 6: Chronic otitis externa with ceruminous exudate in an atopic German Shepherd Dog, showing hyperplasia, thickening and lichenification of the pinnal integument and stenosis of the external auditory meatus

profile in 89.5% of cases. Neurological complications may accompany otitis media (Figures 7 and 8) and the anatomical structure of the middle ear means that progressive pathology (granulation tissue formation, osteomyelitis) and chronic irreversible changes may ensue.

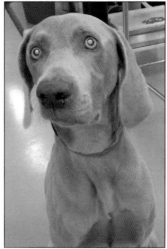

Figure 7: Otitis media in a Weimaraner secondary to chronic otitis externa due to atopic dermatitis, with left-sided facial paralysis

- ■ Deafness
- ■ Horner's syndrome
- ■ Facial paralysis
- ■ Glossopharyngeal damage
- ■ Vestibular disease
- ■ Meningoencephalitis

Figure 8: Neurological complications of otitis

inflammation is accompanied by fibrosis, progressive stenosis and calcification of the cartilage structures of the external ear canal. Ears that have been previously affected by otitis externa are more at risk from future episodes of infection if the inflammatory changes are not fully reversible.

Otitis media is a common complication of chronic otitis externa. Middle ear involvement was noted in 52% of cases of chronic otitis in dogs, compared with 16% of acute cases (Cole *et al.*, 1998). In 82.6% of ears with chronic otitis concurrent otitis media was present, with the tympanum intact in 71% of cases. Bacterial isolates from the horizontal ear canal and tympanic bulla were different in terms of organisms and/or antibiotic sensitivity

Approach to the case

History – Effective client communication is of paramount importance. History relating to the current ear problem is obviously important, but the clinician must not forget to gather information pertaining to the presence of concurrent clinical signs or previous manifestations relating to a more generalised dermatosis (Figure 9). Owners often ignore or misinterpret signs of mild pruritus in dogs,

- Signalment
  Age
  - Parasites and allergies often young animals
  - Tumours and endocrinopathies often older animals
  Breed
  - Predispositions to atopic disease
  - Predispositions to hypothyroidism
- Acute onset or gradual, progressive
- Unilateral or bilateral
- Recurrences
  Time of year, seasonality
- Other dermatological signs
  Pruritus, especially pedal
  Pyoderma
  Scaling/seborrhoea

Figure 9: History in cases of otitis

such as regular foot-licking, an itch–scratch reflex (ticklish spot) and excessive perineal or preputial attention.

Clinical examination of the patient should include general examination, in case of systemic abnormalities and the likelihood of needing sedation or general anaesthesia to assess the ear problem fully, and a complete dermatological examination.

Examination of the ear in the conscious patient may be limited to: an assessment of the pinnae and external auditory meatus, noting the presence and nature of any exudate; and external palpation of the vertical ear canal to assess rigidity and pain. Difficulty or pain on opening the mouth often accompanies middle ear pathology and an assessment of cranial nerve function should be conducted.

Cytological examination of aural exudate should be undertaken in all cases where discharge is evident at the external auditory meatus. Sometimes the outer ear may appear relatively clean, but considerable exudate is present in the ear canal and gentle introduction of a cotton bud will collect material for microscopical examination.

Exudate should be spread on to two microscope slides:

- The first mixed with either liquid paraffin or potassium hydroxide for examination for external parasites
- The second heat fixed and stained with a rapid cytological stain for identification of microbes and cells.

Ceruminous otitis externa is characterised by increased numbers of squames (some of which may be nucleated) increased numbers of yeast organisms (>10 per high power field), a few bacterial cocci and occasional to a few inflammatory cells (Figures 10 and 11).

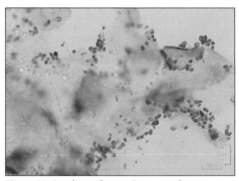

Figure 10: Cytology of ceruminous exudate, showing large numbers of yeast organisms, squames and occasional bacterial cocci, but no inflammatory cells

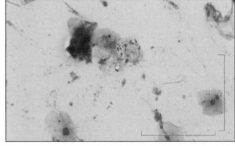

Figure 11: Cytology of aural exudate from a case with mixed yeast and bacterial infection, showing several nucleated squames and moderate numbers of yeast organisms and bacterial cocci, with streaks of chromatin from degenerate neutrophils and clumps of inflammatory debris and some intact neutrophils

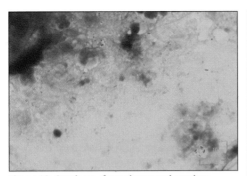

Figure 12: Cytology of purulent aural exudate showing many neutrophils, mostly degenerate, with streaks of chromatin, clumps of inflammatory debris and bacterial rods

Cases of **purulent otitis** may have mainly coccoid bacteria or a mixture of cocci and bacilli, with many neutrophils (both degenerate and band neutrophils) as well as increased squames (Figure 12).

The cytological findings in cases of parasitic otitis, foreign bodies and neoplasia are variable, depending on duration of disease and secondary opportunistic infection.

Significance of bacteria – If bacterial cocci are identified, a presumptive diagnosis of *S. pseudintermedius* infection is justified and empirical selection of antibiotics is appropriate unless the case is long-standing and has failed to respond to appropriate antibiotics previously. All cases in which bacterial rods are identified should have swabs submitted for bacterial culture and sensitivity, preferably by minimum inhibitory concentration techniques rather than by disc diffusion methodology.

Otoscopic examination is likely to need sedation or general anaesthesia. In cases of acute onset of signs of otitis, this should be undertaken at the first presentation in case of the presence of a foreign body, but in cases of chronic or recurrent otitis it may be more appropriate to instigate some initial therapy prior to scheduling this procedure.

Otoscopic examination allows an assessment of the patency of the vertical and horizontal canals and the nature and extent of the inflammatory process, and may allow visualisation of the ear drum. Video-otoscopy allows excellent and detailed visualisation of the ear canal and even the middle ear in larger animals, with accompanying specialised instrumentation. However, a good quality hand-held otoscope is adequate in the majority of cases. If the ear drum cannot be seen, it should be assumed to be ruptured and cleansing agents chosen appropriately. If visible, the tympanum may show evidence of pathology in the middle ear, with loss of transparency, thickening and bulging.

A full assessment of **middle ear involvement** may require imaging by radiography or magnetic resonance imaging, which should be conducted without any attempts to clean the ear canal(s) so that the presence of fluid/soft tissue densities can be evaluated without the prior introduction of cleaning solutions. Considerable information can be obtained by performing myringotomy; the author's preferred instrument is a Spreull's needle rather than a soft catheter, since the rigidity of the needle allows for more accurate manipulation in the middle ear, avoiding the auditory ossicles and round and oval windows, and an assessment of the nature of the lining of the bulla (bony or soft, suggesting the presence of granulation tissue).

In **chronic or recurrent cases**, where flushing under general anaesthesia is planned as part of the therapeutic protocol, and particularly cases where placement of ear wicks is intended, anti-inflammatory therapy should be initiated prior to otoscopy. High anti-inflammatory doses of steroids are indicated (prednisolone 1–2 mg/kg daily). This will give some immediate relief to the animal and controlling the inflammation will enable more effective cleansing both by the clinician and subsequently by the owners. Otoscopic examination can be scheduled for a few days to a week later, depending on whether bacteriology samples have been submitted.

Medical management of otitis

The recent trend in the management of otitis has been towards topical therapy without use of systemic antibiotics. Much higher concentrations of drugs can be achieved by medicating the ear directly rather than by systemic administration of drugs. Some clinicians will still employ systemic medication in some cases of *Malassezia* otitis, particularly when concurrent *Malassezia* hypersensitivity is present, and for cases of streptococcal bacterial otitis. Opinion in the veterinary dermatology field appears to be divided in respect of the use of systemic drugs in cases of otitis media.

Thorough initial and repeated ongoing cleaning of the ear canal(s)

This is an essential prerequisite to allow effective specific topical therapy. Inspissated deposits of wax may require the use of ear curettes or forceps to remove material from the ear canal, but in most cases the exudate can be softened by use of light oils or lubricants (liquid paraffin or propylene glycol), or ceruminolytics (sulphosuccinates, lactic acid or acetic acid). The ear canals can then be flushed and cleansed.

Choosing an ear cleaner – There are many ear cleaners available on the veterinary market and factors to be considered in selecting a suitable cleaner should include irritancy, safety in the middle ear in case the ear drum is ruptured, efficacy at cleaning and antimicrobial effect. Cleaners containing organic acids tend to have better antimicrobial effects, but are more astringent and may not be well tolerated by some patients, particularly in the presence of significant inflammation.

For cleaning under general anaesthesia some clinicians prefer to use water or sterile saline, in order to avoid damage to the middle ear and associated structures, but dilute chlorhexidine (<0.05%) and acetic acid at low concentrations (2.5%) are safe in the middle ear and have antimicrobial properties. TrizEDTA solution is also safe in the middle ear and can be used after an acidic cleanser to neutralise the solution, as well as having a potentiating effect on some antibiotics. However, use of TrizEDTA alone as a cleaner may enhance or encourage the growth of yeast organisms; this can be avoided by using solution with added chlorhexidine or ketoconazole.

Whilst ear flushing under sedation or general anaesthesia is usually without complications, neurological disturbances may ensue in a small number of cases and owners should be warned of the risk at the time of obtaining consent for the procedure.

Treatment of infections

Choosing a medication – Most medicated ear preparations authorised for veterinary use in the UK include:

- *An antifungal agent* (nystatin, tiabendazole, monosulfiram, clotrimazole, miconazole)
- *An analgesic or anti-inflammatory agent:* most include a glucocorticoid, such as prednisolone, betamethasone or dexamethasone
- *An antibiotic:* the antibiotics included in ear drops effective against Gram-positive organisms include fusidic acid, framycetin, neomycin, gentamicin and marbofloxacin. Some of these are also effective against some Gram-negative organisms, with polymixin B another good first choice antibiotic.

In cases of *Pseudomonas* infection, bacterial resistance is a very significant problem, which may arise due to intermittent or incomplete treatment of otitis externa. Some isolates may be sensitive to veterinary labelled drugs, but often the clinician will have to use a drug 'off-label', such as silver sulphadiazine 1%, enrofloxacin solution, ceftazidime, piperacillin, tobramycin or ticarcillin. Whilst some of these drugs are potentially ototoxic and are not recommended for use if the ear drum is ruptured, the risks of ongoing infection and potential extension of pathology into the cranial vault may necessitate the use of one of these drugs. Interestingly for some of these, particularly the aminoglycosides, there may be less ototoxicity with local use in the ear than with systemic use. The toxicity of agents in the middle ear may relate more to the vehicle carrying the drug than to the drug itself. Drugs in aqueous solution are far safer in the middle ear than those in an oily vehicle.

Daily owner care

Cleaning – Where the owner is able to, and the dog permits, the ear canals should be cleaned daily with an appropriate cleaner until there is no further discharge evident. It is vitally important that the client is given suitable instruction in how to clean their pet's ears properly.

Medicating – Medicated drops should be applied at least 15–20 minutes after cleaning, allowing time for the dog to shake out residual cleaner and exudate that cannot be wiped away. This ensures that when the medication is applied it can contact the surface of the integument rather than sit in a puddle of exudate and cleaning solution. In most cases medicated drops should be applied twice daily.

The duration of treatment will depend on the chronicity of the condition, but should continue until beyond cure of infection and will usually be of the order of 1–3 weeks. Response to treatment should be assessed at appropriately scheduled re-examinations. Failure to follow up cases of otitis externa is a clear factor in the development of chronic resistant infections.

Use of ear wicks in case of poor patient compliance or resistant infection

Where patient compliance is poor, or resistant infections are present, the placement of polyvinyl A ear wicks followed by impregnation with antibiotic solution to give a high local concentration of drug is often effective in securing bacteriological cure. The ear wicks are left in place for 7–10 days, with the owner maintaining hydration of the wicks by introduction of antibiotic solution every other day. Ear wicks are usually well tolerated if the dog is on adequate anti-inflammatory doses of glucocorticoid at the same time. At the time of wick removal further cytological assessment and bacterial culture should be undertaken.

Management of otitis media

Surgical intervention is indicated if there are chronic inflammatory changes in the middle ear; in such cases medical management is inappropriate. Those cases amenable to medical therapy may need to have the middle ear flushed on several occasions. A cuffed endotracheal tube is essential to prevent aspiration of material entering the nasopharynx via the auditory (Eustachian) tube.

The tympanic bulla should be flushed with 5–10 ml of warm sterile saline gently introduced in a ventral direction via a Spreull's needle and solution and debris aspirated. The procedure is repeated until the aspirate is clear. Topical antibiotics in aqueous solution chosen on the basis of culture and sensitivity testing and systemic steroid therapy should be employed.

Brainstem auditory evoked response (BAER) studies in patients with otitis media have shown improved hearing in those successfully treated with topical marbofloxacin, gentamicin, clotrimazole and silver sulfadiazine. A profound reduction in BAER was documented after treatment with ticarcillin and tobramycin, more severe with the latter drug. However, if successful treatment obviates the need for total ear canal ablation (TECA), the residual auditory function may be better than after surgery.

Diagnosis and management of underlying disease

Many of the manifestations of otitis observed are secondary; the **primary causes of otitis externa will require appropriate investigations** in order to reach a definitive diagnosis and enable specific therapy to be initiated. The therapeutic requirements of the ear pathology may delay some diagnostic procedures, particularly where steroid therapy would interfere with tests and interpretation of results. However, it may be appropriate to initiate an elimination diet whilst appropriate therapy for the ear disease is conducted. When other diseases have been ruled out, allergen-specific IgE testing can be undertaken at a later date when steroid therapy has been withdrawn.

Managing recurrence – Recurrent episodes of otitis externa are a risk even when the underlying disease process is correctly identified and appropriate treatment regimes initiated. Many cases will require ongoing prophylactic aural care. The atopic Labrador Retriever who enjoys a regular swim is an example of a dog at risk of *Malassezia* overgrowth. The aim of routine treatment is to maintain normal aural health, with a normal, non-inflamed integument over the whole of the external ear and a normal population of microbial flora (i.e. a few yeast organisms and no bacteria). This can be achieved by regular use of an ear cleaner that has antimicrobial and astringent properties, the frequency of use depending on the individual patient's needs, but usually between 1–2 times weekly to 1–2 times monthly.

Some authors advocate the use of topical medicated ear drops on an intermittent, pulse-treatment basis, but this author considers that this may enhance the risk of selecting for resistant bacterial strains and the benefits of this treatment probably lie in the regular use of a topical glucocorticoid.

Since the majority of cases of recurrent otitis externa are due to **underlying atopic dermatitis**, the primary pathological event in these cases is cutaneous inflammation, often starting on the pinnal surface and then extending down the ear canal. If this allergic inflammation can be kept under control, then episodes of otitis and secondary infection will be minimised. Suitable agents to achieve this include prednisolone succinate or phosphate drops applied to the ear canal(s) and hydrocortisone aceponate spray for the pinnal surfaces 2–3 times weekly. More chronic, lichenified changes may require the use of more potent steroids such as dexamethasone or betamethasone in solution for the ear canals or in gel formulation for the pinnae.

Indications for surgery

Some cases will require surgical intervention because of the primary disease process, such as neoplasia or inflammatory polyps. Whilst many cases of otitis externa are suffering from primary medical rather than surgical disease processes, repeated episodes of otitis may result in chronic progressive pathology, sometimes termed 'end-stage' otitis and TECA surgery is

- Neoplasia
- Stenosis of ear canal
- Proliferative/nodular hyperplasia
- Calcification of ear cartilages
- Bony changes to bulla
- Granulation tissue in middle ear
- Neurological deficits, deafness
- Failure to respond to medical therapy

Figure 13: Indications for ear surgery

indicated in such cases (Figure 13). Occasionally the difficulties of ongoing management in uncooperative patients not amenable to regular treatment may indicate the need for surgical intervention, even when irreversible pathology is not present, since removal of the ear canal removes the source of pain and inflammation albeit at the cost of significant hearing loss. ∎

FURTHER READING

Baxter M (1976) The association of *Pityrosporum pachydermatis* with the normal external ear canal of dogs and cats. *Journal of Small Animal Practice* **17**, 231–234

Bensignor E (2003) An approach to otitis externa and otitis media. In: *BSAVA Manual of Small Animal Dermatology, 2nd edn*, ed. A Foster and C Foil, pp. 104–111. BSAVA Publications, Gloucester

Cole LK, Kwochka KW, Kpwalski JJ *et al.* (1998) Microbial flora and antimicrobial susceptibility patterns of isolated pathogens from the horizontal ear canal and middle ear in dos with otitis media. *Journal of the American Veterinary Medical Association* **202**, 534–538

Crespo MJ, Abarca ML and Cabañes FJ (2002) Occurrence of *Malassezia* spp. in the external ear canals of dogs and cats with and without otitis externa. *Medical Mycology* **40**, 115–121

Ginel PJ, Lucena R, Rodriguez JC and Ortega J (2002) A semiquantitative cytological evaluation of normal and pathological samples from the external ear canal of dogs and cats. *Veterinary Dermatology* **13**, 151–156

Hill PH, Lo A, Eden CAN, *et al.* (2006) Survey of the prevalence, diagnosis and treatment of dermatological conditions in small animals in general practice. *Veterinary Record* **158**, 533–539

Mansfield PD, Boosinger TR and Attelberger MH (1990) Infectivity of *Malassezia pachydermatis* in the external ear canal of dogs. *Journal of the American Animal Hospital Association* **26**, 97–100

Mactaggart D (2008) Assessment and management of chronic ear disease. *In Practice* **30**, 450–458

Paterson S and Payne L (2008). Brainstem auditory evoked responses in 37 dogs with otitis media before and after topical therapy. *Veterinary Dermatology* **19**, 30 [WCVD abstract]

How to...

Treat a rabbit with urine scalding

by Brigitte Lord

Urine scalding in rabbits is a clinical sign that is seen frequently in practice. The causes of urine scalding commonly include conditions causing polyuria or urinary incontinence. Unless the cause or causes are investigated, supportive treatment alone is unlikely to be effective.

The causes of polydipsia and polyuria are similar to those in the cat and dog (Figure 1). However, endocrine diseases are less common and, instead, dental disease or oral pain is a common cause of polydipsia in the rabbit. Cystitis is common, may be one of the predisposing factors for urolithiasis in rabbits and can be associated with incomplete voiding. In addition, incomplete voiding may be caused by: lumbosacral vertebral fractures or subluxations; behavioural or neurological micturition disorders (due to trauma or *Encephalitozoon cuniculi*); or excessive production of urinary sediment (due to hypercalcaemia) and cystoliths.

- Renal insufficiency and failure (including *Encephalitozoon cuniculi*)
- Oral pain/dental disease
- Liver disease
- Psychogenic water drinker (boredom)
- Hypercalcaemia
- Pyometra
- Postobstructive diuresis
- Diabetes mellitus

Figure 1: Differential diagnosis list for polyuria/polydipsia in the rabbit

As rabbits have a unique calcium metabolism they are predisposed to excessive urinary sediment if they are fed a diet high in calcium. Rabbits passively absorb all ingested calcium from their digestive system, and then excrete 60% of the excess calcium via the urinary tract; this compares with 2% in most other mammals. If there is chronic excess in dietary calcium or a problem in the urinary tract slowing voiding of urine, precipitation of the calcium ions into crystals and stones will occur.

What clinical signs may be seen?

Alopecia, erythema and secondary pyoderma are all features of urine scalding (Figure 2).

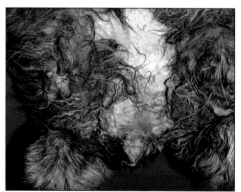

Figure 2: Erythema and alopecia of the perineum and ventral abdomen in a female rabbit with chronic urine scalding. Reproduced from the *BSAVA Manual of Rabbit Medicine and Surgery, 2nd edition*

How can urinary incontinence be distinguished from polyuria?

As both incontinence and PU/PD result in urine scalding, differentiation between these two syndromes is the first step during investigation. Incontinence can be difficult to distinguish from polyuria on history, although careful observation of the rabbit urinating usually aids differentiation, particularly if clinical signs compatible with urinary tract disease are present. Clinical signs that may be found are palpation of a large or small firm bladder, palpation of a cystolith, and discomfort on abdominal palpation. Signs of lower urinary tract disease include stranguria, urine scalding, pollakiuria, anuria, discomfort or pain evident by bruxism or vocalisation during urination, urination outside the rabbit's latrine, haematuria, anorexia, depression and reluctance to move.

What are the causes of urinary incontinence?

Causes of incontinence can be grouped according to the effect on bladder size.

Large distended bladder

Causes include: (a) neurogenic disorders including upper and lower motor neuron lesions and reflex dyssynergia (e.g. *E.cuniculi, Toxoplasma*, lumbosacral vertebral fractures or subluxation); and (b) outflow tract obstruction (paradoxical incontinence).

Clinical signs of outflow tract obstruction are dysuria/stranguria, urine dribbling, haematuria and, on palpation, a distended bladder that is difficult to express and catheterise. 'Paradoxical' incontinence occurs because the intravesicular pressure exceeds pressure within the urethra, resulting in urine leaking past an outflow obstruction. The most common causes of partial outflow obstruction in rabbits are calculi. Other potential causes include bladder or urethral neoplasia, bladder

polyps, urethral strictures, severe urethritis, and (in the male) prostatic disease. The author has seen a case of partial outflow obstruction in a female rabbit due to advanced uterine adenocarcinoma. Rabbits with partial urethral obstuction can be stable in this compensated condition for long periods, but if urethral resistance increases progressively, further hypertrophy of the bladder occurs. Decompensation may finally occur due to the resultant decreased luminal volume and loss of ability of the bladder to contract and empty.

Small or normal bladder size

Causes include: urethral sphincter mechanism incontinence (USMI); detrusor hyperreflexia/ instability; or congenital disorders (e.g. ectopic ureters). Analogous to the case in dogs and cats, oestrogen and testosterone are believed to contribute to urethral muscle tone, and ovariohysterectomised rabbits can develop USMI. Clinical signs that may be observed include dribbling of urine when relaxed or asleep, but otherwise normal voiding of urine. In contrast, detrusor hyperreflexia or instability is the inability to control voiding due to a strong urge to urinate as a sign of cystitis or urethritis.

How can I investigate the cause of urine scalding in a rabbit?

A presumptive diagnosis is often made based on historical and clinical signs and following clinical examination. However, thorough investigation is required to rule in or out common causes, including oral pain from tooth root disease, which would only be found on skull radiography. Hospitalisation is usually required to allow evaluation of urination, including observation of posture and, where possible, urine stream flow and character.

Most rabbits with dysuria tend also to have polyuria, making observation of urination more feasible than in normal rabbits, which are naturally secretive in hospital surroundings. Immediately after the rabbit has attempted to void, the bladder should be palpated to estimate the residual volume. In the healthy rabbit almost all urine, including urine sediment, should be passed with each voiding. If the bladder is still large following voluntary voiding, the rabbit should be sedated for catheterisation. A blood sample should be taken from the lateral saphenous or femoral vein for routine haematology and biochemistry to help rule in or out some of the common causes of polydipsia and polyuria.

Routine urinalysis and bacterial culture should be carried out. Cystocentesis can usually be performed in the conscious rabbit, although sedation is recommended in fractious patients. Free catch urine samples can be obtained relatively easily from litter-trained rabbits, using sterilised aquarium gravel as a replacement for litter in their tray. Urethral catheterisation under sedation or general anaesthesia can be both diagnostic and therapeutic, as removal of sludgy urine sediment and flushing with sterile saline often alleviates the clinical signs.

Haematuria can be differentiated from red urine caused by plant porphyrin pigments by a positive reaction for blood on dipstick testing or >5 red blood cells per high powered field on urine sediment examination, as opposed to fluorescence of plant pigments under the ultraviolet light of a Wood's lamp.

Neurological examination is indicated in all cases with large bladders. Plain and contrast radiography and ultrasonography will reveal bladder wall, neck or urethral abnormalities and identify cystoliths or urethroliths (Figure 3). In addition, ultrasonography has been shown to estimate bladder hypertrophy accurately in rabbits. Cystoscopy has been used in female rabbits and allows further complementary assessment of the lower urinary tract and indirect assessment of the

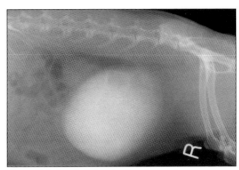

Figure 3: Lateral abdominal radiograph demonstrating a very large bladder filled with radiodense material. The sediment was removed by repeated flushing of the bladder via urethral catheterisation

upper urinary tract, by evaluation of urine production by each ureter.

Serology for *E.cuniculi* infection should be carried out in all cases; a positive titre in addition to neurological signs support the diagnosis. A urine or faecal PCR will also give a definitive diagnosis of *E.cuniculi* infection in those rabbits that are actively shedding the parasite, which usually occurs in the first 3 months of infection. Renal biopsy and parasite identification may also help in diagnosis.

A 24-hour water measurement test is recommended to confirm polydipsia (>120 ml/ kg/day). An average consumption taken over 3 days in the rabbit's home environment is usually representative. Further investigation of the aetiology of the polyuria should then be carried out.

How do I treat urine scalding in a rabbit?

Therapy with broad-spectrum antibiotics such as enrofloxacin (10–30 mg/kg orally or s.c. q24h) or trimethoprim/sulfamethoxazole (co-trimoxazole suspension) (30 mg/kg orally q12h) should be implemented while awaiting urine culture and sensitivity test results. Analgesia, non-steroidal anti-inflammatories and/or partial opioids are recommended, depending on renal function.

Supportive treatment in the initial stage of urine scalding involves careful clipping of fur around the perineum, cleaning the perineum and topical treatment of the pyoderma. Once the pyoderma has resolved, application of a water-resistant barrier spray or cream can be helpful to avoid recurrence of skin scalding and pyoderma. Weight loss is recommended in overweight rabbits, as obesity will exacerbate urine scalding and clinical signs of urolithiasis.

Sedation or general anaesthesia and urethral catheterisation to remove sediment and small cystoliths is indicated if excess sediment is found on radiography.

What specific treatment can be used in rabbits with excessive urinary sediment or uroliths?

Urinary acidification via diet is not practical, as rabbits have naturally very alkaline urine. Urohydropropulsion is a non-surgical technique used in cats and dogs to remove small round urocystoliths, and has been used successfully in rabbits. Pre-anaesthetic diazepam is recommended to relax the urethral smooth muscle, and pre-emptive analgesia is recommended. Once anaesthetised, 4–6 ml/kg sterile saline should be administered through a urethral catheter to moderately distend the bladder, after which the catheter should be removed. The rabbit is held in an upright position and the bladder is manually expressed using steady firm, digital pressure. The procedure is repeated as necessary and then followed up with radiography to ensure removal of all uroliths has been achieved. Haematuria and dysuria are expected for up to 2 days following this procedure. Particular care must be taken in bucks to ensure that uroliths are small enough to pass through the urethra to avoid urethral obstruction.

Cystotomy is recommended for the removal of all medium to large or irregular cystoliths. Reverse urohydropropulsion is recommended to return large urethral uroliths to the bladder for removal by cystotomy.

How do I treat urinary incontinence?

Response to therapy frequently aids the diagnosis of urinary incontinence. A positive response to diethylstilbestrol* (0.5 mg per rabbit orally once or twice a week) is suggestive of USMI. Treatment of urolithiasis and management of urine scalding is required.

What long-term treatment and prevention can be carried out for rabbits with excessive urinary sediment?

Client education regarding dietary modification to reduce dietary calcium is recommended for long-term management and prevention of excess sediment precipitation or retention and the formation of uroliths (Figure 4). Timothy grass-based pellets should be fed, and then only in a small quantity (e.g. one tablespoon/day/rabbit). The majority of the diet should be mixed meadow hay or Timothy hay (a pile of hay equal to the size of the rabbit), some root vegetables and moderate amounts of green leafy vegetables (a small handful daily). In general, items to be avoided include all vitamin and mineral supplements, alfalfa (pellet or hay), excess kale, carrot tops, dandelion and clover.

What prognosis should I give?

Prognosis is dependent on the cause and severity of the lesion. Chronic renal failure carries a poor prognosis. Chronic over-distension or severe hypertrophy of the bladder carries a poor prognosis for recovery. *E.cuniculi* unresponsive to fenbendazole treatment (20 mg/kg orally q24h for 30 days)

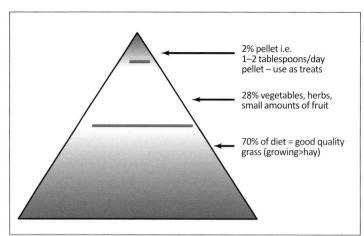

Figure 4: Diagrammatic demonstration of the correct way to feed adult pet rabbits

2% pellet i.e.
1–2 tablespoons/day
pellet – use as treats

28% vegetables, herbs,
small amounts of fruit

70% of diet = good quality
grass (growing>hay)

also carries a poor prognosis. However, a large proportion of rabbits have excessive urinary sediment as a result of being fed excess dietary calcium, and resulting in urinary tract disease. In these cases, once the sediment has been removed and the diet is corrected, the prognosis can be good. ∎

*Editor's comment: Diethylstibestrol may not be readily available; phenylpropanolamine has also been recommended for USMI in rabbits.

How to...
Manage **seizures**
by Mark Lowrie

Epilepsy is a term used to describe recurrent seizures. It can result from any number of causes (Figures 1–4), but regardless of the underlying problem the principles for managing the seizures are usually very similar. This article gives guidance on the management of epilepsy.

When should you start treatment?
Unfortunately the answer to this question is not black and white. The reasons for treatment are: to prevent further damage to the patient's brain; and to provide the best possible quality

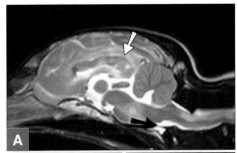

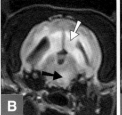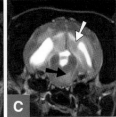

Figure 2: Not all cases of seizures are due to idiopathic epilepsy: MRI scans of a 3-year-old dog with a 3-week history of progressively more frequent seizures. The predominant lesions are seen as hyperintense regions on T2-weighted (A and C) and FLAIR (B) scans throughout the forebrain (white arrows), indicative of inflammation. Further hyperintense regions are seen within the brainstem (black arrows), showing the multifocal nature of this disease. In between the seizures the dog also demonstrated abnormal behaviour including pacing around the house, standing facing the wall and loss of toilet training. The most common cause for this presentation and distribution of lesions is an immune-mediated inflammatory encephalitis, e.g. granulomatous meningoencephalitis

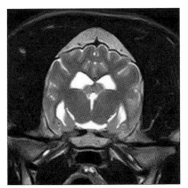

Figure 1: A dog presenting with seizures between 6 months and 6 years of age with normal behaviour and a normal inter-ictal neurological examination is most likely to have idiopathic epilepsy. The diagnosis is obtained by ruling out other causes of seizures and so haematology, serum biochemistry and an MRI scan of the brain will be unremarkable

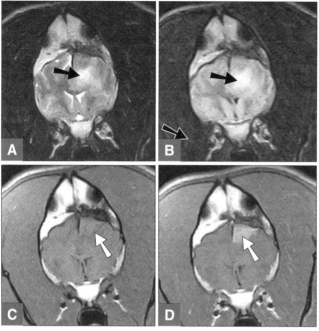

Figure 3: Not all cases of seizures are due to idiopathic epilepsy: MRI scans of a 13-year-old dog that had suffered only three seizures in the previous 6 weeks and had a normal neurological examination and was normal inter-ictally. A dog that first presents with seizures over the age of 6 years is more likely to have an identifiable underlying cause for the seizures. T2-weighted (A), FLAIR (B), and pre- (C) and post-contrast (D) T1-weighted transverse images are presented. The images reveal an ill-defined high signal intraparenchymal lesion of the left parietal lobe on T2-weighted and FLAIR images (black arrows) likely to represent oedema. Following administration of contrast medium (D) an extra-axial homogeneous hyperintense lesion becomes apparent, with a broad-based meningeal association (white arrows). In this case the imaging findings were compatible with an intracranial extra-axial neoplasm, with a meningioma seeming most likely

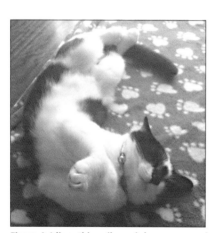

Figure 4: Idiopathic epilepsy is less common in cats than in dogs. It is important to exclude some of the common metabolic causes for seizures in this species, including hepatic encephalopathy, renal encephalopathy, ionic imbalance, hypoglycaemia, polycythaemia, hypertensive encephalopathy and hyperthyroidism

of life for the patient and client. Indications for starting treatment include:

- Status epilepticus or cluster seizures
- An underlying progressive disorder provoking seizures
- Post-ictal signs that are objectionable
- Multiple seizures occurring in a short period
- An increased frequency and/or severity of seizures.

There is much contention concerning whether one seizure leads to another, an effect known as 'kindling'. No convincing scientific evidence exists in favour of early medical management of epilepsy and if only a single seizure has been observed it seems reasonable to withhold therapy until a problem with seizures is observed (i.e. repeated or severe seizures). It seems unlikely that the introduction of antiepileptic medication will alter the long-term prognosis, unless the patient has clusters of seizures or has had an episode of status epilepticus.

What should the owner expect?

Our clients are not a homogeneous population and we may find that one person's perception of adequate seizure control is another owner's nightmare. Therefore, what constitutes an adequate treatment response? Adequate treatment is assessed based on:

- Seizure frequency once steady-state serum drug concentrations are achieved
- Severity of side effects.

The aim of therapy is to restore a normal life for the pet and owner, with no adverse drug effects. However, in reality, achieving this goal is often extremely difficult. A better approach is to aim to reduce seizure severity and frequency to a level which does not substantially compromise the quality of life for the pet and owner, whilst trying to avoid adverse drug effects. Adequate seizure control is defined most commonly in the literature as a reduction in seizure frequency of ≥50% and therefore novel antiepileptic medication is considered successful if it meets this criterion. It is clear to see that this may not be considered acceptable by an owner. Many clients have difficulty in understanding that therapy may not lead to a seizure-free pet, and may still request treatment even if the seizures are very infrequent. These points are crucial to success as further medications can be expensive and require a solid commitment from the owner with the understanding that acceptable control for a patient may only constitute a reduction in seizure frequency of 50%.

Client compliance is also a factor that must be considered in the management of refractory epileptic patients. It is important to ensure the drugs are given appropriately, at the correct time and dosage, and that the client doesn't adjust the dosage based on a short-term assessment of seizure control or side effects. This is a common reason for failure of response to medication.

What treatment options are there?

A. Phenobarbital – Phenobarbital is a good first-line medication, achieving acceptable seizure control in an estimated 60–80% of dogs if serum concentrations are maintained within the therapeutic range. A common mistake is to start on an inappropriately low dosage of phenobarbital and discontinue the medication before it has reached a reasonable therapeutic concentration in the blood. The datasheet recommends a dosage of 1–2.5 mg/kg p.o. q12h, although experience would suggest that this leads to a low or sub-therapeutic concentration in the blood. A more appropriate and acceptable starting dosage in dogs and cats is 3 mg/kg p.o. q12h as this allows a therapeutic concentration to be achieved. Another often overlooked feature of phenobarbital is its ability to cause enzyme auto-induction with long-term use. With time, the body increases its ability to metabolise this medication (hepatic enzyme induction), which results in a quicker clearance and hence lower serum concentration. A clinical manifestation of this phenomenon would be a dog on phenobarbital, which was within the therapeutic serum range and controlling the seizures, that suddenly experiences breakthrough seizures giving the illusion of having become refractory to medication. Indeed, to maintain the therapeutic serum concentration, subsequent increases in dose may be required. This auto-induction means that many patients may eventually require an oral dose of phenobarbital that is much higher than the starting dose; hence it is important to remember that it is the serum concentration we are interested in and not the oral dosage. The half-life of this drug is very variable (between 40–90 hours), meaning it takes 10–14 days to reach a steady state. Thus, blood samples to determine the serum concentration of phenobarbital should be taken 2 weeks after any dose change. The main factor to consider when obtaining these samples is to ensure that the specimen is always collected at the same time of day, to avoid comparing peak and trough serum levels within the same individual. In summary, serum concentrations should be measured approximately 10–14 days after starting treatment. Additionally, they should be repeated every 3–6 months to monitor for auto-induction. Further indications for monitoring serum concentrations include: poorly controlled seizures; following any dose change; or if there are suspected drug-related adverse effects. Sedation and ataxia are common adverse effects seen with this medication, although they are usually transient and only persists in some cases. Polyphagia, polydipsia and polyuria are also frequently encountered and are usually dose-related. Other side effects that occur with phenobarbital are classified as idiosyncratic, as they seem to be related to neither dose nor prolonged administration. These include hyperexcitability, acute hepatotoxicity, blood dyscrasias (e.g. thrombocytopenia, anaemia or leucopenia) and superficial necrolytic dermatitis. Hepatic toxicity is one of the more serious side effects and can be difficult to detect. Given that phenobarbital induces hepatic enzymes, it is not unexpected to see elevations in liver enzymes suggesting that the hepatic

structure has been altered. However, hepatic function is more important in a patient on phenobarbital therapy and should be assessed by monitoring albumin, urea, cholesterol and glucose levels as well as performing a bile acid stimulation test. It is recommended that these tests are performed every 6 months as routine.

KEY POINTS

Loading phenobarbital

- When presented with a patient suffering status epilepticus or severe cluster seizures it may be desirable to achieve a steady state more rapidly than the standard 10–14 days.
- The dosage for achieving this is 4 mg/kg phenobarbital intravenously or intramuscularly every 10–30 minutes either until the seizures stop or until a total dose of 18–24 mg/kg has been given.

KEY POINTS

Monitoring for hepatotoxicity

- **Liver structure** can be crudely assessed by monitoring alanine transaminase (ALT), aspartate transaminase (AST), alkaline phosphatase (ALP) and gamma-glutamyl transpeptidase (GGT).
- **Liver function** can be crudely assessed by monitoring glucose, urea, albumin and cholesterol. A bile acid stimulation test is the best test to assess liver function.
- Given that phenobarbital affects ALP, ALT, cholesterol and GGT, monitoring AST, bile acids, albumin and urea is acceptable to assess for hepatotoxicity.

B. Potassium bromide (KBr) – This drug may be used as a monotherapy or in conjunction with phenobarbital. A big advantage of this medication is that it is excreted exclusively by the kidneys, so is an appropriate choice in dogs with liver dysfunction. One of the disadvantages of using KBr is its long elimination half-life (24–46 days). A steady state is achieved only after 3–6 months from initiating therapy and, therefore, when changing the dose in order to alter the serum concentration, it is important to remember that it can take around 3–6 months to reach a steady state. In some patients this means a loading dose may be necessary if seizures are frequent and severe, or when phenobarbital must be withdrawn because of liver disease. The major limitation of loading KBr is that there is no time for tolerance to the sedative effects of the drug to develop. Thus, lethargy and ataxia may be severe and vomiting may occur; hospitalisation of the patient during the loading period is recommended. If loading is performed, a blood sample may be taken 24 hours later to assess the serum concentration. The loading dose is 600 mg/kg p.o. divided over 5 days. This medication is not a suitable choice for cats as they develop an idiosyncratic allergic pneumonitis, which is fatal in a large number of cases. Given that KBr is a salt, any change in serum sodium osmolality can alter the excretion of bromide. Therefore, dogs that have a sudden intake of salt (e.g. due to an altered diet or swallowing sea water) can increase the elimination of bromide, resulting in lower serum concentrations. Diuretics can also increase the elimination of bromide and this should be considered if epileptic patients are given the two medications concurrently. The starting dose of KBr is approximately 30 mg/kg/day p.o. given once daily or divided twice daily. It is advisable to give KBr with food as it can irritate the oesophageal and gastric walls, causing vomiting. Side effects are similar to phenobarbital and include vomiting, ataxia, weakness, polyuria, polyphagia, polydipsia, pancreatitis and pruritus. If side effects are suspected, then the serum levels should be measured, although the timing of sampling is not important due to the long half-life of the drug.

KEY POINTS

Loading potassium bromide
- The loading dose for KBr is 600 mg/kg p.o. divided over 5 days.
- In severe cases this dosage can be divided over fewer days, although this will result in more severe side effects and therefore should be reserved for cases in which the seizures are causing major concern (e.g. continued status epilepticus despite appropriate management).

C. Rectal diazepam – Rectal diazepam can be extremely useful, particularly in dogs with severe cluster seizures. Rectal absorption is comparatively faster than oral or intramuscular absorption, occurring within 10 minutes. The recommended dose is 0.5–2 mg/kg for a maximum of three treatments within 24 hours. This is usually used as an adjunct to the above medications as opposed to an alternative.

D. Levetiracetam (Keppra): This is a relatively new medication that is reserved for those patients who fail to respond to phenobarbital and KBr or, in the case of cats, phenobarbital alone. It has a unique mechanism of action, which is a potential advantage when the drug is used in combination with other antiepileptic medications. The half-life of this drug is 4–6 hours, meaning that a steady state is achieved within 48 hours, but also that frequent administration is necessary. It is primarily excreted by the kidneys, making it a suitable choice in patients with liver disease. Its efficacy is initially excellent and the recommended starting dosage is 20 mg/kg p.o. q8h. In a study of 14 dogs with refractory idiopathic epilepsy, 9 dogs responded to the addition of levetiracetam to the drug regimen (i.e. seizure frequency decreased by >50% in these patients). The drug was well tolerated by all dogs in the study and sedation was the only side effect reported in just one of the 14 dogs. However, of the 9 dogs that responded to levetiracetam, two-thirds experienced an increase in seizure frequency after 4–8 months. Therefore, some dogs that initially improve on levetiracetam therapy may return to the baseline seizure frequency after 4–8 months (the so-called 'honeymoon effect'). Thus, this drug may be useful for dogs demonstrating cluster seizures who have numerous seizure episodes within 24–72 hours but a relatively long inter-ictal period between clusters (usually weeks to months). The short-term addition of levetiracetam for the duration of the cluster can reduce the number of seizures during the episode. The drug can be used at a dose of 10–30 mg/kg p.o. q8h for the duration of the cluster (usually 2–3 days) and then stopped again until the start of the next cluster. No study has proven the efficacy of 'pulse-dosing' but anecdotally it has been useful in patients and appears to offset the 'honeymoon effect'. The main factor limiting the use of levetiracetam in dogs and cats is its expense, although it is slowly becoming more affordable, particularly in small dogs and cats.

PRACTICAL TIP

Using levetiracetam

Occasionally a patient may present suffering from very severe clusters of seizures within a short period of time (e.g. 24–48 hours) followed by a long inter-ictal period of weeks or months. Levetiracetam may be given during these severe clusters to reduce the number and severity of the seizures. Following cessation of the seizures, the medication can be discontinued and restarted next time a severe cluster occurs. In this way, some of the high costs of the drug are avoided as well as reducing the possibility of tolerance. The drug can be used at a dose of 10–30 mg/kg p.o. q8h for the duration of the cluster (usually 2–3 days) and then discontinued when the patient has been seizure-free for 24 hours.

In summary, phenobarbital remains a good first-line drug in the majority of patients. Potassium bromide is useful when phenobarbital alone does not control the seizures sufficiently or when hepatotoxicity is a problem. Levetiracetam is reserved for those patients where potassium bromide and phenobarbital are found to be inappropriate, either due to their side effects or due to continued frequent and/or severe seizures. However, the owners of all patients should be provided with rectal diazepam regardless of the severity or frequency of the seizures. ∎

Editor's note: Readers are reminded to follow the cascade when considering use of medications not authorised for use in veterinary species.

How to...

Perform a **CSF tap**

by Mark Lowrie

C erebrospinal fluid (CSF) bathes the brain and spinal cord, which are ensheathed by the meninges. Any disease within this compartment has the potential to alter the characteristics of this fluid, thus analysis of CSF is extremely sensitive for the diagnosis of central nervous system (CNS) disease but is rarely specific as to the cause. It is especially useful in inflammatory diseases of the brain, the surrounding meninges and nerve roots that result in meningitis, encephalitis or myelitis.

When to collect CSF

Collection of CSF should be performed in any disease in which CNS involvement is suspected. If an encephalopathy or myelopathy is considered, CSF analysis can give a clearer indication of whether an inflammatory or non-inflammatory process is present and, in the light of signalment, history and other findings (e.g. imaging, serology), lead to refinement of the diagnosis.

Features that should alert the clinician to perform a CSF analysis include:

- **Multifocal or diffuse CNS disease** – when a neurological examination is performed and the abnormalities identified cannot be explained by a single anatomical site, the localisation is said to be multifocal. This is typical of inflammatory or infiltrative neoplastic diseases

- **Focal or generalised pain** – this can be indicative of meningeal involvement (manifesting as head or neck pain), particularly in dogs of less than 2 years of age in which disc disease is an unlikely diagnosis. Diseases involving the meninges may be painful, with meningitis presenting either as a primary condition or occurring secondary as a common sequela to many inflammatory, infectious and neoplastic conditions. Common clinical signs include a low head carriage, neck pain, pyrexia and lethargy. These symptoms may wax and wane during the course of the disease

- **The presence of systemic inflammatory disease** – an inflammatory leucogram suggests the presence of an inflammatory process and, in cases where the origin of this inflammation has not been readily identified and neurological signs are present (e.g. deficits or pain), the CNS must be considered as a possible focus. Pyrexia of unknown origin is one of the key indications for CSF analysis, particularly in the presence of pain

- **Myelography** – contrast agents used in myelography can alter CSF characteristics for prolonged periods of time. Therefore CSF should be routinely collected prior to myelography.

Contraindications to CSF collection

As with any test, CSF sampling is not a benign procedure and should be undertaken with caution in every patient. However, there are some circumstances in which it should be completely avoided:

- **Atlanto-axial instability** – this disease can be of congenital or traumatic origin. A good rule of thumb is always to suspect cervical instability in any small-breed dog with neck pain (whether trauma was reported or not) and to perform a neutral cervical radiograph as the first step in investigation. If instability is found then a CSF tap should not be performed
- **Dermatitis** – CSF should not be collected from a site if the overlying skin is infected
- **Critically ill** – CSF should not be collected in a patient for whom general anesthesia is contraindicated
- **Raised intracranial pressure (ICP)** – this may be suspected on the basis of a combination of clinical signs. These signs are discussed below:
  - Mentation – any alteration in consciousness should alert the clinician to raised ICP. These patients may be dull or obtunded but in severe situations they can become stuporous or comatose
  - Vestibular eye movements – moving the head from side to side provokes a physiological jerk nystagmus in a normal animal that stops when the head is still. If this reflex is absent it would suggest abnormal brain function and raised ICP
  - Pupil size – anisocoria is a frequent finding early on in the pathogenesis of raised ICP. This is thought to be due to pressure on cranial nerve III and its nucleus. As ICP rises, small pin-prick pupils (miotic) result (possibly due to facilitation of cranial nerve III) and as the

pressure increases pupils may become large (mydriatic) and unresponsive to light (due to compression of cranial nerve III)
  - Motor function – initiation of motor function is often abnormal in these patients and an assessment of proprioception is important. This is due to compression and subsequent disruption of the higher pathways of the pyramidal and extra-pyramidal motor system within the brain
  - Advanced imaging – given access to magnetic resonance imaging then herniation secondary to raised ICP may be seen. This may be seen as foramen magnum herniation (the caudal vermis of the cerebellum herniates through the foramen magnum) or trans-tentorial herniation (compression of the caudal parts of the cerebral hemispheres beneath the tentorium cerebelli).

How to collect CSF

When performed routinely CSF collection is a straight forward procedure with few complications. CSF can be collected from either the cerebellomedullary cistern (CMC) or the caudal lumbar subarachnoid space. CSF flows in a cranial to caudal direction and therefore it is advisable to collect the sample from a site caudal to the suspected lesion. It is therefore recommended to sample CSF from the CMC in brain disease, whereas a lumbar sample is preferred in patients with spinal lesions. Collection is performed under general anaesthesia and the site must be clipped and aseptically prepared. Many texts recommend that no more than 1 ml per 5 kg should be taken from the patient and the sample should be collected into a plain sterile plastic tube.

Cerebellomedullary cistern CSF collection

Positioning is essential to successful and safe collection, so time should be taken to ensure the patient is held correctly. The patient is held in lateral recumbency with the head ventroflexed at an angle of 90 degrees and the muzzle parallel to the table (Figure 1A). The cuff of the endotracheal tube should be deflated and, if possible, a non-collapsible tube should be used. Palpate the dorsal spinous process of the axis vertebra (C2) and the occipital protuberance on the midline of the skull (Figures 1B and 1C).

A spinal needle (a standard hypodermic needle may be used in smaller patients) is placed midway between these two points, directly in the midline at the level of the cranial border of the atlas vertebra (C1). Once the skin has been punctured the stylet is removed and the needle is advanced slowly, taking a course towards the ramus of the mandible, parallel to the muzzle and the table top. Varying degrees of resistance are encountered as the needle is advanced through the muscle and fascial planes. If an area of fluid accumulation is encountered, it will usually flow freely from the hub of the needle as it does not contain a stylet. It is good practice to stop for a few seconds after penetrating any area of altered resistance to see if CSF flows from the needle. Three scenarios are possible when CSF collection is attempted:

■ If frank blood is seen in the needle hub then it is likely that the needle is positioned too far off midline or the patient is not positioned appropriately

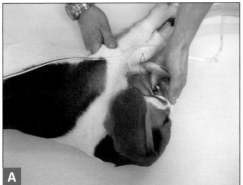

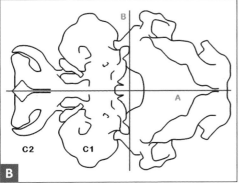

Figure 1: The correct positioning for collection of cerebellomedullary cisternal cerebrospinal fluid is shown in (A). (B) shows a diagrammatic representation of the atlanto-occipital junction with landmarks indicated. Line A marks the midline between the dorsal spinous process of axis (C2) and the occipital protuberance of the skull. Line B marks the atlanto-occipital space found by palpating the cranial border of atlas (C1). The needle is placed directly where these two lines intersect. (C) shows these landmarks on the live dog

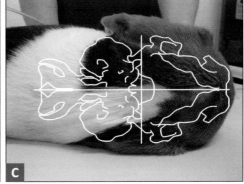

- If the needle hits bone then the needle must be positioned more cranially or caudally depending on its current location
- When the subarachnoid space is entered there is often a small degree of resistance followed by a 'pop'. As this occurs the needle should be held in position and CSF allowed to drip into the tube. Do not aspirate CSF from the needle as this can cause severe damage to the neural structures.

Lumbar CSF collection

This is technically more difficult, although it carries less risk of iatrogenic CNS trauma than does CMC puncture. The patient is positioned in lateral recumbency. The spinous processes of L5 and L6 are palpated (L6 is usually the most caudal spinous process that can be palpated) and the needle is inserted at the level of L6, aiming at the space between the fifth and sixth lumbar vertebrae (Figures 2A and 2B).

Keeping to the midline, the needle should be 'walked' cranially off the edge of the L6 process until it punctures the ligamentum flavum (also known as the interarcuate or yellow ligament). This is usually accompanied by a change in resistance and as the needle passes through the cauda equina or caudal spinal cord a slight twitch of the tail and/or pelvic limbs is seen. If the patient is a dog then the spinal cord will usually terminate at the level of L4/L5; in a feline patient this is further caudal, at L5/L6. The stylet must be kept in place until the needle is fully inserted in the ventral subarachnoid space. The stylet is removed and the hub of the needle is observed for CSF. It may be necessary to withdraw the needle slightly if no CSF is seen (Figure 2C). ■

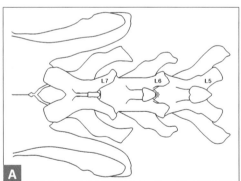

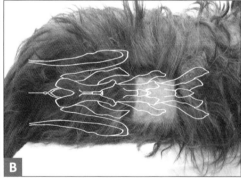

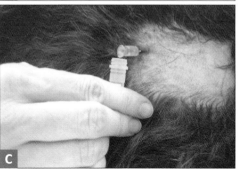

Figure 2: A diagrammatic representation of the lumbosacral junction is shown in (A). The site of puncture for a lumbar tap is marked with an X (between the fifth and sixth lumbar vertebrae). The correct positioning for collection of lumbar cerebrospinal fluid is shown in (B), with successful collection demonstrated in (C)

Editor's note: Readers are reminded that CSF collection is not a benign procedure and owners should be warned of the inherent risks involved. Ideally CSF collection is a technique which should be taught by an experienced clinician in addition to the operator being familiar with the technique as outlined in this article. Iatrogenic trauma to the brainstem caused by excessive advancing of the needle is a possible complication of CMC puncture. Should it occur, patients may show signs of opisthotonus, even under GA, changes in breathing and heart rate and should they recover from anaesthesia, tetraparesis and cranial nerve deficits. Full recovery is unlikely but does occur.

CMC puncture should be employed with caution in Cavalier King Charles Spaniels, due to the incidence of Chiari-like malformations in this breed. As such CMC puncture may lead to needle penetration into the cerebellum and/or brainstem. Lumbar CSF collection is therefore advisable in the absence of advanced imaging evidence that the cerebellum is not caudally displaced.

How to...

Perform a **surgical extraction** of a canine tooth

by Lisa Milella

What is a surgical extraction?

An extraction technique involving raising a flap of tissue to remove bone that forms part of the socket, to allow access to the root and facilitate its extraction (Figure 1).

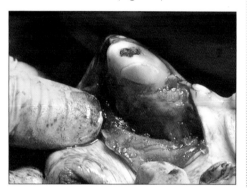

Figure 1: Surgical extraction of a tooth

INDICATIONS FOR TOOTH EXTRACTION

- Severe periodontal disease (mobility, furcation exposure, periodontal probing depths)
- Complicated crown fracture (pulp exposed)
- Worn tooth with pulp exposure
- Crown root fracture
- Odontoclastic resorptive lesion
- Non-vital tooth
- Persistent deciduous teeth
- Teeth involved in a jaw fracture
- Unerupted teeth causing pathology
- Teeth causing malocclusions
- Supernumerary teeth
- Chronic gingivostomatitis

When should this technique be used?

This technique should always be used for extraction of canine teeth, but the same principles can be applied to extraction of any tooth in the mouth. A surgical extraction technique is also used for retrieval of root remnants and if any abnormal tooth morphology exists. It may also be the surgeon's preference to use a surgical technique if multiple adjacent teeth need to be extracted as in Figure 2.

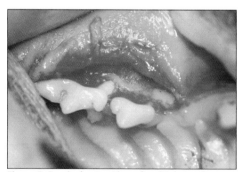

Figure 2: Surgical extraction of multiple teeth

Equipment required to perform a surgical extraction

(Author's preference – Figure 3A)

- Scalpel handle and blade (No.11).
- Periosteal elevator (Goldman Fox).

- Dental luxators and elevators (sharp and of a suitable size) (Couplands No.1 and No.3) – Figure 3B.
- Extraction forceps (Pattern 76 and 76N).
- High-speed water cooled dental drill with a selection of round and tapered burs (No.2 and No.4 round and a 701 tapered fissure bur) – Figures 3C and 3D.
- Small surgical scissors.
- Rat tooth forceps.
- Needle-holders.
- Monofilament absorbable suture material (poliglecaprone 25 – size 5/0).

All equipment should be sterile as tooth extraction is considered a surgical procedure.

Patient preparation
- General anaesthesia – a cuffed endotracheal tube and throat pack are recommended to secure the airway. Local anaesthesia should also be considered.
- Pre-emptive analgesia.
- Perioperative antibiotics should be given in selected cases only. These include debilitated animals, immunocompromised animals, animals with severe local or

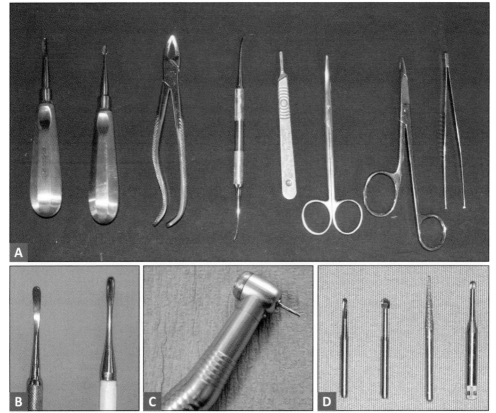

Figure 3: (A) Author's preferred equipment for surgical extraction (see text). (B) Dental luxator and elevator. (C) Dental drill. (D) Burs for dental drill

systemic infection, animals with organ disease or endocrine disorders.

- Scale and polish all teeth prior to performing any extractions. Tooth extraction, by whatever technique, is a surgical procedure and should be performed in as clean a field as possible. The surgical site should also be irrigated with a chlorhexidine-based mouthwash.
- Preoperative radiographs should be taken. Radiographs will enable the surgeon to assess any abnormal root morphology and the integrity of the surrounding bone. Postoperative radiographs can be taken to ensure complete tooth root removal (Figure 4).

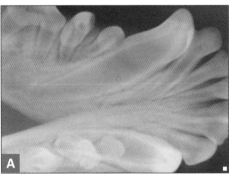

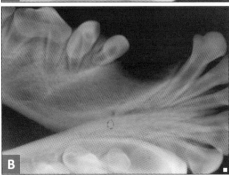

Figure 4: (A) Preoperative radiograph.
(B) Postoperative radiograph following surgical removal of a mandibular canine

TECHNIQUE

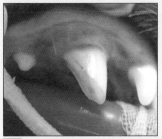

A This upper canine tooth has a complicated crown fracture (the pulp cavity is exposed). There is a vertical fracture extending on to the root. This tooth cannot be salvaged by root canal treatment and extraction is the only option.

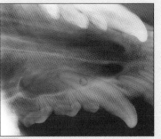

B A pre-extraction radiograph of an upper canine tooth showing the length of the root. As a general rule the apex of the canine tooth finishes at the mesial root of the second premolar. This should be taken into consideration when designing the flap. The flap should enable unimpeded access to the whole root if necessary.

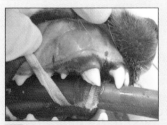

C Vertical releasing incisions are made between the upper canine and lateral incisor rostrally and at the mesial line angle of the second premolar. The blade is also run in the gingival sulcus around the tooth, being careful not to perforate the gingiva. The vertical releasing incisions should extend beyond the mucogingival junction (the junction between the attached gingiva and the alveolar mucosa). The incisions can be slightly divergent to allow adequate blood supply to the flap. They should also be made so that there is bone support for the sutured wound and thus incisions should not lie over a void.

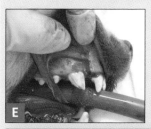

D A sharp periosteal elevator is used to raise a full thickness mucoperiosteal flap. The elevator is positioned at an angle to the bone – if too flat, accidental perforation of the flap can occur. The tissue is tightly adhered at the mucogingival junction and care must be taken not to perforate the flap here. The flap raised should give good exposure to the alveolar bone overlying the tooth root (Figures E and F).

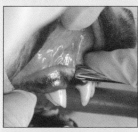

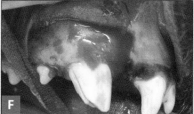

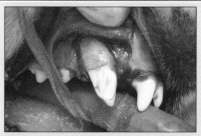

G Using a high-speed water-cooled round bur*, a gutter is created on either side of the canine tooth root. Some overlying buccal bone can be removed to enable the mesial and distal edges of the tooth root to be seen. The gutters should be half the width of the tooth root and extend up to 2/3 of the length of the root. The gutters are then connected on the buccal aspect, so that the bone plate overlying the root is removed together with the root.

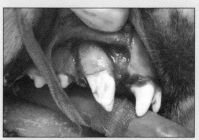

H A dental elevator is positioned in the groove created on either the mesial or distal aspect of the tooth. Elevators should not be used on the palatal aspect of the upper canine tooth to avoid iatrogenic oronasal communication. The elevator should be rotated slowly to tear the periodontal ligament attachment. Tension should be held for about 10 seconds to allow the ligament to tear. The elevator is then moved to the opposite groove and the motion repeated until the tooth starts to loosen. When the tooth is loose, extraction forceps are positioned as far apically as possible and the tooth rotated along its long axis, pulling gently at the same time. The extracted tooth should be checked to ensure that the whole root has been extracted (a postoperative radiograph should be taken if there is any doubt).

TECHNIQUE

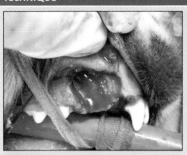

I The empty socket should be debrided if there is any granulation tissue or debris. The socket is checked for any loose bone fragments. The edges of the socket should then be smoothed using either a diamond-coated bur or with rongeurs. The extraction site can be lavaged with lactated Ringer's solution to remove any remaining debris. The air–water syringe on the dental machine should not be used as air may cause an embolism or emphysema and water is cytotoxic to connective tissue cells.

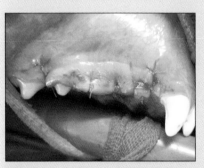

J The flap is then replaced and sutured in position using a monofilament absorbable suture material and a simple interrupted suture pattern. The flap should be sutured with no tension. Releasing incisions can be made in the periosteum on the underside of the flap to release tension if necessary. Care must be taken not to perforate the flap.

*High-speed burs should be used with extreme caution. Complications include soft tissue trauma, thermal bone necrosis, emphysema and fatal air embolisms.

Applying the principles to the lower canine tooth

The basic principles described above are used for the mandibular canine with the following exceptions (Figures 5 and 6):

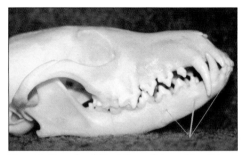

Figure 5: Care should be taken when making the vertical releasing incisions and raising the flap to avoid damaging the inferior alveolar blood vessels and nerve exiting the middle mental foramen

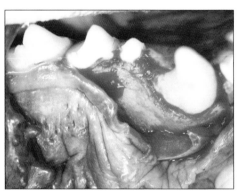

Figure 6: A longer releasing incision can be made rostrally creating more of a triangular flap. Dental elevators should not be placed directly mesially and distally but rather on the mesolingual and distolingual aspects of the tooth. This is to avoid fracture of the rostral mandible

KEYS TO SUCCESS

- Knowledge of the correct root morphology
- Correct technique
- Appropriate tools
- Practice and patience

Complications

The complications encountered with surgical extractions are summarized in Figure 7. ■

Complication	Cause and avoidance
Tooth fracture (crown/root/both)	Incorrect technique – careful use of elevators and luxators. Extraction forceps should not be used before the tooth is adequately loosened
Oronasal communication (Figure 8)	May be due to infection or iatrogenic damage – avoid excessive force during the extraction
Jaw fracture	Preoperative radiographs should be taken to assess bone loss in advanced periodontal disease. Incorrect technique (placement of luxators and elevators especially associated with lower canine) must be avoided
Haemorrhage	Accidental damage to neurovascular bundle during surgery. Haemorrhage may occur as a result of a root fracture. Pre-existing disease should be identified before surgery if possible
Displaced root fragments	Avoid downward force in cats as the root fragment may be displaced into the mandibular canal. Avoid excessive force on the palatal root of the upper carnassial in dogs to avoid pushing the root into the nasal turbinates ➡

Figure 7: Complications of extractions (continues)

Complication	Cause and avoidance
Thermal bone damage	Adequate cooling of high-speed bur when used
Emphysema	Incorrect use of the high-speed handpiece. Avoid blowing air into soft tissue or bone
Soft tissue injuries (gingiva, tongue, frenulum, lip, eye)	Use spatulas to avoid accidental damage when using the high-speed bur. Controlled force when using elevators and avoid slippage by correct holding of instrument and stabilisation of the patient's head
Wound breakdown	Avoid tension when suturing in the mouth. Periosteal releasing incisions can be made on the surface of mucoperiosteal flaps to release tension. Careful flap planning prior to extraction is required

Figure 7 (continued): Complications of extractions

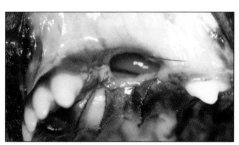

Figure 8: Oronasal communication can be a complication of surgical extraction

How to...

Treat **hyperthyroid cats** with radioactive iodine

by Carmel Mooney

Although a wealth of data are available on the consequences and outcome of feline hyperthyroidism, the exact cause remains unclear. Prevention is therefore not possible but because of the benign nature of the lesions in most affected cats, the disease carries a favourable prognosis with effective therapy.

Treatment of hyperthyroidism is achieved by removing or destroying the abnormally functioning thyroid tissue or inhibiting thyroid hormone synthesis and release. Surgical thyroidectomy and thyroid ablation using radioactive iodine (Figure 1) are the only

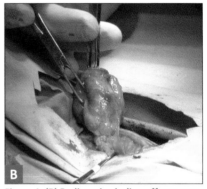

Figure 1: (B) Radioactive iodine offers a non-surgical, curative therapy for hyperthyroidism

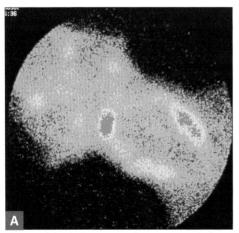

Figure 1: (A) Scintigram revealing asymmetrical, bilateral disease (continues) ➡

curative methods. Medical management controls thyroid hormone production but has no effect on the underlying disorder. Although an option long-term, medical management is also often used to stabilise patients prior to surgical thyroidectomy or to control clinical signs until radioactive iodine administration.

Each treatment method carries its own specific advantages and disadvantages that must be taken into consideration for each individual case. Few studies exist that directly compare the outcome of each of the different treatment methods in hyperthyroid cats. However, radioactive iodine therapy, if available, is considered by most to be the optimal treatment in terms of safety, simplicity and efficacy.

How does radioactive iodine work?

Radioactive iodine as ^{131}I, like stable iodine, is actively concentrated by the thyroid gland. It has a half-life of eight days and emits both β-particles and γ-radiation. The β-particles cause over 80 per cent of tissue damage, and are locally destructive, travelling a maximum of 2 mm with an average penetration of 400 μm. The radiation therefore destroys abnormally functioning thyroid tissue, but carries minimal risk of significant damage to adjacent parathyroid tissue, atrophic thyroid tissue or other cervical structures.

How is the dose of radioactive iodine calculated?

The overall aim of radioactive iodine therapy is to restore euthyroidism with a single dose whilst minimising the risk of hypothyroidism. The smallest dose possible should be used – radiation exposure should be kept 'as low as reasonably achievable' (ALARA principle) to decrease potential risk for humans. Various methods have been used to calculate the optimum dose for individual cats. In initial reports, tracer kinetic studies were performed with low doses of intravenous radioactive iodine.

Data were collected on percentage iodine uptake, effective half-life and estimation of thyroid gland weight (all factors known to influence therapeutic dose) and the therapeutic dose subsequently calculated. However this method requires access to sophisticated computerised nuclear medicine equipment, is time-consuming, expensive, involves repeated sedation of the patient and it has been shown to be a poor predictor of actual therapeutic dose kinetics. It is therefore rarely used today. Another method is to use a relatively high fixed dose of between 150 and 250 MBq in all cats regardless of their clinical presentation. Although this method is successful and simple, it potentially results in the under- or overtreatment of a significant proportion of cats.

Markedly elevated pretreatment serum thyroid hormone concentration, the size of goitre and the severity of the clinical thyrotoxicosis all have potentially adverse effects on the eventual response to radioactive iodine therapy. These factors can be used in a scoring system to calculate the therapeutic dose – an example is presented in Figure 2. When such a scoring system is used, doses range from approximately 50 to 250 MBq allowing titration to each individual cat, avoiding unnecessary under- or overtreatment. It is a simple method that does not require access to sophisticated nuclear medicine equipment. Success is comparable to dose estimation by tracer kinetic studies. Although some variations are applied, it is the principle method used by most centres offering radioactive iodine today.

Score	Severity of clinical signs	Total T4 (nmol/L)	Size of goitre	Total score	Dose ^{131}I (MBq)
1	Mild	< 80	Barely palpable		
2	Mild – moderate	< 100	1.0 x 0.5 cm	3–9	< 120
3	Moderate	100–150	1.5 x 0.5 cm	9–12	120–150
4	Moderate–severe	150–400	>1.5 x 0.5 cm	> 12	160 or more
5	Severe	> 400	Visible to naked eye		

Figure 2: Estimating the dose of radioactive iodine from clinical signs, total thyroxine (T4) and size of goitre as estimated by palpation. (Data adapted from Mooney, 1994)

How is radioactive iodine administered?

Traditionally, ^{131}I was administered intravenously. Oral administration has been attempted but higher doses are generally required, the risks of radiation spillage are greater, and vomiting may occur. Subcutaneous administration is equally effective, simpler to administer, safer for personnel and less stressful to cats, and is currently preferred. Although not strictly required, patients are usually lightly sedated prior to injection to avoid any risks to those handling the cat.

How successful is radioactive iodine therapy?

Whatever method of dose calculation or route of administration, attainment of euthyroidism is expected in approximately 95 per cent of cases with a single dose. A small percentage of cats remain persistently hyperthyroid. In some of these cases, serum total T4 concentrations continue to decline after treatment and euthyroidism is eventually attained up to 3 months later. Those that remain persistently hyperthyroid are usually the most severely affected but will respond to a second treatment. Recurrent hyperthyroidism can develop but appears to be rare and other side effects are minimal. Serum total T4 concentrations may become subnormal after treatment but the development of clinical signs of hypothyroidism is rare, and there is eventual reactivation of normal or ectopic thyroid tissue with time.

Renal failure may develop or worsen as glomerular filtration rate declines when cats become euthyroid. This may occur in up to 25 per cent of treated cats. Generally the decline in renal function becomes evident within one month of therapy and then remains relatively stable for up to 6 months. It is an unavoidable consequence of any treatment modality but should not preclude treatment of the hyperthyroidism. To date, there is no simple biochemical test capable of predicting cats at risk. However, it is prudent to assess renal function one month after treatment and institute renal support as necessary.

How do I prepare cats and their owners for radioactive iodine therapy?

Currently within the UK there are six centres offering radioactive iodine therapy:

- Animal Health Trust, Newmarket, Suffolk (www.aht.org.uk)
- Barton Veterinary Hospital, Canterbury, Kent (www.barton-vets.co.uk)
- Bishopton Veterinary Group, Ripon, North Yorkshire (www.bishoptonvets.co.uk)
- Glasgow University Veterinary School, Glasgow, Scotland (www.gla.ac.uk)
- Langford Veterinary Services, Langford, North Somerset (www.langfordvets.co.uk)
- Queen Mother Hospital, Royal Veterinary College, London (www.rvc.ac.uk).

Capacity at each centre is limited to 1 to 2 cases per week and isolation times vary from a minimum of 2 weeks to a maximum of approximately 4 weeks. Shorter isolation periods necessitate greater restrictions in the home environment (limited close contact, no children, etc.) Waiting lists vary but can be up to 6 weeks. Only Langford Veterinary Services (Figure 3) can use the extremely high doses required for the treatment of thyroid carcinoma.

Most hyperthyroid cats can be treated with radioactive iodine. However, given the prolonged period of boarding and restrictions on handling, the presence of any concurrent

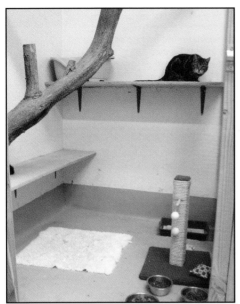

Figure 3: Patient quarters following ¹³¹I treatment at Langford Veterinary Services. Courtesy of University of Bristol Veterinary School

illness that adversely affects appetite or necessitates frequent medications usually precludes radioactive iodine therapy. Most centres require full haematological and biochemical screening, often with cardiac ultrasound, before accepting patients for treatment.

The effect of prior antithyroid medication on efficacy of radioactive iodine therapy is controversial. Prior methimazole (and therefore carbimazole) therapy has been variably suggested to enhance, worsen or have no effect on radioiodine treatment outcome. Overall prior therapy probably has a minimal effect if at all. However, concurrent administration adversely affects effective half-life of radioactive iodine and is not recommended. Therefore, such drugs are withdrawn for at least 5 days and up to 2 weeks prior to administration of radioactive iodine. While some centres accept untreated hyperthyroid cats, others require assessment while euthyroid on antithyroid medication in order to assess renal function accurately.

How can I establish a radioactive iodine unit at my practice?

The main drawback to widespread establishment of radioactive iodine units is the requirement for special licensing, specific personnel training and suitable premises for receipt, administration and disposal of radioactive iodine. A dedicated isolation unit and a means of storing radioactive waste (for up to 3 months) are required. In addition, an attainable source of radioactive iodine is required. Many centres are supplied by local hospitals but not all hospitals use radioactive iodine. Obtaining radioactive iodine direct from manufacturers can be difficult and erratic. Advice should first be sought from your local radiation protection adviser (**www.hpa.org.uk**).

Most of the requirements will be dictated by national and local ionising radiation protection legislation. However, consideration must also be given to minimising the adverse effects of prolonged hospitalisation through appropriate environmental management. This may include, but is not confined to, using larger cages with separate areas for feeding and sleeping and of a size that allows some movement, in a room with some form of stimulation. It may be worth checking out the USA website www.hypurrcat.com for an example of one of the most successful large scale dedicated radioactive iodine units together with its webcam system for owners to look in on their pet. ■

FURTHER READING

Boag AK, Neiger R, Slater L *et al.* (2007) Changes in the glomerular filtration rate of 27 cats with hyperthyroidism after treatment with radioactive iodine. *Veterinary Record* **161**, 711–715

Milner RJ, Channell CD, Levy JK *et al.* (2006) Survival times for cats with hyperthyroidism treated with iodine 131, methimazole, or both: 167 cases (1996–2003). *Journal of the American Veterinary Medical Association* **228**, 559–563

Mooney CT (1994) Radioactive iodine therapy for feline hyperthyroidism: efficacy and administration routes. *Journal of Small Animal Practice* **35**, 289–294

Peterson ME and Becker DV (1995) Radioiodine treatment of 524 cats with hyperthyroidism. *Journal of the American Veterinary Medical Association* **207**, 1422–1428

Slater MR, Geller S and Rogers K (2001) Long-term health and predictors of survival for hyperthyroid cats treated with iodine 131. *Journal of Veterinary Internal Medicine* **15**, 47–51

Slater MR, Komkov A, Robinson LE et al. (1994) Long-term follow-up of hyperthyroid cats treated with iodine-131. *Veterinary Radiology and Ultrasound* **35**, 204–209

Van Hoek I, Lefebvre K, Peremans K et al. (2009) Short and long term follow up of glomerular and tubular markers of kidney function in hyperthyroid cats after treatment with radioiodine. *Domestic Animal Endocrinology* **36**, 45–56

How to...

Handle **bats**

by Liz Mullineaux and Matt Brash

Why might bats have to be handled?

There are sixteen species of bats in the UK, with the possibility of other non-resident migrant species as well. All resident UK species are of the suborder *Microchiroptera*, and are either vesper bats (vespertillionids) or horseshoe bats (rhinolophids). Bats increasingly come into contact with people as a result of their roosting in houses and other buildings. Although bats will generally avoid contact with humans, injury, entrapment and disease may all result in their being brought into contact with veterinary surgeons. In particular, domestic cats are a major risk to low-flying bats leaving their roosts in the summer months. Puncture wounds, wing tears (Figure 1) and fractures resulting from cat attacks and other causes are the most common reasons for presentation.

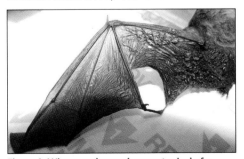

Figure 1: Wing membrane damage typical of a cat-induced injury. Courtesy of James Aegerter

What are the legal considerations when dealing with bats?

Bats are protected under the Wildlife and Countryside Act 1981, and in common with other British wildlife species their care is covered by both the RCVS Guide to Professional Conduct and the BVA/RSPCA memorandum of agreement, requiring veterinary surgeons in practice to provide emergency care to these species.

Bat conservation is very well represented by the Bat Conservation Trust (BCT), which has active members throughout the UK and is able to offer help and advice to both the general public and veterinary surgeons. BCT produced and distributed the excellent 'Bat Care Guidelines' to veterinary surgeons in 2008.

What are the risks of handling?

In common with handling any wild species, bats can be a danger to handlers through bites and scratches. Unfortunately the danger is increased in bats as a result of the risk of these animals potentially carrying European Bat lyssavirus (EBLV).

What are European Bat lyssaviruses?

European Bat lyssaviruses (EBLVs) are strains of rabies-related lyssaviruses found in bats across Northern Europe. Two strains are recognised, EBLV1 and EBLV2, the lyssavirus serotypes 5 and 6. The viruses are generally bat-specific, but on rare occasions EBLVs have been known to infect other animals and humans, although the risk of infection is very low. The Veterinary Laboratories Agency (VLA) carries out routine surveillance of UK bats for evidence of EBLVs. EBLV2 has been found on 8 occasions out of more than 6,000 cases since 1996, most recently in October 2008. All the cases of EBLV2 have been in migrant Daubenton's bats (*Myotis daubentonii*). Two VLA cases have additionally tested positive for EBLV1 antibodies: a serotine bat (*Eptesicus serotinus*) (Figure 2) in 2005 and a Natterer's bat (*Myotis nattereri*) in 2007. Although the risks to humans are low, it is possible that five human deaths have occurred in Europe as a result of EBLVs since 1977 (three confirmed, two unconfirmed) including the death of an unvaccinated Scottish bat worker in 2002.

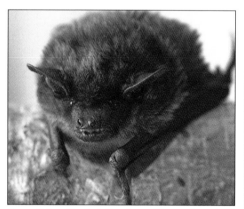

Figure 2: Serotine bat. Courtesy of James Aegerter

The risk to other species is also thought to be very low, with no recorded cases in the UK and transmission to domestic livestock limited to two cases in Denmark in sheep, in wildlife to one case in a stone marten in Germany, and in pets, two cases of EBLV1 in cats in France.

Only Daubenton's bats have been found carrying EBLV2 in the UK. Up to 8% of this species carry antibodies to the virus; special care when handling these bats should therefore be taken. Daubenton's bats tend to roost in trees, bridges and unoccupied buildings rather than homes so human contact is less likely than with some of the other species. Daubenton's bats are slightly larger than the more commonly presented pipistrelle bats (*Pipistrellus pipistrellus*) but are smaller than other species vets may be familiar with, noctules (*Nystalus noctula*) and serotine bats.

A good bat guide is needed to ensure correct identification or advice can be obtained from BCT members. As most vets will be unfamiliar with bat species and because there is a risk that EBLVs may move across bat species, precautions should be taken when handling all bats.

The VLA surveillance scheme provides ongoing surveillance of all dead bats (not just suspect rabies cases) for routine rabies screening. Veterinary surgeons dealing with bats are encouraged to send all fresh carcasses to the VLA for this purpose. The BCT run a postage paid service for the general public to submit carcasses.

What precautions should be taken in practice before handling bats?

Ideally veterinary practice policy should discourage members of the public from handling or approaching sick, injured or trapped bats unless trained and suitably equipped. This policy should ideally be extended to all clients handling wildlife species and practices should have a list of local telephone numbers for trained help and advice in dealing with casualties. In the case of bats, assistance should be sought through the Bat Conservation Trust, Scottish Natural Heritage or SPCA.

A health and safety risk assessment should be in place in all veterinary practices and wildlife centres to cover the risks to staff and volunteers handling bats (and other wildlife). These should include limitations as to which staff are allowed to handle bats, necessary training of these staff and suitable protection mechanisms in place for the safe handling of bats including: provision of prophylactic vaccination against rabies; provision and use of suitable gloves for handling; and known action in case of bites and scratches from bats.

Prophylactic vaccination of staff handling bats frequently should be implemented. Vaccines can be obtained free of charge from each staff member's own general practitioner (GP). Such vaccination is outlined in the Department of Health's 'Information on Immunisation against Infectious Diseases' known as the 'Green book' and GPs questioning the need for free vaccination should be directed to this publication or to the Department of Health's website. Employers should ensure that booster vaccinations are kept up to date. Ideally, blood tests to confirm sero-conversion following vaccination should be carried out.

Transmission of EBLVs (and other infections) from bats is likely to occur via bites, scratches and contact with mucous membranes. Contamination is best avoided by always wearing suitable gloves to handle bats. If anyone is bitten or scratched by a bat, any wounds should be cleaned with soap and water or a suitable disinfectant, and medical advice sought immediately, regardless of rabies vaccine status. Medical advice on the need for post-exposure protection against rabies can be obtained from the Central Public Health Laboratory.

Special care should be taken to consider EBLV infections if bats seem especially agitated or show neurological signs or aggression on handling. As with all wildlife species, the need for an animal to come into captivity means that there is the potential for an increased risk of disease. If signs or suspicion of rabies are seen in bats the local Animal Health Office of the Department for Environment Food and Rural Affairs (Defra) should be contacted immediately. Bats should initially always be kept in isolation in captivity to prevent the transmission of EBLVs and other infections between individuals.

How to handle bats safely

Despite the risks described above, bats are usually some of the easiest British wild mammal species encountered in practice to handle. Their behaviour is usually quite passive and their relatively small size makes them easier to deal with than larger species. Towels are not suitable for handling as the animals easily become tangled in the fabric, making gloves most suitable. The type of glove is important, maintaining dexterity as well as ensuring safety. Thin latex gloves are really only suitable for the very small species (Figure 3). Leather driving gloves have been suggested for handling the larger species but are hard to keep clean. A range of modern materials such as that found in gardening gloves are available in a range of thicknesses and provide cleanable fabrics. Particularly useful are those with an abrasion-resistant nitrile rubber palm (e.g. Showa®). Care should be taken to ensure that all personnel handling bats are gloved and have suitable rabies protection.

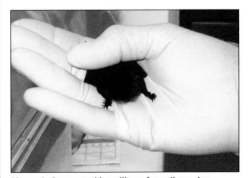

Figure 3: Suggested handling of small species. Courtesy of Secret World

Minimal gentle handling of bats should be employed. Many grips are possible but two general principles should be adhered to:

- Grip around the whole animal so that the wings are kept close to the side of the animal. Distress and injury are most likely to occur if the bat can free its wings and attempts to flap or fly; restrained, they often remain calm
- Ensure that only sufficient pressure is placed on the chest or abdomen to restrain movement, though a digit placed underneath the chin or neck is often a good way to limit the range of head movements and the chances of a bite. Care should be taken not to hold the animal too tightly and interfere with respiration.

Most people find it easiest to hold the bat dorsoventrally between the thumb and index finger, supporting the body on the palm (Figures 3, 4 and 5). A full introduction to handling can be found in the 'Bat Workers' Manual'. It is possible to hold the bat with one hand and examine the wings with the other, though some people may find it easier to have an assistant hold the bat so they have both hands free for examination. A full systematic examination should take place to avoid further or repeated handling being necessary. General anaesthesia with a

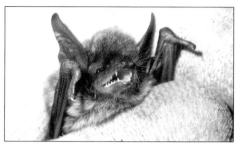

Figure 5: Handling a whiskered bat. Courtesy of James Aegerter

gaseous agent may be useful but should not be used as a reason to remove gloves and ignore health and safety considerations.

For further information on medical conditions and treatment of bats see the *BSAVA Manual of Wildlife Casualties*. ■

USEFUL INFORMATION

Bat Conservation Trust
15 Cloisters House, 8 Battersea Park Road, London SW8 4BG
www.bats.org.uk Helpline 0845 130 0228

If BSAVA members were not sent a copy of 'Bat Care Guidelines' and would like one they should email Helen at **hmiller@bats.org.uk** and she will send them a copy.

Assistance with Bats in Scotland
Scottish SPCA: 0870 7377722
Scottish Natural Heritage Batline: 01738 458663

Veterinary Laboratories Agency bat rabies surveillance
Rabies Diagnostic Unit, Veterinary Laboratories Agency, New Haw, Addlestone, Surrey KT15 3NB

Fresh carcasses of all dead bats (not just those suspected of having rabies) should be sent to the address above.
Packaging should observe postage guidelines for pathological specimens. Submission forms can be downloaded at:
www.defra.gov.uk/corporate/regulat/forms/vla/bat1.htm

Vaccination and medical advice
For information on prophylactic rabies vaccination and post-exposure advice contact:
Central Public Health Laboratory (0208 200 4400)

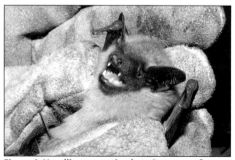

Figure 4: Handling a serotine bat. Courtesy of James Aegerter

How to...

Collect a diagnostic
bone marrow sample

by Kate Murphy

I t has been said that with practice, collecting bone marrow becomes as easy as placing an intravenous catheter. That may be a slight exaggeration but once a clinician gets over the 'fear factor', collecting bone marrow is not difficult. Making good smears from the bone marrow sample can be more challenging, however! If the practitioner does not perfect the art of making good smears then the interpretation of the bone marrow sample may be rendered meaningless.

Benefit

The first step in collecting a diagnostic bone marrow sample is selecting a patient that will benefit from the technique.

There are many indications for performing bone marrow aspiration (Figure 1). Some are immediately obvious (e.g. non-regenerative anaemia after excluding extra-marrow suppression); others are less clear (e.g. in patients with fever of unknown origin but without obvious haemopoietic disease).

In most patients it is preferable to collect both an aspirate and a core biopsy sample. Suitable sites include the iliac wing, proximal humerus and proximal femur.

Anaesthesia

The author's preference is to use general anaesthesia and to sample from the proximal humerus (Figure 2), although aspirates from a

- Pancytopenia
- Non-regenerative or poorly regenerative anaemia
- Neutropenia or thrombocytopenia where the cause is not obvious (not usually performed in suspected immune-mediated thrombocytopenia)
- Suspected haemopoietic neoplasia, myelodysplasia, or marrow dysfunction as indicated by ineffective cytopoiesis or erythropoiesis
- To evaluate iron stores when other information is inadequate
- Fever of unknown origin
- Evaluation of lytic bone lesions
- Staging of neoplasia, e.g. lymphoma, mast cell tumours, histiocytic disease
- Investigation of hyperglobulinaemia
- Investigation of hypercalcaemia
- Evaluation of unexplained leucocytosis or thrombocytosis

Figure 1: Indications for performing bone marrow sampling

number of sites including the iliac crest (Figures 3 and 4) can be taken under sedation with local anaesthetic. The author prefers performing bone marrow aspiration under general anaesthesia for a number of reasons:

- The procedure can be performed quickly and without pain during the technique
- If a 'dry tap' is obtained, aspiration can be attempted from the other humerus or another of the sites listed above.

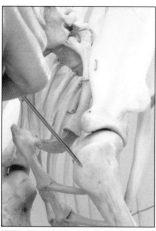

Figure 2: Site for bone marrow sampling from the proximal humerus

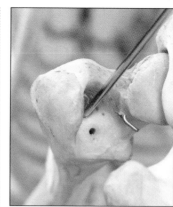

Figure 4: Site for bone marrow sampling from the proximal femur

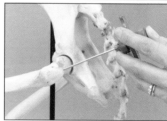

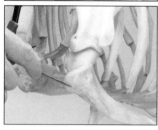

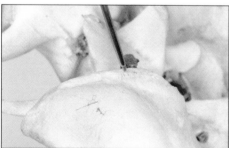

Figure 3: Site for bone marrow sampling from the iliac wing

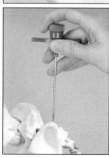

Premedication and anaesthetic agents/protocol may be influenced by the patient's primary disease and the reader is referred to more specialised texts such as the *BSAVA Manual of Canine and Feline Anaesthesia and Analgesia, 2nd edition* for advice on this aspect.

Equipment required

- Jamshidi bone marrow needle, e.g. bone marrow aspiration/biopsy needle (11 G x 4 inches).
- 20 ml syringe.
- Local anaesthetic (without adrenaline).
- No. 11 scalpel blade.
- Anticoagulant (sterile) – CPDA/ACD (collect from transfusion bag) or EDTA (prepared from a standard EDTA blood tube; see below).
- Microscope slides (>10).
- EDTA pot and formalin pot.
- Surgical drape and sterile gloves.
- Strong assistant.

Preparation

Bone marrow interpretation is a challenge but this can be reduced if a blood sample is taken into an EDTA tube on the day of the bone marrow collection. This allows the bone marrow to be interpreted in the light of 'current' peripheral haematological status.

Before starting the bone marrow collection it is important to coat the aspiration needle and syringe with anticoagulant to avoid clotting during sample collection.

1 Remove the stylet and attach the 20 ml syringe to the needle.

2 Aspirate the ACD/CPDA or EDTA anticoagulant in a sterile fashion and roll anticoagulant around the syringe before squirting the excess out – this should leave the syringe and needle 'coated' (Figure 5).

3 Remove the syringe and carefully replace the stylet, ensuring it is properly sited and fully locked.

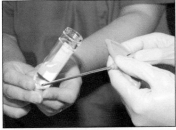

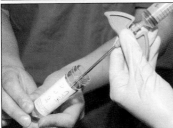

Figure 5: Coating the needle and syringe with anticoagulant

If you do not have blood transfusion bags in the practice it is possible to make EDTA anticoagulant by adding sterile saline or water to an EDTA tube and mixing well. This solution can then be used to coat the needle and syringe. Since bone marrow aspiration is rarely an emergency procedure, the practitioner is advised to order in some commercial anticoagulated blood bags to improve the success of their bone marrow aspiration as, in the author's experience, using EDTA for this purpose is not as effective at preventing clotting of the marrow sample.

Procedure using a Jamshidi biopsy needle

This needle is designed to take both aspirates and core samples. General anaesthesia is induced and once the patient is stable:

1 Position the patient in lateral recumbency.

2 Widely clip the area around the scapulohumeral joint.

3 Surgically prepare the biopsy site.

4 Position the leg with the humerus flexed (parallel to the patient's thorax) (Figure 6). Ensure a strong colleague is holding the leg for you and prepare them for the pressure you will be applying to the leg – they will need to apply counterpressure.

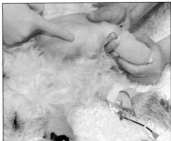

Figure 6: Position of the limb for obtaining a bone marrow aspirate from the proximal humerus

5 Instil local anaesthetic to the level of the periosteum over the greater tubercle of the humerus.

6 Re-scrub the area.

7 Make a small stab skin incision with the No. 11 scalpel blade (Figure 7).

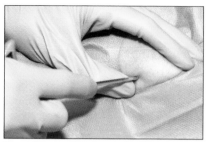

Figure 8: Use a firm forward drilling pressure to advance through the cortex and into the marrow cavity

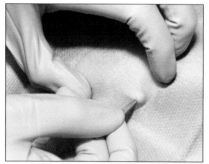

Figure 7: Make a small stab incision with the scalpel blade

8 Insert the Jamshidi needle with the stylet firmly in place (check the stylet has been firmly replaced after the aspiration of anticoagulant described earlier).

9 Humeral samples are taken by palpating the most proximal facet of the humeral head (greater tubercle) and inserting the needle into the craniolateral aspect of the greater tubercle (slight flattened area). Gradually advance into the marrow cavity (heading towards the elbow and parallel to the humeral shaft) using a drilling/firm 'forward rotating' action and steady pressure (Figure 8).

Counterpressure from an assistant holding the limb can be helpful (they push with all their might against you pushing from the other end!). Initially it can be hard to get the bone marrow needle to get a purchase into the bone, and occasionally it slips off. If this is happens, start again and recheck your anatomical landmarks.

Once you are happy the needle is in the correct position, retry going very slowly and with controlled forward pressure.

Reduced resistance is usually felt as the needle enters the medullary cavity. If correctly placed, the needle should feel solidly 'fixed' in place, and moving the needle should result in moving the bone itself. If the needle is placed too medially over the humeral head, it is easy to penetrate the joint capsule. This does not pose a significant danger to the patient but can render the bone marrow sample non-diagnostic if contaminated by joint fluid and may cause mild joint inflammation.

10 Once the needle is believed to be correctly sited, remove the stylet. Attach the 20 ml syringe (previously coated with anticoagulant) and aspirate firmly (Figure 9).

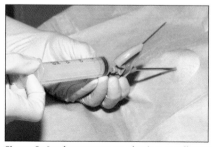

Figure 9: Apply pressure to obtain a small quantity of marrow

As soon as bone marrow (which looks like thick blood) is noted in the hub of the syringe, stop aspirating – you do not need more than 0.2 ml of bone marrow (Figure 10). Excessive suction will result in haemodilution of the sample. There are no prizes in the technique for the biggest sample collected – just for a diagnostic one!

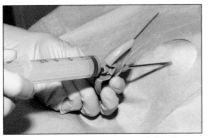

Figure 10: A small marrow sample has been collected

11 Detach the syringe but leave the needle in place and replace the stylet whilst smears are prepared.

12 Smears are prepared by angling multiple slides at 45 degrees (Figure 11) and placing a drop of marrow at the top of each. There are a number of alternative techniques. It may be helpful for practitioners to discuss the technique of preparing the slides with the clinical pathologist who will evaluate the bone marrow sample.

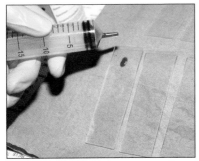

Figure 11: Transfer the marrow sample on to glass slides

a. Excess blood is allowed to run down the slide on to absorbent paper, leaving flecks of marrow attached to the glass.

b. A clean slide is then backed on to the remaining marrow and the marrow is allowed to spread along the edge of the spreader slide, which is then swiftly pushed forward to provide a thin smear with a feathered edge (Figure 12).

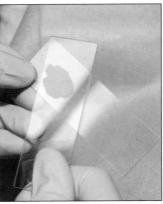

Figure 12: Technique for spreading bone marrow on the slide

It is essential that smears are prepared and air-dried immediately. It is important to assess whether a diagnostic marrow sample has been obtained grossly by looking at the slides as they dry. If the slides look like blood smears – they probably are. Marrow smears should look like blood but with fatty bits and refractile spicules.

13 Obtain a core biopsy sample by removing the stylet and advancing the needle approximately 1–2 cm further into the bone. Move the needle swiftly sideways a few times to break off the distal part of the sample and then retract the needle. Use the blunt probe supplied with the needle to push the core sample out (from tip through the handle) (Figure 13). The core sample can be gently rolled along a slide to produce an impression smear (Figure 14) which can be

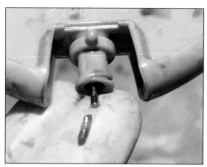

Figure 13: Core sample pushed out of the needle

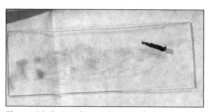

Figure 14: Preparing an impression smear from the bone marrow core sample

helpful to provide more rapid results if the bone marrow aspirate is non-diagnostic. The core is then placed in a pot of formalin.

14 Submit samples for cytology and histopathology. A concurrent blood sample should be submitted to aid interpretation, as discussed above.

Additional investigations may be performed on bone marrow samples, e.g. infectious disease tests, iron profile and Coombs' test.

Problems

Common problems in obtaining diagnostic bone marrow aspirates and core biopsy samples are:

- Haemodilution of the sample
- Poor smear preparation – too thick or inadequately spread material. ■

How to...

Approach canine mammary tumours

by Gerry Polton

Mammary tumours arise from the glandular epithelium of the mammary glands. Various histological forms are described. Other non-epithelial neoplasms can arise in the mammary region; these are uncommon and will not be discussed here.

The prevalence of mammary neoplasia varies remarkably between different countries. This variation is linked to cultural behaviour with respect to neutering practices. The incidence in entire bitches is approximately 71%, so in countries where neutering is not routinely practised this is easily the most significant neoplastic consideration affecting adult dogs, despite the fact that the disease is almost never seen in adult males. In a recent study from Italy, mammary neoplasia in bitches accounted for 45% of all cancer diagnoses over the course of 17 years.

The various canine epithelial mammary tumours are listed in Figure 1. Mammary tumours are classified first according to their tissue of origin and secondly on whether they are benign or malignant. Unfortunately, the distinction between benign and malignant is not always clear. Furthermore, to a non-pathologist the terminology is bewildering.

Originating tissues include glandular (adenoma/adenocarcinoma), ductular (papilloma/carcinoma), myoepithelial and pluripotential (mixed) cells, though some uncertainty about the histogenetic origin of many mammary tumour types remains. In addition to the histogenetic and benign/malignant classification, additional descriptive terms can be used (Figure 2). The distinction between tumours demonstrating tubular/papillary differentiation and those exhibiting solid/anaplastic histology is considered to be prognostically significant.

In entire bitches, the ratio of benign to malignant tumours is approximately 50:50. Neutering, however, preferentially reduces the incidence of benign mammary neoplasia. Therefore, while neutering reduces the overall incidence of mammary cancer in bitches, it does result in an increased proportion of mammary tumours that are diagnosed as malignant. In addition there are significant data indicating that neutering at the time of mammary tumour resection affords no benefit to the patient.

Aetiology

Physiological mammary development occurs under the influence of the somatotrophic and gonadal hormones. The earliest study to recognise an increased risk of mammary neoplasia associated with remaining sexually entire was performed in 1969 and indicated that the relative risk of mammary neoplasia development was as low as 0.5% for bitches undergoing ovariohysterectomy before their

	Tumour type	Histological features
Benign	Ductal papilloma	Simple or complex
	Adenoma	Simple or complex
	Benign mixed tumour	Epithelium plus mesenchymal tissue
	Fibroadenoma	
	Myoepithelioma	
Malignant	Adenocarcinoma	Solid, tubular or papillary Simple or complex
	Ductular carcinoma	Intra- or inter-lobular Simple or complex
	Spindle cell carcinoma	
	Anaplastic carcinoma	
	Squamous cell carcinoma	
	Mucinous carcinoma	
	Malignant myoepithelioma	
	Carcinoma or sarcoma in a mixed tumour	Epithelial and mesenchymal tissue; one is neoplastic
	Carcinosarcoma	Epithelial and mesenchymal tissue; both neoplastic

Figure 1: Epithelial mammary tumours in the dog

Histological term	Definition
Simple	Single (epithelial) tissue type present
Complex	Lesion with both epithelial and significant myoepithelial proliferation
Mixed	Contains both epithelial and/ or myoepithelial tissue and a mesenchymal component such as fat, cartilage or bone
Solid	Solid sheets or cords of cells without evidence of tubular lumens
Anaplastic	No indication of cellular differentiation
Tubular	Tubular lumens present
Papillary	Frond-like epithelial projections

Figure 2: Histological terms in canine mammary neoplasia

first oestrus when compared to bitches that remained entire (Figure 3). It must be stated that the conclusions drawn from these data were based upon remarkably few cases from the younger neutering age groups.

As we grow to understand the non-neoplastic complications of early

Age at neutering	Relative risk of mammary neoplasia
Before 1st season	0.5%
Between 1st and 2nd seasons	8%
Between 2nd and 3rd seasons	26%
After 3rd season	100%

Figure 3: Age of neutering and relative risk of the development of mammary neoplasia in the bitch compared to intact individuals. Data from Schneider *et al.*, 1969

ovariohysterectomy (e.g. incontinence), these data must be examined critically; there is an urgent need for this study to be revised. Intriguingly, bilateral oophorectomy has been shown to reduce the incidence of breast cancer by up to 80% in women carrying high-risk germline mutations in certain breast cancer susceptibility genes and some veterinary surgeons use this technique in preference to the more usual ovariohysterectomy.

A model of canine mammary neoplasia development has been proposed in which the malignant phenotype develops within an otherwise benign tumour. It has been observed that the proportion of tumours exhibiting characteristics of malignancy increases with increasing tumour size (Figure 4).

Tumour size (max diameter)	Benign cases (%)
<1 cm	98
1–1.9 cm	97
2–2.9 cm	85
3–3.9 cm	45
>4 cm	42

Figure 4: Proportion of canine mammary tumours exhibiting benign histology; cases separated according to tumour size

Presentation

Mammary neoplasia can be presented as a solitary mammary mass or, frequently, as multiple lesions. In cases with infiltrative disease, the abnormal tissue is not necessarily confined to the mammary line.

Mammary tumours primarily undergo metastasis to the regional lymph nodes (superficial inguinal and axillary) or to the lungs. Examination of the lymph nodes is mandatory in the physical examination of a patient. Presenting signs that should alert the wary clinician to a high probability of malignant behaviour include diffuse swelling, ulceration, marked erythema, serous or bloody discharge, pain, lymphadenopathy, discoloration and an irregular nodular appearance.

Inflammatory carcinoma is an unusual manifestation of mammary neoplasia typified by large erythematous and painful mammary swellings, frequently occupying all of the mammary tissues. Sometimes these lesions will spontaneously discharge a serous exudate. Patients are typically extremely depressed.

Diagnosis

The use of cytology to diagnose mammary neoplasia presents a point of great controversy amongst veterinary oncologists, as marked heterogeneity can be seen histologically within a single tumour. This variation represents more than histological pedantry. There is a subset of cases that present with an overtly benign tumour, for example a simple adenoma, with microscopic evidence of a malignant tumour *in situ*. These lesions exhibit malignant behaviour; survival times may correlate with the size of the malignant element.

Proponents of the use of diagnostic cytology in mammary neoplasia would therefore advocate the collection of at least four samples from distinct areas within the mass in question, with the ultimate diagnosis being determined by the sample that yields the most malignant cytological appearance.

Histological evaluation of an incisional or excisional biopsy, which includes the apparent junction between normal tissue and the mass, remains the gold standard recommendation for mammary tumour diagnosis. It is not practical to perform biopsy on all mammary masses, particularly on those that are <1 cm in diameter. For solitary small nodular masses, marginal (~2 mm) excision will be diagnostic and may be curative. Importantly, the conservative margin obtained is unlikely to complicate a subsequent surgical procedure if one is indicated.

Histological grade

Multiple strategies for assigning histological grade to canine mammary tumours have been presented. Features considered relevant to tumour grade include: degree of cellular differentiation; nuclear pleomorphism; and degree of invasiveness. A simplified system incorporating elements of histological grade and clinical stage is given in Figure 5. It is important to note that the inflammatory carcinoma does not fit into other histological grading schemes and should be regarded as a separate entity in this context.

Clinical stage determination

In oncology, definition of the clinical stage, or the anatomical extent of disease, is critical to good decision making. Since malignant mammary tumours are recognised to be associated with metastasis in a number of cases, simple evaluations to define clinical stage are advised prior to performing surgery.

Therefore, close examination for multiple mammary masses and fine needle aspiration of enlarged regional lymph nodes must be performed. Thoracic radiography is recommended for all but the smallest lesions. Abdominal ultrasonography allows evaluation of the deep inguinal lymph nodes and the parenchyma of the abdominal viscera. For small lesions (<1 cm diameter) it would be hard to justify the expense of radiography or ultrasonography, as the likelihood of malignancy is so low.

Clinical stage also defines local invasiveness. Increasing tumour size is known to be associated with increasing probability of

Histological "stage"	Features	Prognosis	Prognosis simplified	Notes
Stage 1	Lesions are non-infiltrative and resemble the tissue of origin. Tubular structures are evident	High probability of surgical cure	Curable	Occasional cases develop metastatic disease
Stage 2	Loss of tubular lumen and/or invasion of the surrounding stroma but no evidence of vascular or lymphatic invasion	Median survival time 380 days	1 year	6-monthly re-evaluations recommended (adjuvant chemotherapy or surgery considered in the face of progressive disease)
Stage 3	Presence of lymphatic or vascular invasion	Median survival time 108 days	3 months	3-monthly re-evaluations recommended. Adjuvant chemotherapy may be justified in the face of progressive disease based on present knowledge
Stage 4	Evidence of metastasis	Median survival time 108 days	3 months	Occasionally patients with regional LN metastasis do enjoy prolonged periods of good-quality life. Lymphadenectomy and advanced surgical techniques required

Figure 5: Histological 'stage' of canine mammary tumours and prognostic implications following appropriate surgery

significant local invasion. In canine mammary tumours, the TNM classification separates tumours (Figure 6), where T relates to tumour size and whether it has invaded nearby tissue, N describes the involvement of regional lymph nodes and M describes metastasis. In a survey of 54 cases, two-year survival percentages were 62% for T1 tumours and 23% for T2 and T3 tumours. Figure 7 shows a mammary mass exhibiting extreme local infiltration and invasiveness.

T stage	Tumour size
Tis	Tumour *in situ*
T1	<3 cm diameter
T2	3–5 cm diameter
T3	>5 cm diameter

Figure 6: T stage classification of canine mammary tumours

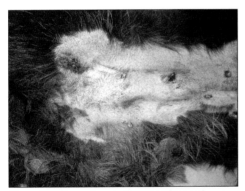

Figure 7: Diffuse, ulcerated locally advanced mammary adenocarcinoma. The local extent of the tumour is such that it is no longer limited to the mammary tissue. It can be appreciated that the tumour tissue extends down the medial aspect of the right thigh (caudal is to the left)

Management

The mainstay of management for canine mammary tumours is surgery. Historically, recommendations have been made to perform surgery according to a notional distribution of lymphatic drainage. With recognition of the variability of lymphatic drainage, this is now recognised to be an oversimplification. Instead, best management is now considered to be to perform the simplest surgery that allows the job to be done.

For example, a small mass associated with a single mammary gland may, in theory, be removed by partial mammectomy (removal of part of a single gland) if a 1 cm margin were required. However, it would be considerably less traumatic to simply remove the entire gland. If a superficial inguinal lymph node and gland 4 on the same side need to be removed, it would be less traumatic to remove glands 4 and 5 as well as the lymph node than it would be to attempt to dissect these structures free from the surrounding tissues (Figure 8).

For benign mammary tumours, marginal excision can be curative. For most well circumscribed malignant mammary tumours a 1 cm margin will also be curative, and attempting to obtain a closer margin may introduce additional surgical complications.

In situations where previous advice may have been simply to monitor a mass because it had been behaviourally benign, or because an owner would not accept alternative management, it is important to remember that mammary tumour behaviour can change with the passage of time.

Prophylactic surgery by means of a bilateral mammary strip can, of course, prevent mammary neoplasia developing in the future. This is, however, an extremely aggressive surgical procedure. An alternative approach, preferred by the author, is to undertake regular re-examination and to perform prompt intervention if a new mass is recognised. There are no data to suggest that prior malignant mammary neoplasia exposes a bitch to a higher risk that subsequent *de novo* mammary masses will be malignant.

Chemotherapy use has been described sporadically in the management of canine

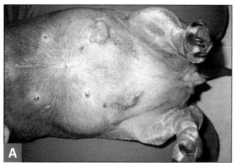

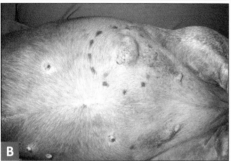

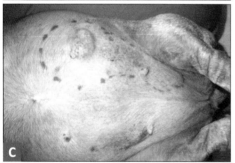

Figure 8: Solitary discrete mammary nodule and options for removal. (A) Well circumscribed, mobile mammary nodule affecting gland 4 on the left-hand side of a 12-year-old entire Miniature Dachshund bitch. (B) Dashed line indicates surgical margin for single mammectomy. (C) Dashed line indicates surgical margin for removal of glands 4 and 5 with superficial inguinal lymph node, which is invariably associated with gland 5. This procedure is likely to be less traumatic than simple mammectomy of gland 4 as in many bitches the caudal mammary glands are confluent. The risk of postoperative complication would then be reduced as a result

mammary neoplasia but the results have, historically, been disappointing. A recent innovative formulation of paclitaxel has shown favourable responses in initial drug trials but this product is currently not available. The author has used chemotherapy prior to definitive surgery (neoadjuvant therapy) with encouraging results.

A simple flow chart for management of canine mammary tumours is shown in Figure 9. While it is hoped that this is helpful, it must be acknowledged that there are numerous controversies and uncertainties in this field, as highlighted in the figure.

X-ray beam radiotherapy is contraindicated in mammary neoplasia due to the risk of radiation-induced hepatic necrosis or gastrointestinal perforation.

Unfortunately, unlike in the human field, introduction of selective oestrogen receptor modulating agents such as tamoxifen have failed to demonstrate benefits in canine patients. This is probably because many canine malignant mammary tumours of the spayed bitch do not express oestrogen receptors and due to the induction of unpleasant oestrus-like side effects.

Prognosis

While it is important to emphasise that histological evaluation of an excised specimen may not identify a microscopic nest of malignant cells within an otherwise benign nodule, benign mammary tumours should be cured by simple surgery.

For malignant mammary tumours, prognosis is related to histological grade and clinical stage as noted above and detailed in Figure 5.

Inflammatory carcinoma carries a poor prognosis, with most patients succumbing to their illness within 4–8 weeks. Preliminary data have demonstrated improvements in clinical signs with the administration of COX inhibitors, in particular the COX-2 selective antagonist

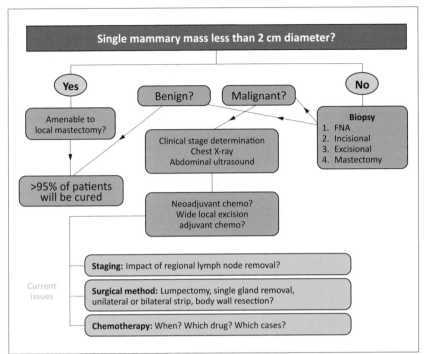

Figure 9: Flow chart indicating simplified approach to canine mammary tumours and highlighting current controversies and uncertainties

firocoxib; these data need to be validated before being accepted.

Follow-up

After diagnosis of a malignant mammary tumour, consideration should be given to the indications or otherwise for further monitoring or therapy. Since chemotherapy has largely proved to be unrewarding, the author's recommendation instead is that patients undergo serial monitoring by means of thoracic radiography and abdominal ultrasonography on a regular, initially quarterly, basis. Accurate recording of lymph node size and definition of the state of the hepatic and splenic parenchyma allow early changes due to the development of metastatic disease to be recognised.

At this time, further surgery may be indicated. Alternatively, chemotherapy can be justified once the presence of gross disease has been confirmed, as response to therapy can then be quantified.

Pitfalls

As noted above, not all mammary tumours that are considered to be benign on the basis of histological evaluation subsequently demonstrate benign behaviour. The best histological service is obtained by providing your laboratory with all of the relevant clinical detail that you can. There is no substitute for open communication between you and your histopathologist.

The surgical margins obtained are typically defined by the surrounding mammary anatomy rather than by oncological principles. Many mammary tumours would be appropriately managed by a skin incision reaching 1–2 cm from the apparent edge of the tumour. If a mass appears to require skin resection beyond the anatomical limit of the mammae, then it may be best to assume that surgical removal will prove incomplete. In this situation, it may be better to perform an incisional biopsy and discuss the case with a surgical oncologist before proceeding with definitive mass removal.

The fibrous sheath of the rectus abdominis muscle presents a reasonably good barrier to deeper tumour invasion. Masses exhibiting any degree of fixation to the underlying tissues will definitely not be completely removed by simple surgery, and advanced imaging should be considered mandatory before a radical or compartmental surgical excision is considered. Should intramuscular invasion become evident during surgery, the damage limitation strategy is to proceed no further, perform tissue biopsy if appropriate, then close the surgical field and discuss the case with an oncologist.

In these cases, abdominal wall resection would be required to achieve complete local tumour eradication, as the first surgery will inevitably have introduced tumour into deeper tissue planes. However, as tumour invasiveness is associated with metastasis, thorough investigations for metastasis are now mandatory. Only if these fail to reveal evidence of tumour spread should abdominal wall resection be considered. Advanced imaging would be advised as part of treatment planning.

Histologically confirmed complete resection of canine mammary tumours should only be regarded to be likely to be predictive of clinical cure in cases of benign or histological Stage 1 malignant cases. In all other cases, consideration should be given to embarking upon a course of subsequent monitoring and/or adjuvant therapy. There is little or no value in subsequent monitoring if no further action would be taken in the event that progression of disease (recurrence or metastasis) is recognised.

Conclusion

Historically, we may have been guilty of treating all mammary tumours as the same and being surprised when local recurrence or metastasis develop. Treatment recommendations should be based primarily upon tumour behaviour rather than anatomy. It is increasingly widely accepted that the degree of malignancy is associated with size of the primary tumour in canine mammary neoplasia. While it is acceptable to perform excisional biopsy of small mammary nodules, incisional biopsy to define grade is appropriate for lesions exhibiting any hallmark features of non-benign disease. In this way appropriate treatment can be planned, an equal number of patients will be cured and surgical morbidity will be minimised for patients with advanced disease. ∎

FURTHER READING

Schneider R, Dorn CR and Taylor DO (1969) Factors influencing canine mammary cancer development and postsurgical survival. *Journal of the National Cancer Institute* **43**(6), 1249–1261

How to...

Manage the systemically unwell, substage b, case of canine lymphoma

by Gerry Polton

It has long been recognised that prognosis in cases of canine lymphoma is significantly affected by the apparent state of systemic health at the time of diagnosis. This reflects more than the simple fact that moribund cases are fewer steps from mortality. The management of these cases is not something that receives attention in the veterinary literature. The purpose of this article is to help clinicians to consider the management of those cases systemically unwell at presentation, so called substage b. While some cases of substage b lymphoma sadly do show little or no response to the management offered, others achieve complete remission and a full quality of life for prolonged periods.

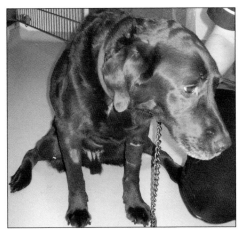

Figure 1: Substage b patients may present without peripheral lymphadenopathy

Presentation

Affected cases can be divided into two groups, those with obvious multicentric lymphoma and those without (Figure 1). The importance of this distinction is that the former are usually diagnosed promptly, and speed may be of the essence in regaining control of the disease.

The aetiology of the substage b status is varied (Figure 2). Efforts should be made to understand the pathophysiology of the patient's ill health in order to optimise management. Pathogenesis is often multifactorial.

It has long been recognised in human haemato-oncology that lymphoma represents

a broad umbrella classification of lymphoproliferative disease. Refinements in diagnostic capacity have led to the development of a classification system that incorporates clinical, histomorphological, cytomorphological, flow cytometric and cytogenetic characteristics to define subtypes of disease. This extensive classification effort is rewarded by more accurate prediction of biological behaviour and responses to therapy. Similar efforts have been made in veterinary oncology with a landmark study by Frédérique Ponce et al. (2004) demonstrating significant survival implications for six different canine lymphoma subtypes.

Pathogenesis		Notes
Metabolic derangements	Hypercalcaemia	Varied causes, including PTHrP, IL-6, OAF
	Hypoglycaemia	Consumption by tumour
	Uncoupling of energy transduction pathways	Due to aberrant cytokine elaboration
Organ dysfunction due to infiltration	Renal insufficiency	Chemotherapy doses may require adjustment
	Hepatic insufficiency	Chemotherapy doses may require adjustment
	CNS involvement	Neurological signs may be generalised or focal
	Respiratory compromise	Widespread pulmonary infiltration is unusual
	Bone marrow	See haematological aberrations
Haematological aberrations	Neutropenia Thrombocytopenia Anaemia	Failure of production or immune-mediated destruction of blood cells
Mass effect	Partial airway obstruction Vascular occlusion	Typically only in advanced cases without other systemic compromise

Figure 2: Causes of failure of systemic health seen in substage b lymphoma. IL-6 = interleukin 6; OAF = osteoclast activating factor; PTHrP = parathyroid hormone related peptide

Diagnostic considerations: definitive diagnosis

Cytology

Cases of suspected lymphoma should undergo appropriate diagnostic testing to make a definitive diagnosis. For patients with generalised lymphadenopathy (Figure 3), fine needle aspiration and cytology can yield a robust diagnosis and spare the need for chemical restraint for biopsy. Further refinements of the diagnosis can be obtained by immunocytochemistry or flow cytometry. These should be discussed with your laboratory prior to sampling, in case specific sample-handling practices must be observed.

Across a population of cases, histological evaluation of an entire lymph node remains a more reliable means of diagnosis of lymphoma. However, in addition to issues of anaesthetic

safety, both time and cost factors merit consideration. A competent cytologist could make a diagnosis of lymphoma in minutes; the author advises that practitioners interested in managing lymphoma cases obtain lymph node aspirates and perform in-house cytological evaluations regularly to gain confidence with the techniques. While a diagnosis of lymphoma may be best made by an experienced cytologist, practitioners can do both themselves and their cases a tremendous service by confidently defining that sample quality is adequate for diagnosis and that the appropriate target has been sampled prior to submission.

Lymphoid cells are easily disrupted by forceful aspiration or smearing. The author advises that samples are obtained without suction and that only the weight of the spreading slide is used to disperse cells in the expelled sample.

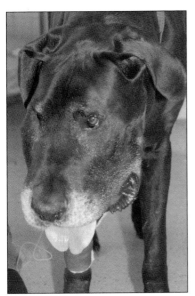

Figure 3: Cranial vena caval syndrome as a consequence of lymphadenopathy. Courtesy of Mark Goodfellow

Diagnostic considerations: supporting data

Haematological evaluation

Haematological aberrations can arise for numerous reasons. Cytopenias arise due to bone marrow infiltration, immune-mediated destruction of mature cells or precursors, anaemia of chronic disease (lymphoma or chemotherapy for lymphoma) and significant haemorrhage. Significant neutropenia predisposes patients to sepsis, so broad-spectrum antibiotic therapy is indicated. Thrombocytopenia can result in spontaneous haemorrhage that is really only responsive to prophylaxis by transfusion of fresh whole blood. Clinicians must be aware that administration of chemotherapy in these instances may precipitate a lethal complication.

Anaemia due to haemorrhage is best managed by diagnosis and treatment of the inciting cause, and whole blood transfusion if indicated. Anaemia of chronic disease is usually mild to moderate and is typically not addressed. In cases with other significant signs of ill health, anaemia with a PCV of 20% or greater does not warrant intervention. If PCV is less than 20% and the patient is symptomatic, transfusion should be considered as a short-term measure while other health parameters are given a chance to improve.

Biochemical evaluation

Hypercalcaemia and indicators of renal and hepatic compromise are readily identified on serum biochemical profiles. Hypercalcaemia frequently responds promptly to the administration of lymphocytolytic therapy, such as corticosteroids. It is critical that diagnostic quality samples are obtained prior to steroid administration, however, as the chances of harvesting diagnostic samples subsequently are reduced. Hypercalcaemia induces cardiovascular and neuromuscular compromise, and uncontrolled hypercalcaemia precipitates renal failure. This effect is exacerbated by reduced renal perfusion, for example under anaesthesia.

Renal compromise may be due to pre-renal effects, such as hypovolaemia due to hypercalcaemia, or it may reflect renal disease. Renal lymphoma can be diagnosed on renal aspirate biopsy. If a diagnosis has already been made, ultrasonographic changes consistent with lymphoma are adequate.

Hepatic compromise has far-reaching implications. Frequently these cases are anorectic, hypoproteinaemic, icteric and vomiting. Dramatic weight loss can be seen. Both renal and hepatic disease can lead to marked alterations in metabolism of chemotherapeutic agents. Usually this results in increased plasma drug concentrations due to failure of elimination, and dose reductions are critical. Patients with hepatic compromise

Imaging studies

Thoracic radiography is indicated to identify the presence of intrathoracic masses (Figure 4). Hypercalcaemia is more common among cases with cranial mediastinal lymphoma and there may be no evidence of lymphoma affecting other sites. Massive intrathoracic lesions can compromise respiratory function. A single lateral thoracic radiograph is often adequate to define the presence or absence of mediastinal disease.

Abdominal radiography is rarely helpful. Significant lymphadenopathy can be missed whereas hepatomegaly and renomegaly may be recognised. Ultrasonography yields more valuable information and, if a diagnosis remains in doubt, aids biopsy of abnormal structures. Clinicians must be aware of the potential for biopsy-induced haemorrhage, which is of greater concern in hepatic or renal compromise.

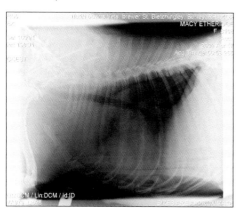

Figure 4: Pretreatment lateral thoracic radiograph revealing mediastinal lymphadenopathy in a severely hypercalcaemic Boxer

Bone marrow sampling

Lymphoma can reside solely in the bone marrow, so the diagnosis should not be ruled out on the basis of absence of evidence of disease in other body systems. If haematological parameters indicate bone marrow involvement and a diagnosis has already been made, there are few indications for marrow sampling. If the diagnosis remains in doubt, however, or if immune-mediated destruction of blood cell precursors is suspected, sampling can be of benefit for subsequent management.

Other considerations

Nutrition

Inappetence or anorexia, vomiting, infiltrative intestinal disease and hepatopathy will all contribute to a negative energy balance. The metabolic demands of advanced lymphoma are great; adequate and balanced nutrition can make the difference between success and failure in these cases.

Risk of sepsis

Neutropenia due to bone marrow infiltration and/or chemotherapy, exposes patients to risk of bacteraemia and sepsis. Extra attention to infection control measures is warranted. In addition, lymphoma can induce vasculitis, with consequential systemic inflammatory response syndrome (SIRS), mimicking changes associated with septicaemia. Sepsis promotes inappropriate cycles of coagulation and thrombolysis; concurrent thrombocytopenia exacerbates risk of disseminated intravascular coagulation (DIC).

Water and electrolyte turnover

Substage b patients typically fail to consume adequate water to compensate for insensible losses. An attempt should be made to quantify losses so that appropriate replacement therapy can be provided. Medications to limit losses through vomiting and diarrhoea are advised.

Most patients are significantly hypokalaemic. Plasma potassium concentration may not accurately reflect total body potassium depletion, as potassium is primarily an intracellular cation. Hypomagnesaemia is also recognised. Potassium and magnesium deficiencies can result in inappetence or anorexia.

Hypercalcaemia can be managed by saline diuresis. Excessive volume replacement should be avoided as cases with significant renal insufficiency are unable to excrete significant water loads; cerebral oedema may result.

Case management

When a diagnosis of substage b lymphoma has been made, priority must be given to:

1. Supporting the patient.
2. Controlling the disease process.

In order to support the patient, basic nutrition, warmth, fluid and electrolyte needs must be attended to (Figure 5). Inappetent or anorexic patients should not be supported on intravenous fluids alone. Assisted feeding is mandatory; this can be greatly aided by the placement of an appropriate feeding tube. Investigations should be undertaken to obtain supporting data, as presented earlier, so that potential problems can be anticipated and prevented or managed.

Control of the disease requires the judicious use of chemotherapy. Hypoalbuminaemia, hepatopathy and renal insufficiency can all lead to apparent overdose of chemotherapy due to reduced plasma protein drug binding or relative deficiencies of excretory metabolism. Biochemical and haematological parameters must be known prior to chemotherapy so that appropriate dose adjustments can be made.

Clinicians are strongly advised not to embark upon unfamiliar chemotherapy protocols when presented with a case of

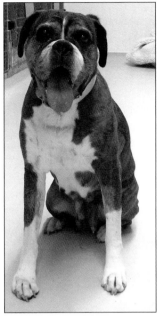

Figure 5: Dramatic clinical improvement following treatment and resolution of hypercalcaemia (same dog as in Figure 4)

lymphoma that is complicated by systemic illness. Good decision-making in these cases requires confident and timely identification of progressive changes, whether those changes represent improvement or deterioration.

Prognosis

At the current time, knowledge of the behaviour of distinct canine lymphoma subtypes is rudimentary. Historically, B or T cell immunophenotype has been regarded to be predictive of outcome but this is an oversimplification. In fact, in the Ponce *et al.* study (2004), the group of cases exhibiting the best survival outcome were a subgroup of T cell immunophenotype whilst the cases exhibiting the poorest prognosis were a subgroup of B cell immunophenotype. Such a pattern would not be predicted by the traditional interpretation of effect of immunophenotype on prognosis. This is a rapidly developing field of veterinary oncology; an experienced veterinary haemato-oncologist should be consulted to offer insight into the prognostic information provided by flow cytometry and detailed cytomorphological evaluations.

Conclusion

As a group, cases of substage b lymphoma carry a poor prognosis. While in part this is simply a reflection of their ill health, it is unclear whether their prognosis would remain poorer than comparable substage a cases if complete remission were achieved. Initial management of these cases can be intensive and, with no guarantee of a successful outcome, not all owners would choose to pursue such an approach. It is the author's experience, however, that many of these cases can enjoy a normal-for-lymphoma quality and length of life if appropriate management is implemented at an early stage. ■

FURTHER READING

Ponce F, Magnol J-P, Ledieu D *et al.* (2004) Prognostic significance of morphological subtypes in canine malignant lymphomas during chemotherapy. *The Veterinary Journal* **167**, 158–166

How to...

Perform reliable veterinary haematology in practice

by Roger Powell

Sampling

Venepuncture should be clean and quick, using as large a needle as possible with minimal suction. Typically use the jugular vein with a 21–23 gauge needle and 2.5–5 ml syringe. A peripheral vein (e.g. cephalic) can be used in large dogs if it is easier to locate and sample, for example in overweight animals. A clean and quick sampling is better than repeated attempts at any single vein. If the first attempt fails, it is advisable to use a new needle and change the site slightly or use a different vein.

These guidelines minimise trauma to the cells which risks artefact and cell lysis. Lysis reduces red cell numbers and PCV and can artificially elevate the haemoglobin concentrations. A clean technique minimises tissue damage and activation of platelets during sampling. Therefore platelet clumping and clot formation is prevented which will artificially reduce platelet numbers and potentially white cells as well, especially neutrophils.

The blood is typically placed into EDTA (ethylenediamine tetra-acetic acid) anticoagulant for many veterinary species. Anti-coagulant **tubes should always be filled, without the needle attached, to the correct level** because:

- Underfilling results in a relative anticoagulant excess. This excess EDTA shrinks the cells and alters their morphology. It can therefore also artificially affect the MCV and PCV. **If the tube is less than half full, the PCV can be reduced by 5%.** This effect is compounded if the animal is actually anaemic
- Overfilling can allow clotting, which can prevent automated analysis and alter cell numbers
- If the needle is still in place the cells are traumatised (Figure 1) and more likely to lyse.

The blood should be gently mixed by inversion and rolling in your hand, not shaking. **At least one fresh blood smear should now be made from the EDTA anticoagulated blood,** especially if the sample is posted to an external laboratory. Blood cells begin to degenerate as soon as they leave the body, with significant changes being seen after 12 hours. Morphological features are then often lost, artificial features created or clinical interpretation severely hampered. As such, smears made after postage may not be representative. Smearing straight from the syringe typically creates platelet clumps and uneven smearing as the blood clots (Figure 1). The reader is referred to Elizabeth Villiers' excellent previous "How to..." **companion** article (December 2008) for more detailed information on blood smearing and examination.

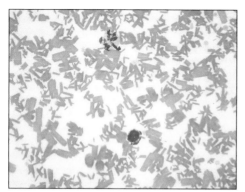

Figure 1: Fresh blood smear showing significant *in vitro* artefact, with red cell lysis and haemoglobin crystals alongside a damaged neutrophil (top) and lymphocyte (bottom). ©Roger Powell

Once smeared, the sample is processed or stored in the fridge if being posted externally. The slides should be stored at room temperature, **not** the fridge, as condensation can damage the cells.

If chemical restraint or sampling occurs under general anaesthesia, this must be noted. Changes in blood pressure will have significant effects on circulating cell numbers. This is seen naturally/physiologically in animals that are agitated during sampling. Agitation results in an increased blood pressure and splenic contraction, increasing numbers of circulating white cells, especially neutrophils and red cells. Conversely, sedation or anaesthesia lowers blood pressure and causes splenic sequestration, reducing the number of circulating cells, both red cells (falsely low PCV) and white cells (false leukopenia).

Performing a complete/full blood count (CBC/FBC)

Ideally, the blood sample should be processed at least 5–10 minutes after filling the EDTA tube to prevent artefacts, such as cell shrinkage, being introduced before the blood and EDTA have time to equilibrate.

Analysis varies from a simple spun microhaematocrit measurement to a full analysis–five part white cell differential.

Packed cell volume (PCV)

This is the volume of red cells produced after high speed (11–15,000 rpm) centrifugation of resuspended whole blood in a microhaematocrit tube for 5 minutes. Whilst not identical to the haemocrit (HCT) it is, or should be, equivalent to the calculated HCT (see later) produced by the analyser. It is worth noting that the PCV is affected by excess EDTA, whereas the HCT can be less affected.

When performing a manual PCV, the microhaematocrit tube **must be 2/3 to 3/4 full**; too little exaggerates red cell packing on centrifugation, whereas too much reduces the force and prevents packing. Whilst this is often not clinically significant, it can be significant when compounded by changes in cell numbers, such as in anaemia.

Automated analyser cell counting

This forms the cornerstone of veterinary haematology, with three main types of analyser being available. Before any blood is run through an analyser, it should be:

- Stirred thoroughly and checked for clots using either a microhaematocrit tube or cocktail stick. If this is not performed and clots are present, cell counts can be unknowingly affected or the analyser blocked/damaged
- Gently and evenly resuspended, by inverting and rolling for at least 1 minute, especially if the tube has been left standing for a period of time. If not performed, cell counts can be artificially affected depending on the degree of cell settling.

There are a large number of haematology analysers available, capable of producing erythrocyte parameters (RBC, Hb, HCT/PCV,

MCV, MCH and MCHC) with a three or five part white cell differential (neutrophils, lymphocytes, monocytes, eosinophils and basophils) and platelet count. These machines vary in accuracy from correct measurements through to misleading or even inaccurate results. A laser flow cytometer calculates the leukogram and erythrogram; the basic principles are described below.

Generating a leukogram

In general, newer impedance and laser cytometer analysers can be accurate in many healthy and some diseased situations. Even haematology analysers in commercial referral laboratories, costing many thousands of pounds more, can and do make differential errors. As such, confirming white cell differentials and assessing cell morphology in a blood smear is a vital part of the complete blood count. Staining in practice typically will be achieved using a rapid based kit and the reader is referred to Kathleen Tennant's "How to…" article on (page 235) for further information.

However, a good analyser counts thousands of cells resulting in a numerical precision superior to any manual count (typically this involves counting 100–500 cells). Therefore the analyser leukocyte differential count is only altered if the manual smear differential is significantly different. Other analysers that cannot reliably differentiate cells should only be used to provide total cell counts; the differential count should be provided by smear examination.

Understanding the methods that these machines use for cell counting help understand circumstances in which manual correction of the differential count might be required.

■ **Presence of nucleated erythrocytes** – The white cells are often counted after the red cells have been lysed; however, immature nucleated red cells are resistant to lysis. The analyser 'assumes' that all cells counted following lysis are leukocytes which may not be true. Therefore most 'white cell counts' are in fact a nucleated cell count. Therefore if nucleated red cells are present (in significant numbers) when examining the smear, the white cell count needs correcting as follows:

corrected (true) white cell count =

$$\frac{100}{(nRBC + 100)} \times \text{nucleated cell count}$$

Generating an erythrogram

Once the cells are counted (RBC), size (MCV) and haemoglobin (Hb) measured, the analyser calculates several red cell parameters: HCT, mean cell haemoglobin concentration (MCHC) and mean cell haemoglobin (MCH).

$$HCT\ (l/l) = \frac{MCV\ (fl) \times RBC\ (\times 10^{12}/l)}{10}$$

$$MCHC\ (g/dl) = \frac{Hb\ (g/dl) \times 100}{HCT\ (l/l)}$$

$$MCH\ (pg) = \frac{Hb\ (g/dl) \times 10}{RBC\ (\times 10^{12}/l)}$$

MCHC is a useful parameter for monitoring the analyser's red cell performance. It is calculated from the Hb and HCT in most machines using two independent techniques. Values less than 28 are likely artefactual, as diseases such as iron deficiency rarely produce values this low. Conversely if the value is elevated, artefact, such as agglutination, haemolysis or lipaemia, is likely. If the MCHC falls outside the reference values, assessing for potential artefact is recommended initially, before ascribing the value to a disease. A good general check to perform on all erythrograms to ascertain the analyser is working correctly is to check that the Hb value is about one third the HCT/PCV (± 3).

Types of analyser commonly used in veterinary practice

Quantitative buffy coat (QBC) analysers

These machines use two separate methods to determine the erythrogram and leucogram.

- The PCV and MCHC are measured, and the other red cell parameters are then all calculated.
- The white cell counts are determined from the width and fluorescence of various cell layers/bands in a centrifuged buffy coat artificially expanded by a float. The layer width and degree of fluorescence reflect cell numbers, assuming that the cells are all normal size. The differentiation of white cell types is based on the variable fluorescence of leukocytes when stained to create a differential of mononuclear cells (lymphocytes and monocytes) from granulocytes (neutrophils and eosinophils). This fluorescence is very reliant on an absence of background interference and healthy normal cells. Often in disease the size, nature and RNA content of the cells changes, and thus the discrimination is lost. Similarly if the distinction

between the bands is lost, counting can be inaccurate or simply wrong. **Therefore whilst these analysers typically give an accurate total white cell count in healthy animals, the differential count is often unreliable and misleading in clinical patients.** Figure 2 provides an illustrative example.

Impedance counters

These analysers sort cells using impedance. The cells are diluted in an electrolyte solution and then drawn through an aperture within an electrode. As each cell passes through, it creates a pulse of resistance – the more pulses, the more cell there are (Coulter principle). The size of each resistance (impedance) pulse is proportional to the size of cell. The size of cell types (platelet *versus* red *versus* white) differs between species so these machines must be set and calibrated to the appropriate species. If there is overlap in size between two cells types, impedance counters fail to distinguish the cells and will ascribe them to the wrong type. Most commonly platelets will be miscounted as red cells if their size overlaps (Figure 3), or platelet and red blood cell clumps as white blood cells.

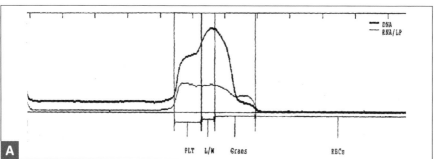

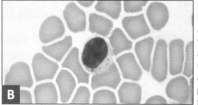

Figure 2: (A) Buffy coat profile from a 1-year-old neutered male Labrador with pyrexia of unknown origin. The automated analysis reported a signficant eosinophilia (with no flags) for which the dog was investigated. (B) Blood film examination by a haematologist revealed a significant lymphocytosis. The majority of these cells were granular lymphocytes, which the analyser was mis-classifying as eosinophils due to their granularity. The dog had an idiosyncratic and eventually self-resolving reaction to a booster vaccination. ©Roger Powell

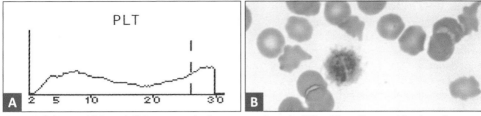

Figure 3: (A) Dog with iron-deficient anaemia due to gastrointestinal blood loss. The combination of microcytosis and a thrombocytosis with macroplatelets prevents accurate automated differentiation, as the platelet histogram merges into the red cells on the right side, the set discrimination threshold (dotted line) not being applicable in this instance. (B) The macroplatelet (left) is the same size as adjacent red blood cells. ©Roger Powell

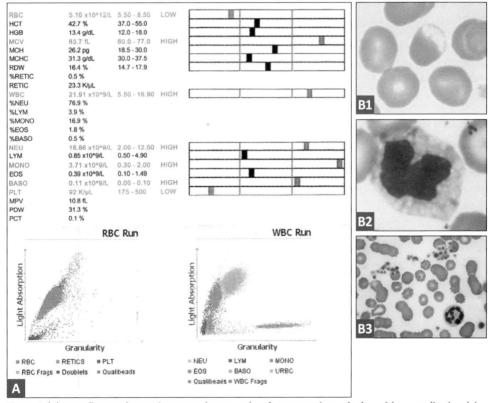

Figure 4: (A) Laser flow analyser print out and scatter plots from an entire male dog with generalised malaise and hyperglobulinaemia. The red cell numbers are discordantly low and the MCV high due to rouleaux red cell clumping and scattered platelet clumps (B2), with eccentrocytosis (B1). White cell differential checking showed no basophilia or monocytosis but there was a left-shifted moderately toxic neutrophilia (B3) with reactive lymphocytes (B2). The dog had an infected prostatic abscess. ©Roger Powell

Laser flow cytometers

These are more recently available as affordable bench top analysers but still remain much more expensive than impedance or QBC analysers. A stream of single file cells is passed through a laser beam, resulting in scattering of the light. This scatter is both forward (related to the size of the cell) and to the side (related to the complexity/granularity of the cell). This scattering effect can be enhanced by use of certain lysing solutions to leave only a few cell types for analysis, and the use of dyes which cause cellular granules of fluoresce under laser light. A number of graphical plots are produced to aid analysis and interpretation. These produce reliable red and white cell analysis in some situations, but are still subject to artefacts or problems during many diseases (see Figure 4).

How are the results reported?

Graphical displays

When counting and assessing the cells, all the above methods produce one or more graphical displays, histograms or scatter plots, both of cell size and also various cellular constituents. Without doubt, using and visually assessing these displays enhances the information that is gained from the analysis. Whilst this does not replace the need to look at a fresh blood smear, it can identify potential artefacts and significant changes in cell populations that would otherwise be misdiagnosed or not identified if only numerical values are assessed. For example, red cell indices are typically reported as mean values. A significant change in the red cell population has to occur before the mean value changes. The red cell and platelet distribution width values (if provided) are a numerical indicator of the histogram's or scatter plot's 'width' so can show such changes more readily (Figure 5).

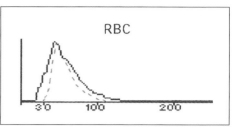

Figure 5: Impedance RBC histogram from a dog with iron-deficient regenerative anaemia (black line); and a healthy dog (red line). The peaks are similar and therefore the MCV was within reference limits, but the histogram clearly shows increased numbers of small cells (microcytosis), as well as macrocytosis due to regeneration. ©Roger Powell

All analyser problems are more significant and dramatic the more diseased an animal is. Automated flags and comments are often misleading, especially if the disease is haematological (e.g. leukaemia). Abnormally large cellular material can however be identified on these graphical displays. This prompts analysis of the smear as it is expected that the automated differentiation will likely have ascribed them to the wrong cell line (Figure 6).

There is as yet no good way for these analysers to detect or report morphological changes such as toxicity in neutrophils that would be evident in a blood film to the trained eye (such as in Figure 4).

In summary

1. Check the sampling information for significant pre-analytical factors.
2. Check the RBC, Hb and HCT/PCV values are relatively similar within their reference intervals. Also check the Hb value is approximately 1/3 of the PCV/HCT.
3. Check the MCHC value is not elevated nor 'inappropriately' low.
4. If these criteria are not met, look for significant artefactual factors and correct by repeat analysis where possible.

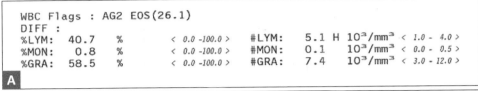

```
WBC Flags : AG2 EOS(26.1)
DIFF :
%LYM:   40.7   %      < 0.0 -100.0 >   #LYM:   5.1 H  10³/mm³  < 1.0 - 4.0 >
%MON:    0.8   %      < 0.0 -100.0 >   #MON:   0.1    10³/mm³  < 0.0 - 0.5 >
%GRA:   58.5   %      < 0.0 -100.0 >   #GRA:   7.4    10³/mm³  < 3.0 - 12.0 >
```

A

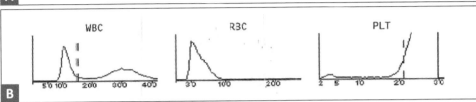

B

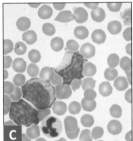

C

Figure 6: (A) Numerical values from an impedance analyser suggesting a mild lymphocytosis. (B) The graphical display clearly shows an abnormal WBC pattern with very large cellular material peaking at about 300 whereas white cells in health are much smaller (<300). (C) This was an acute lymphoblastic leukaemia, the cells shown here being enlarged and accounting for the graphical pattern. ©Roger Powell

5. Check the white cell graphical print out for abnormal or irregular areas and blurring coalescing of cell groups or histograms. If present, the film must be examined and potentially the sample re-analysed.

6. If the platelet count is low, check the smear for large platelets and/or clumps. Resampling may be required for accurate counting.

7. Examine or send away a blood smear to identify artefacts and significant cell morphology.

8. Repeat the haematology as required to assess shifts in pattern and disease, potentially from day to day.

Accurate and precise veterinary haematology or a complete blood count always requires both automated analysis and blood smear examination. With a few minutes spent examining a blood smear and the numerical and graphical output of in house haematology machines, reliable results are readily achievable. ∎

How to...

Perform a successful joint tap

by Alasdair Renwick

A joint tap, or more correctly arthrocentesis, refers to the surgical puncture of a joint cavity for aspiration of synovial fluid. It is a vital tool in the investigation of joint disease allowing gross examination, cytology and bacterial culture of synovial fluid. It can be used in the investigation of any arthropathy, but should be considered to exclude sepsis in cases with chronic osteoarthritis presenting with an acute deterioration, in cases presenting with single inflamed joints, and is essential in the diagnosis of immune-mediated polyarthritis. In addition, arthrocentesis allows instillation of contrast media for contrast arthrography and also allows injection of medications directly into the joint cavity.

In most cases heavy sedation or general anaesthesia is required. The joint to be aspirated should be clipped of hair and prepared aseptically. The operator should scrub their hands and wear sterile surgical gloves. A variety of needles should be available: 21 G 1 inch or 1.5 inch needles are appropriate for most joints; 23 G needles may be needed for smaller joints such as the carpus or tarsus and may be needed for smaller dogs and cats; and 3 inch spinal needles may be required for the hip joint in large dogs. Glass slides should be available to make direct smears, and fluid collection tubes are required if samples are to be submitted to an external laboratory. These tubes should be either plain or with EDTA, depending on the individual laboratory's preference. If sepsis is suspected, blood culture medium should be available as synovial fluid frequently shows no bacterial growth in the presence of infection when cultured directly on agar plates.

Shoulder joint

The needle is inserted approximately 5–10 mm distal to the acromion (for a medium sized dog) and aimed slightly proximally until it is felt to enter the joint (Figure 1). If no fluid is obtained, an assistant can apply gentle traction on the distal limb to open up the joint space.

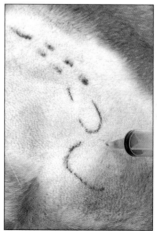

Figure 1: Arthrocentesis of the left shoulder joint. The dotted line outlines the scapular spine and the solid line the greater tubercle

Elbow joint

Technique 1: Extend the elbow to allow the capsule to distend caudally. The needle is inserted lateral to the olecranon or triceps tendon and aimed into the olecranon fossa (Figure 2). Alternatively, with the elbow flexed, the needle can be inserted into the caudolateral aspect of the joint between the olecranon and the lateral epicondylar ridge.

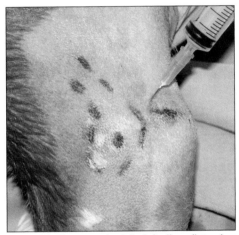

Figure 2: Arthrocentesis of the left elbow (lateral view). The dotted line outlines the lateral aspect of the humeral condyle. The solid line outlines the proximal extent of the olecranon and the dot marks the position of the lateral epicondyle

Technique 2: With the medial surface of the elbow uppermost, palpate and then draw an imaginary line from the greater tubercle and through the medial epicondyle of the humerus. The caudodistal edge of the medial aspect of the humeral condyle can be palpated approximately 1 cm (for a medium sized dog) on this line distal to the medial epicondyle. A neurovascular bundle (ulnar nerve and recurrent ulnar artery) can usually be palpated subcutaneously and avoided. The needle is inserted at this point and aimed in the same line about 30–45 degrees from vertical until the needle is felt to enter the joint (Figure 3).

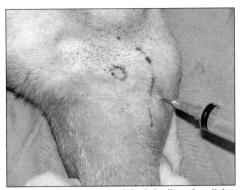

Figure 3: Arthrocentesis of the left elbow (medial view) using the alternative technique. The broken line marks the medial aspect of the humeral condyle and the circle marks the position of the medial epicondyle

Carpus

By palpating the dorsal aspect of the distal radius, the level of the radiocarpal joint can be identified on flexion and extension of the joint. With the joint flexed the needle is inserted into the radiocarpal joint (Figure 4). Tendons and vascular structures on the dorsal aspect of the carpus should be avoided.

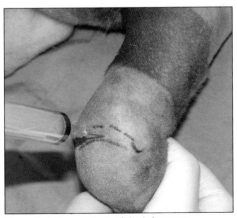

Figure 4: Arthrocentesis of the left carpus (craniolateral view). The dotted line outlines the distal aspects of the radius and ulna and the solid line marks the cranioproximal aspect of the radial carpal bone

Hip

Technique 1: The needle is inserted cranial and proximal to the greater trochanter and directed slightly ventrally and caudally (Figure 5). This technique can be difficult in large, well muscled breeds due to the distance of the joint from the skin.

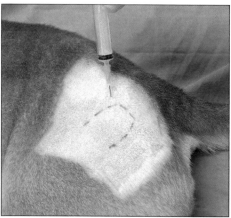

Figure 5: Arthrocentesis of the left hip (lateral view). The dotted line outlines the greater trochanter

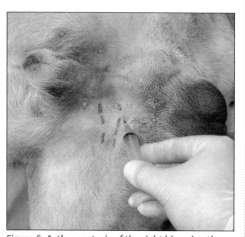

Figure 6: Arthrocentesis of the right hip using the alternative technique (ventral view). The dotted line outlines the pectineus muscle. Great care must be taken with this technique

Technique 2: With the animal in dorsal recumbency allow the hindlimbs to abduct. The ventral aspect of the hip joint can be palpated caudal to the band of the pectineus muscle. The femoral artery and vein can be palpated cranial to this muscle. The needle is inserted in line with the long axis of the femur, with the tip of the needle angled slightly medially from the sagittal plane (Figure 6). Care must be taken with this technique to identify the femoral artery. There is a slight risk of injury to the deep femoral artery and vein.

Stifle joint

Technique 1: With the stifle partially flexed, the needle is inserted medial or lateral to the patellar tendon half way between the patella and tibial tuberosity and is directed caudally (Figure 7). Fluid frequently cannot be obtained with this method as the needle tip lies within the fat pad or cruciate ligaments.

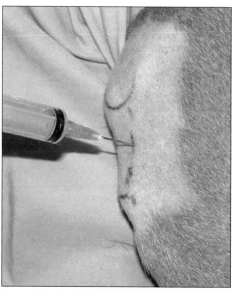

Figure 7: Arthrocentesis of the left stifle (craniolateral view). The solid lines outline the patella and the tibial tuberosity and the dotted line outlines the lateral aspect of the patellar tendon

Technique 2: With the stifle partially flexed, digital pressure is applied either medial or lateral to the patellar tendon. The needle is inserted on the opposite side of the patellar tendon and directed proximally towards the patella, aiming to enter either the medial or lateral recess (Figure 8). Alternatively, the needle can be directed into the femoropatellar space. Fluid can often be more reliably obtained with this method.

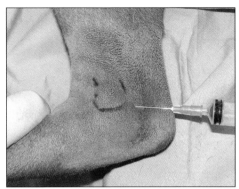

Figure 9: Arthrocentesis of the left hock (lateral view). The solid line outlines the lateral malleolus of the fibula

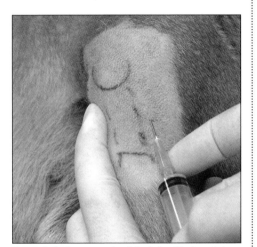

Figure 8: Arthrocentesis of the left stifle (cranial view) using the alternative technique. The solid lines outline the patella and the tibial tuberosity and the dotted line outlines the patellar tendon

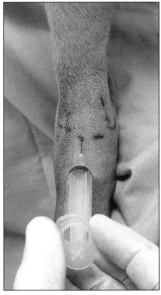

Figure 10: Arthrocentesis of the left hock (cranial view). The dotted line outlines the talocrural joint

Hock

Technique 1: Hyperflex the hock joint. The needle is inserted perpendicular to the long axis of the tibia, medial to the lateral malleolus of the fibula (Figure 9). If the joint is more effused dorsally, try technique 2.

Technique 2: Palpate the talocrural joint space on its cranial aspect and insert the needle perpendicular to the long axis of the tibia (Figure 10). It is best to insert the needle slightly off the midline so that it enters the medial or lateral tibial sulcus.

Collection and analysis

Once the needle has been inserted into the joint space, apply gentle suction via a 2.5 or 5 ml syringe. Once fluid is obtained, release the negative pressure and remove the needle. If blood is obtained withdraw the syringe immediately and try again with a new syringe and needle at an adjacent site. Blood contamination is unavoidable in some cases. While this will increase the cell counts, a relative increase in leucocytes can usually be appreciated when present. Once the needle is withdrawn a visual estimate of viscosity can be made by the string test (Figure 11), with a normal joint giving a 2.5–5 cm or more string. In diseased joints this may be reduced to 1–2 cm. Viscosity is related to hyaluronan concentration or hyaluronan chain length, which can vary with dilution due to effusion or

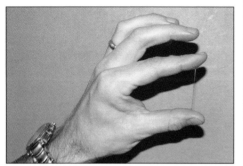

Figure 11: Visual estimate of viscosity of synovial fluid from a normal joint

reduced production due to synovitis. However, normal viscosity can be maintained in some osteoarthritic joints. In cats and small dogs, only a few drops of synovial fluid may be obtained, which should be used to make direct smears. If greater volumes are obtained these should be placed into collection tubes as above. A visual estimate of fluid quality can be made; fluid should be clear and colourless or very pale straw coloured. Abnormal synovial fluid may be turbid or contain visible clots of purulent exudate (Figure 12). Inability to read printed text through a sample indicates increased turbidity.

Cytology of synovial fluid is often the most useful test. This can be done in house, on stained smears, for example with Diff-Quik, or by an external laboratory. External

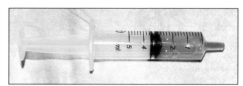

Figure 12: Synovial fluid from a septic joint. The fluid is turbid

laboratories offer the advantage of accurate cell counts as long as sufficient volumes of fluid have been obtained. Normal synovial fluid contains $<3 \times 10^9$ cells/l, which should be >90% monocytes (Figure 13). Osteoarthritic joints usually contain $<5 \times 10^9$ cells/l which contains >90% monocytes (Figure 14), but effusion often allows

	Cell count (x 10^9) cells/l	Cell types
Normal	<3	>90% monocytes
Osteoarthritis	<5	Usually >90% monocytes
Immune-mediated polyarthritis	Variable	Predominantly polymorphonuclear cells
Septic	>5–10	Predominantly polymorphonuclear cells

Figure 13: Typical cell counts from various arthropathies

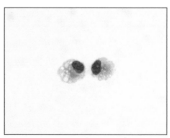

Figure 14: Macrophages in synovial fluid from a joint with osteoarthritis. Courtesy of CytoPath Ltd, Diagnostic Veterinary Pathology Laboratory

aspiration of greater volumes of fluid; in addition, the fluid is often slightly more discoloured than normal fluid. In some cases, such as traumatic arthritis, a greater proportion of polymorphonuclear cells may be seen (20–30%); however, total cell counts are generally <5 x 10^9/l in these cases. Septic joints will have increased numbers of leucocytes (>5–10 x 10^9/l) with a high proportion (usually >90%) of polymorphonuclear cells, and bacteria may be visualised (Figure 15). Cases of immune-mediated polyarthritis have variable total white cell counts (generally >5 x 10^9/l) but those present are predominantly polymorphonuclear cells (Figure 16). It is important to realise that there is considerable

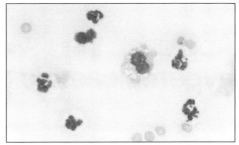

Figure 16: Synovial fluid from a dog with immune-mediated polyarthritis. The cells are predominantly polymorphonuclear leucocytes

overlap of these values between different conditions. Thus a normal and an osteoarthritic joint can be very similar. Likewise septic joints and those affected by immune-mediated polyarthritis can be difficult to differentiate on cytology. Correlation with clinical findings is thus important. A single joint with increased polymorphonuclear cells is more likely to be septic, whereas multiple joints with similar cytology are more likely to be associated with immune-mediated polyarthritis. If sepsis is suspected, synovial fluid should be placed in blood culture medium for transport to an external laboratory. In this situation it is especially important that aseptic technique is used as sample contamination and false positive cultures may be seen.

In summary, arthrocentesis is a quick and relatively straightforward procedure that can provide vital information in obtaining a definitive diagnosis and should be considered in any animal presenting with an arthropathy. ■

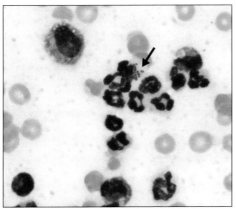

Figure 15: Mixed cells but predominantly neutrophils in synovial fluid from a septic joint. Intracellular bacteria can be seen (arrowed). Courtesy of CytoPath Ltd, Diagnostic Veterinary Pathology Laboratory

How to…
Approach the
hypercalcaemic patient

by Kirsty Roe

Hypercalcaemia can be an unexpected abnormality on a biochemistry profile and although it can be a fortuitous finding in a patient displaying non-specific clinical signs, it is often difficult to decide how to proceed. When developing a diagnostic and treatment plan consideration must be given to the magnitude of the hypercalcaemia, the rate of its development, progression and the clinical state of the patient. Animals with rapid and progressive increases in calcium require aggressive therapy, which is discussed at the end of the article.

Calcium is required for many intracellular and extracellular functions including enzyme reactions, transport of substances across membranes and membrane stability, nerve conduction, neuromuscular transmission, muscle contraction, smooth muscle tone, blood coagulation, hormone secretion, control of hepatic glycogen metabolism, bone formation, and cell growth and division. A basic knowledge of calcium metabolism within the body is essential to help develop a logical approach to the hypercalcaemic dog or cat.

Calcium metabolism

99% of body calcium is contained in the skeleton as hydroxyapatite. Serum calcium is found in three fractions: ionised calcium (55%), protein-bound calcium (35%) and complexed calcium bound to citrate, lactate, bicarbonate and phosphate (10%). Ionised calcium (iCa) is the biologically active form and protein-bound calcium acts as a storage pool or buffering system for iCa.

Regulation of calcium concentration requires the integrated action of parathyroid hormone (PTH), vitamin D metabolites and calcitonin. PTH and calcitriol (1,25-dihydroxyvitamin D3) are the main regulators, with PTH regulating minute-to-minute iCa concentration and calcitriol regulating the day-to-day iCa.

Parathyroid hormone is synthesised and secreted by the chief cells of the parathyroid gland when iCa decreases. PTH increases serum calcium concentration via:

- Increased renal tubular reabsorption of calcium, resulting in decreased calciuria
- Increased bone resorption and number of osteoclasts on bone surfaces
- Accelerated formation of active vitamin D (calcitriol) by the kidney through the synthesis and activation of 1-alpha-hydroxylase.

PTH secretion is inhibited by increasing serum iCa and calcitriol (Figure 1).

Vitamin D is absorbed in the intestine and converted to 25-hydroxyvitamin D3 (calcidiol) in the liver. This is further hydroxylated to

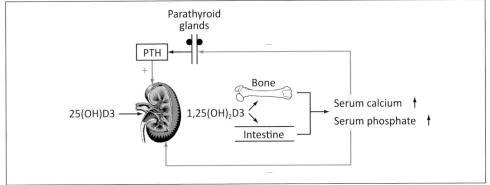

Figure 1: Feedback control of the formation of 1,25-dihydroxyvitamin D3 (1,25 (OH)₂D3) from 25-hydroxyvitamin D3 (25(OH)D3)

1,25-dihydroxyvitamin D3 (calcitriol) in the kidney via 1-alpha hydroxylase. Decreased phosphorus and iCa (via PTH) increase calcitriol formation, which acts to:

- Increase calcium and phosphorus absorption from the intestines
- Stimulates renal reabsorption of calcium and phosphorus from the glomerular filtrate.

Calcitriol secretion is inhibited by calcitriol, hypercalcaemia and phosphate loading.

Calcitonin is synthesised by the C cells of the thyroid gland when iCa increases. Calcitonin inhibits osteoclastic bone resorption and at high doses may enhance renal calcium excretion.

Clinical signs associated with hypercalcaemia

Hypercalcaemia most commonly affects the kidneys, central nervous system, neuromuscular system, gastrointestinal tract and heart. The most common clinical signs are polydipsia, polyuria, lethargy, weakness and anorexia. Signs vary depending upon the underlying cause, magnitude of hypercalcaemia, rate of development and duration: rapid development and increased

magnitude of hypercalcaemia results in more severe clinical signs. Soft tissue mineralisation, in particular the heart and kidneys, is a serious complication of hypercalcaemia and the extent is dependent upon serum phosphorus in addition to the magnitude of hypercalcaemia. Figure 2 lists the clinical signs and conditions associated with hypercalcaemia.

Common
- Polydipsia
- Polyuria
- Anorexia
- Dehydration
- Lethargy
- Weakness
- Vomiting
- Pre-renal azotaemia
- Chronic renal failure

Uncommon
- Constipation
- Cardiac arrhythmia
- Seizures
- Twitching
- Death
- Acute renal failure
- Calcium oxalate urolithiasis

Figure 2: Clinical signs and conditions associated with hypercalcaemia

Upper and lower urinary tract effects:
Polyuria occurs due to impaired renal tubular response to antidiuretic hormone and impaired tubular reabsorption of sodium and chloride, which results in a dilute urine and compensatory polydipsia. It is worth remembering that poor renal concentrating function can not be diagnosed from hyposthenuric urine in a hypercalcaemic patient. Renal failure can occur as a consequence of hypercalcaemia and there is a higher risk of this if the calcium (mmol/l) x phosphorus (mmol/l) product is >6 due to progressive renal mineralisation, vasoconstriction and depletion in extracellular fluid volume.

Chronic renal failure is a more common consequence of hypercalcaemia than is acute renal failure. Dysuria, haematuria and pollakiuria may be observed in patients with calcium oxalate urolithiasis. Urinary tract infection may occur secondary to urolithiasis or polyuria.

Central nervous system and neuromuscular effects: Lethargy and weakness may result from decreased excitability of the central and peripheral nervous systems and muscular tissue. Seizures and muscle twitching may occur as a result of cerebral microthombi or secondary to neuromuscular depression.

Gastrointestinal tract effects: Decreased excitability of gastrointestinal smooth muscle may result in anorexia, vomiting and constipation. Decreased renal clearance of gastrin may contribute to gastric hyperacidity and vomiting.

Cardiac effects: Clinically significant effects on the heart are uncommon. On an ECG P–R interval prolongation and Q–T interval shortening can occur. Severe hypercalaemia may induce serious arrhythmias.

Conditions associated with hypercalcaemia

Common (the most common causes in dogs *versus* cats are listed in Figure 3):

Dogs
■ Neoplasia: lymphoma and anal sac adenocarcinoma
■ Primary hyperparathyroidism
■ Chronic renal failure

Cats
■ Chronic renal failure
■ Idiopathic
■ Neoplasia: lymphoma and squamous cell carcinoma

Figure 3: Most common causes of hypercalcaemia in dogs *versus* cats

- Lymphoma
- Anal sac adenocarcinoma
- Primary hyperparathyroidism
- Chronic renal failure
- Hypoadrenocorticism
- Physiological in young growing animals.

Uncommon:
- Multiple myeloma
- Hypervitaminosis D
  - Iatrogenic, cholecalciferol rodenticides, calcipotriol/calcipotriene psoriasis creams, plants containing cardiac glycosides (*Cestrum diurnum* (Day-blooming Jessamine), *Solanum malacoxylon* (South American eggplant), *Trisetum flavescens* (Oat grass))
- Idiopathic (cats)
- Haemoconcentration/dehydration.

Uncommon to rare:
- Carcinoma
  - Lung, pancreas, mammary gland, nasal, thyroid, skin, testicle, thymus, vaginal
- Spurious
  - Laboratory error, lipaemia, haemolysis
- Granulomatous disease
  - *Angiostrongylus vasorum*, (+ other conditions such as blastomycosis or histoplasmosis which are not present in UK)

- Acute renal failure
- Nutritional secondary hyperparathyroidism
- Hyperthyroidism
- Melanoma
- Skeletal lesions (malignant)
  - Metastatic or primary bone neoplasia, myeloproliferative disease
- Skeletal lesions (non-malignant)
  - Osteomyelitis, hypertrophic osteodystrophy, disuse osteoporosis.

Diagnostic approach to the hypercalcaemic patient

1. Confirm the result with an external laboratory.

- Ensure the hypercalcaemia is not spurious before pursuing a costly investigation by rechecking the total serum calcium and measuring ionised calcium.
- If total hypercalcaemia is present but ionised calcium is within or below the reference range, laboratory error or chronic renal failure should be considered.
- Correction formulae to 'correct' the total calcium relative to albumin concentration have been described but this is less accurate than measuring ionised calcium and use of these formulae are not recommended.

2. Review the signalment and history.

- In young dogs renal failure, lymphoma and hypoadrenocorticism are the most common causes of hypercalcaemia.
- Dogs with primary hyperparathyroidism are often quite bright, whereas dogs with neoplasia, renal failure, vitamin D toxicity and hypoadrenocorticism are more likely to be systemically ill.
- Primary hyperparathyroidism is more common in Keeshonds and dogs older than 8 years; malignancy (other than lymphoma) is more common in older patients.

- A waxing and waning history of illness may occur with hypoadrenocorticism.
- Ensure no access to rodenticides or psoriasis creams and check that calcium-containing supplements are not being administered.
- Check for any possible ingestion of toxic plants that contain glycosides of calcitriol such as Day-blooming Jessamine (*Cestrum diurnum*).
- Check for the possibility of mollusc ingestion, the dog's endoparasiticide regime and its geographical location to determine whether angiostrongylosis is a possibility.
- Check for any history of lameness suggestive of bone pain.
- Idiopathic hypercalcaemia is more common in long-haired cats.
- Cats with idiopathic hypercalcaemia commonly have no clinical signs.

3. Physical examination.

- Remember to palpate all peripheral lymph nodes for enlargement suggestive of lymphoma, although it is important to note that hypercalcaemic dogs with lymphoma can have a mediastinal mass and unremarkable peripheral lymph nodes. No single anatomical location of lymphoma has been found to be more likely to cause hypercalcaemia in cats.
- Perform a rectal examination to palpate for anal sac masses.
- Palpate the long bones and spine for evidence of pain.
- Parathyroid masses are not usually palpable and the physical examination in dogs with primary hyperparathyroidism is usually unremarkable. In contrast, the presence of a palpable cervical mass in cats is suggestive of (though not pathognomonic for) hyperparathyroidism in a hypercalcaemic patient.

- Perform a fundic examination to look for retinal lesions. For example, increased blood vessel tortuosity or retinal haemorrhage could occur due to hyperviscosity syndrome (multiple myeloma) or due to hypertension secondary to chronic renal failure.

4. Routine database.
- Perform complete haematology including blood smear examination, biochemistry and urinalysis.
- Normocytic, normochromic non-regenerative anaemia may occur with chronic renal failure, hypoadrenocorticism and various neoplasms.
- If serum phosphorus is normal or low, renal failure, vitamin D toxicity and hypoadrenocorticism are less likely. Low, low normal or normal phosphorus are more consistent with primary hyperparathyroidism or malignancy.
- Azotaemia is rare in primary hyperparathyroidism as phosphate is often low or low normal.
- Hyperglobulinaemia should raise suspicion for multiple myeloma.
- Remember that hypercalcaemia itself results in decreased ability to concentrate urine by causing nephrogenic diabetes insipidus and that dehydrated vomiting patients may have a prerenal azotaemia. Consequently azotaemia and isosthenuria does not necessarily imply intrinsic renal failure.
- Determining whether renal failure is primary or secondary to hypercalcaemia caused by another disorder when hyperphosphataemia and hypercalcaemia coexist with azotaemia is difficult. Serum ionised calcium concentrations are typically normal or decreased in renal failure and increased in hypercalcaemia caused by other disorders.
- Hyperkalaemia and hyponatraemia are suggestive of hypoadrenocorticism. An

ACTH stimulation test should be performed if these abnormalities are detected.
- Urine may be isosthenuric or hyposthenuric in hypercalcaemic patients.

NOTE
Both hypoadrenocorticism and hypercalcaemia can result in azotaemia and isosthenuria where the azotaemia is prerenal. Following intravenous fluid therapy the azotaemia will improve if it is prerenal.

5. Aspirate any enlarged lymph nodes (even if not significantly enlarged).

6. Radiography of thorax and abdomen.
- Performed primarily to search for a neoplastic focus.
- Mediastinal lymphoma more commonly causes hypercalcaemia than other forms of lymphoma in dogs. Mediastinal masses can be subtle and good quality thoracic radiographs are needed (Figure 4), with or without thoracic ultrasonography. If a mediastinal mass is present, fine needle aspiration or Tru-cut biopsy should be

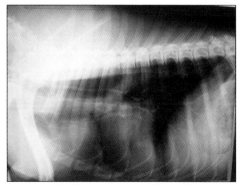

Figure 4: Right lateral thoracic radiograph showing a cranial mediastinal mass and megaoesophagus. Differential diagnoses include lymphoma with paraneoplastic polyneuropathy causing megaoesophagus or thymoma and secondary myasthenia gravis

performed, as hypercalcaemia has also been reported secondary to thymoma.

- Remember to assess the spine and ribs for lytic lesions caused by multiple myeloma or neoplasia with bone metastasis. A core biopsy of a lytic lesion may be necessary if the diagnosis cannot be achieved by other less invasive tests.
- Thoroughly evaluate the lungs for metastases or patterns suggestive of *Angiostrongylus* infection: a peripheral alveolar to diffuse interstitial pattern (Figure 5) is most common. Submit a pooled faecal sample for Baermann testing if suspicious of angiostrongylosis (a single faecal Baermann test is only 50% sensitive).
- Metastasis to sublumbar lymph nodes by an anal sac adenocarcinoma may be visible on abdominal radiographs.
- Soft tissue calcification is rare but is most common with renal failure or hypervitaminosis D.
- Calcium oxalate uroliths are radiodense and their presence should not be overlooked as medical dissolution is not possible. Owners of male dogs and cats with cystic calculi should be warned of the risk of urethral obstruction.

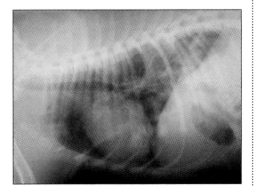

Figure 5: Left lateral thoracic radiograph showing a peripheral alveolar lung pattern in a dog with angiostrongylosis

7. Abdominal ultrasonography.
- May reveal enlarged mesenteric lymph nodes, hepatomegaly or splenomegaly from which fine needle aspirates can be taken.

8. Measure parathyroid hormone (PTH) and parathyroid hormone-related protein (PTHrp) concentrations.
- PTH concentration should be interpreted relative to the calcium concentration. Serum PTH may be increased with primary hyperparathyroidism but a PTH concentration in the upper part of the reference range in a hypercalcaemic patient is inappropriate and therefore is also consistent with primary hyperparathyroidism. Dogs with renal failure may have increased PTH concentrations; therefore, to distinguish this from primary hyperparathyroidism, the result should be interpreted in the context of urea, creatinine, phosphorus and ionised calcium concentrations (Figure 6) and other pertinent information.

NOTE

PTH concentration within the reference range is not normal in a hypercalcaemic patient and does not rule out primary hyperparathyroidism.

- PTHrp measurement is helpful if malignancy is suspected, although PTHrp concentrations are not always increased in malignancy. PTHrp should be negligible if hypercalcaemia is not due to a PTHrp-secreting malignancy. Lymphoma and anal sac adenocarcinoma are the most common PTHrp-secreting malignancies.

9. Cervical ultrasonography.
- If primary hyperparathyroidism is still suspected, ultrasound examination of the parathyroid glands should be performed. Results are highly dependent upon operator skill, experience and equipment. Parathyroid

	Total calcium	Ionised calcium	Phosphorus	PTH	PTHrp	Calcidiol
Primary hyperparathyroidism	↑	↑	↓ or Normal	↑ or Normal	Normal	Normal
Nutritional secondary hyperparathyroidism	Normal or ↓	Normal or ↓	Normal or ↑	↑	Normal	↓ or Normal
Renal secondary hyperparathyroidism	Normal or ↓ or ↑	Normal or ↓	↑ or Normal	↑	Normal	Normal or ↓
Humoral hypercalcaemia of malignancy	↑	↑	↓ or Normal	↓ or Normal	↑ or Normal	Normal
Osteolytic hypercalcaemia of malignancy	↑	↑	Normal or ↑	↓ or Normal	Normal or ↑	Normal
Hypervitaminosis D (cholecalciferol)	↑	↑	↑ or Normal	↓	Normal	↑
Hypoadrenocorticism	↑	↑	Normal or ↑	↓ or Normal	Normal	Normal
Idiopathic (cat)	↑	↑	Normal or ↑	↓ or Normal	Normal	Normal

Figure 6: Serum total and ionised calcium, phosphorus, PTH, PTHrp and calcidiol levels in diseases causing hypercalcaemia

masses are usually hypoechoic, round to oval masses >4 mm in diameter in dogs (Figure 7). Occasionally more than one parathyroid gland can be affected and the absence of a visible mass does not rule out primary hyperparathyroidism.

10. Vitamin D metabolites.

NOTE

In dogs, if the diagnosis still hasn't been made by this point, aspiration or biopsy of lymph nodes, spleen, liver and/or bone marrow should be considered to try to rule out lymphoma. If the hypercalcaemia is mild and there are only mild clinical signs without azotaemia, another option is to recheck the patient in 4–6 weeks. Inconclusive test results may become more conclusive with time or an occult neoplasm may become more evident. In cats, if all investigations have been unremarkable, idiopathic hypercalcaemia is most likely.

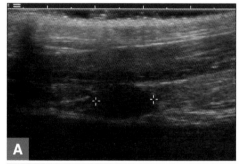

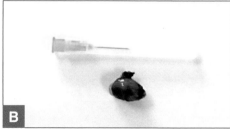

Figure 7: (A) Cervical ultrasonogram showing a 12 mm diameter parathyroid nodule in a dog. (B) Parathyroid gland adenoma following surgical excision

- Measurement of 25-hydroxyvitamin D3 (calcidiol) in cases of suspected vitamin D toxicity can be helpful.

11. Further imaging.
- In dogs, if the underlying cause of hypercalcaemia has still not been found, more advanced imaging such as CT may help detect lytic bone lesions (Figure 8) not evident on radiographs. However CT is rarely necessary in the investigation of hypercalcaemia as the diagnosis will often have been made following initial investigations.

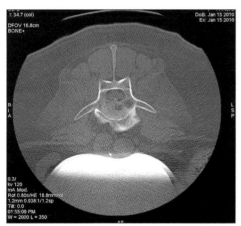

Figure 8: Transverse bone-window CT image of the fifth lumbar vertebra, showing well defined regions of lysis in a dog with multiple myeloma

Emergency management of hypercalcaemia

Hypercalcaemia is regarded as a medical emergency when there is concurrent hyperphosphataemia due to the risk of progressive renal failure. The most important points to remember are to treat the underlying cause and not to administer glucocorticoids without a diagnosis as they can mask the clinical signs by reducing the size of lymph nodes and complicating the

interpretation of fine needle aspirates in patients with lymphoma. Pre-treatment with glucocorticoids reduces the likelihood of successful induction of remission with chemotherapy for lymphoma.

- **Treat the underlying cause.**
- **Intravenous fluids:** Correct any fluid deficits then administer diuresis with 0.9% NaCl at 4–6 ml/kg/h (unless contraindicated e.g. congestive heart failure or hypertension). Fluid supplementation with potassium chloride may be necessary to prevent hypokalaemia (see below). Monitor carefully for signs of volume overload.
- **Diuretics:** Give furosemide 2 mg/kg i.v. q4–12h to promote calciuresis if calcium is not decreasing with fluid therapy alone. Adequate hydration must have been achieved before starting diuretics. Monitor potassium, as furosemide is a loop diuretic and there is a risk of hypokalaemia. Potassium chloride supplementation of fluids is usually necessary (no more than 0.5 mmol K^+/kg bodyweight/h).
- **Glucocorticoids:** These should be given only following confirmation of a diagnosis and at a dose of prednisolone 1–2 mg/kg orally q12h. Glucocorticoids decrease intestinal calcium absorption, decrease bone resorption of calcium and promote renal excretion of calcium. Hypercalcaemic disorders that are often steroid-responsive are listed in Figure 9.

- Lymphoma
- Leukaemia
- Anal sac adenocarcinoma
- Multiple myeloma
- Thymoma
- Vitamin D toxicity
- Granulomatous disease
- Hypoadrenocorticism
- Idiopathic hypercalcaemia

Figure 9: Hypercalcaemic disorders that may be steroid-responsive

- **Calcitonin:** This decreases osteoclast activity and formation of new osteoclasts. It is reserved for cases with severe hypercalcaemia and marked clinical signs where rapid normalisation of calcium is desired. Calcitonin 4–6 IU/kg s.c. q8–12h often decreases calcium within a few hours but hypocalcaemia can occur. Long-term use is not recommended as a lack of response to subsequent treatments can occur within a few days.
- **Bisphosphonates:** These inhibit osteoclast function and therefore decrease bone resorption. Intravenous administration is more effective than oral and, as nephrotoxicity can occur as a side effect, good hydration must be achieved prior to administration. Serum calcium should normalise after a few days. The most commonly used bisphosphonate is pamidronate at a dose of 1 mg/kg in dogs and cats given over 2 hours with a saline infusion every 4–6 weeks, as needed. Oral bisphosphonate therapy can be prescribed for maintenance treatment in patients with recurrent hypercalcaemia where intravenous bisphosphonates have previously normalised calcium. Oesophagitis can occur as a side effect of oral bisphosphonate treatment. ∎

How to...

Approach the anorexic rabbit

by Richard Saunders

norexia is a very common presenting sign in the rabbit, and it is exactly that, a clinical sign. It is not a single disease entity nor, generally, the primary issue. Identifying the reasons for the development of anorexia is vital, in order to approach and successfully treat such a case. Successful management of the anorexia is needed during the diagnostic process to avoid the anorexia becoming a fatal problem in its own right.

Anorexia, in its strictest sense, refers simply to inappetence. This may be total or there may be a reduction in general food intake or an alteration in food preferences, with some items still being eaten and others not. The lack of food intake may go hand in hand with altered gastrointestinal motility, and may or may not include an alteration in faecal consistency and/or volume.

Recognising the early signs

The onset of clinical signs may have been subtle and gradual, or acute. Whilst some rabbits are extremely well cared for by highly attentive and observant owners, many rabbits are poorly observed due to their outdoor lifestyle. Thus the premonitory signs of a problem developing may not always be noted. Furthermore the ideal grouping for rabbits is as a pair housed together. Whilst this is perfect from a social and welfare perspective,

it can obscure the initial subtle stages of a gradually reducing food intake and faecal output. Finally, rabbits are a prey species; this has given them an evolutionary incentive to hide signs of illness, as predators select the potentially weakest animal.

Initial examination

The initial approach to any anorexic rabbit involves taking a detailed history, bearing in mind the possibility that the problem is longer standing than the owner may imagine. In fact, it is important to recognise this potential and ensure that anorexic rabbit cases are seen with greater urgency than the equivalent domestic carnivore case.

Current and past husbandry, with particular emphasis on diet, should be evaluated. Quantitative descriptions of the diet are necessary to avoid inaccurate assumptions. It is common for owners to describe a diet superficially as being ideal, and only on further investigation is it apparent that the hay and grass given is inadequate in quantity and/ or quality, and that the amount of concentrate diet is in vast excess of what is necessary.

The physical examination is an extremely important part of the diagnostic evaluation of any anorexia case, as a wide range of disorders may cause anorexia. The aim is to identify clues as to primary cause(s) as well as the degree and consequences of anorexia.

The mouth is the most common site of problems leading to anorexia (Figure 1). It is vitally important to examine the mouth, and particularly the teeth, carefully and thoroughly. Simple lack of prehension of food, due to incisor malocclusion, is common, and easily identified. More subtle cheek tooth abnormalities are equally likely, but will require more thorough evaluation using otoscopic or other visualization. Anaesthesia or sedation, sufficient to fully open and examine the mouth, is necessary for complete assessment (Figure 2). Oral endoscopic examination facilitates visualization of the interdental spaces, and the very caudal area of the mouth. Imaging is vital to assess lesions involving reserve tooth crown, or boney structures, and is also helpful in diagnosing nasal cavity lesions (see Further diagnostics).

Although dental causes of anorexia are common, the entire rabbit should be thoroughly assessed. Attention should be paid to the signs of respiratory disease (Figure 3). Rabbits with upper respiratory problems may find eating difficult due to their anatomical preference for nasal breathing, and so nasal

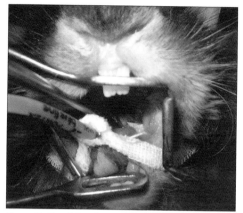

Figure 2: Cheek tooth spurs may cause significant mouth pain and prevent eating

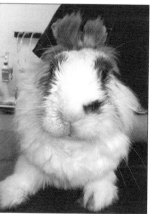

Figure 3: Upper respiratory tract disease makes eating and breathing at the same time difficult

cavity lesions (tumours, abscessation or infection) may lead to inappetence. In particular, the abdominal cavity should be gently but thoroughly palpated. As well as detection of abnormal masses or identification of painful foci, the general degree of gut fill and tympany gives clues as to the chronicity and severity of the problem.

Any source of pain may initiate anorexia; common pain sites (apart from the mouth) include the abdomen, perineal region and feet. Remember that gastrointestinal stasis,

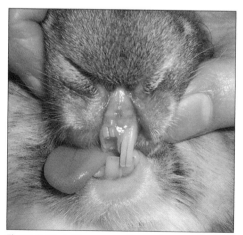

Figure 1: Dental trauma or disease is a common cause of anorexia

causing gas to accumulate in the intestine, leads to distension and painful stimulation of stretch receptors. This pain further depresses appetite and activity, reducing gut motility and perpetuating the problem.

Other common sources of abdominal pain include the urogenital tract. In the un-neutered female, uterine adenocarcinoma is a common finding, and should be considered high on the differential list. In the neutered female, adhesion formation following spaying may lead to (often intermittent) episodes of gastrointestinal stasis, occurring several months or even years afterwards. In either sex, the presence of large amounts of crystalline material in the bladder, so called 'sludgy urine' syndrome, may lead to waxing and waning anorexia due to the discomfort of passing urine, and the associated secondary cystitis. Passage of large amounts of thick, toothpaste-like urine from time to time may occur, giving temporary relief from clinical signs.

The presence of urine scalding around the perineal region (Figure 4) is a common consequence of urinary tract disorders. As well as being a direct source of pain from

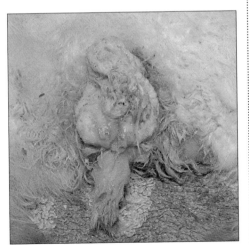

Figure 4: Urine scalding is a common source of pain in the rabbit, potentially leading to anorexia

inflamed and infected skin, this will predispose to fly strike. Indeed, fly strike may be the first indication of a problem. It is therefore vitally important when presented with a fly strike case to investigate the underlying cause.

Further diagnostics

A differential list should be constructed and will include sources of stress or pain and changes of environment or food. Transient stress or pain may be sufficient to initiate anorexia, but unless it is of significant duration the problem should be easily identified and should rapidly resolve once treated. More chronic cases may require further diagnostic investigation.

Radiography is invaluable for the further investigation of dental disorders, particularly those occurring at the very caudal areas of the mouth, or under the gum line. It therefore complements the physical examination (with or without endoscopy). It also allows assessment of the nasal cavity for investigation of upper respiratory disease.

Survey radiography is helpful for evaluating the thorax and abdomen, identifying musculoskeletal problems and assessing the urinary tract for crystalluria and urolithiasis. Abdominal radiography is also helpful for distinguishing between obstructive and non-obstructive ileus, the former typically characterised by a build-up of gas proximal to the site of obstruction, and the latter showing a typical halo-shaped accumulation of gas around ingesta in the stomach, with intestinal gas either largely absent, or relatively evenly distributed throughout the rest of the gastrointestinal tract. In extreme cases, gut rupture will be evident, with free gas and/or fluid (a ground-glass appearance) in the abdomen.

Ultrasonography is an incredibly helpful technique, complementing radiography. Although the presence of gas limits the information that may be obtained, it is superior to radiography in evaluating the liver and uterus, and is often more sensitive than radiography in detecting urinary tract disorders.

More advanced imaging modalities have a place, with CT and MRI being increasingly utilised. CT provides high quality images of the skull and teeth, in particular, and MRI is highly effective at identifying soft tissue lesions within the skull, such as nasal cavity masses.

Haematology and serum biochemistry have a role in identifying underlying disorders such as chronic renal failure, and are probably under-utilised in practice.

Treatment

Treatment of the specific underlying problem obviously depends on a specific diagnosis. It should be noted that rabbits commonly have multiple problems, often arising from a common cause; dental disease, urinary scalding, and caecotroph accumulation around the perineum may all be interlinked, with an inappropriate diet as the initiating cause, and all aspects must be addressed. However in addition to specific therapies, inappetence requires supportive and general treatment, including fluid therapy, nutritional support, analgesics and gastrointestinal prokinetics.

Fluid may be supplied parenterally, but the old adage 'if the mouth works, use it', applies particularly well to rabbits, as hydration of the gut and its contents is especially important. During inappetence a mixture of food material and fur (often present to some degree in the stomach, and usually a sign of slow motility rather than its cause) becomes dehydrated and forms a solid matrix, which further impedes stomach emptying. Rehydration of gastric contents is vital to reverse any effect on appetite.

Nutritional support is vital (Figure 5). Rabbits, especially those suffering from obesity (which is common and under-

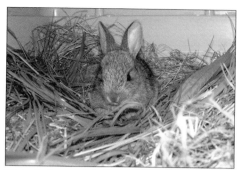

Figure 5: Appropriate fibre rich items such as grass and hay should be offered to all in-patients

recognised), rapidly develop hepatic lipidosis following starvation (Figure 6). As well as fluid, a source of energy to maintain enterocyte viability and prevent hepatic lipidosis developing is important (Figure 7). Commercial products, such as Oxbow Critical Care Formula and Supreme Science Recovery, are palatable and widely available.

Gut distension is painful and, even if no other source of discomfort is present, analgesia is indicated. This may be in the form of opioids (e.g. buprenorphine) or NSAIDs (e.g. meloxicam), or both. Concerns over opioid effects on gut motility are generally unfounded at the doses and durations used, and poorly controlled pain is a far more potent gastrointestinal motility depressor.

Gastrointestinal prokinetics definitely have a place in the management of anorexia and

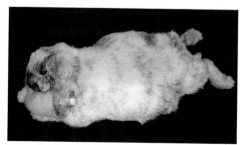

Figure 6: Obese rabbits are at particular risk of hepatic lipidosis developing with starvation

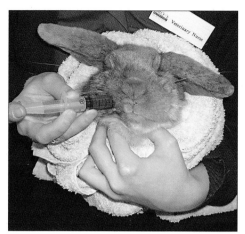

Figure 7: Syringe feeding a commercially available recovery diet is helpful in anorexic rabbits

uses ranitidine syrup as a first line treatment, with domperidone a useful adjunctive or alternative option in more severe cases. Suggested doses are given in Figure 8.

Drug	Dosage
Ranitidine	3–5 mg/kg orally q8–12h
Metoclopramide	0.5–1.0 mg/kg s.c. or orally q6–12h
Domperidone	0.25–0.5 mg/kg q12h
Buprenorphine	0.05–0.1 mg/kg i.m. q6–8h. Anecdotally, this drug appears efficacious given across the oral mucosa
Meloxicam	0.3–0.6 mg/kg s.c. or orally q24h

Figure 8: Author's suggested drug doses

ileus in rabbits. Their use, as with most pharmaceuticals in the rabbit, is based on a small amount of scientific trial data (often performed on laboratory rabbits, with little individual variation in size and breed), and mainly on anecdotal experience. There are few licensed products available for the rabbit (as is also the case with analgesics), and fully informed, written, owner consent is therefore required, following the Cascade appropriately. This author has used metoclopramide, ranitidine and domperidone, and generally

Prognosis

Prognosis depends on the precise diagnosis, and the likelihood of full resolution of the underlying cause. In addition, the duration of clinical signs is an important prognostic indicator, with every day of anorexia bringing with it an increasingly dehydrated gut content, and a more and more bloated and painful abdomen, reducing the chances of a successful resolution. Early intervention is always better than late! ◼

Perform a **cystotomy**

by Chris Shales

C ystotomy can be indicated as part of a diagnostic investigation or to offer either temporary or permanent therapeutic benefit for several relatively common diseases affecting the urinary tract. The prevalence of disease processes that affect the bladder and frequent lack of access to cystoscopy requires that the general practitioner interested in surgery is able to offer cystotomy to their patients. Whilst a straightforward cystotomy should not present a significant obstacle to either the surgeon or patient, complications have the potential to be serious and are often avoidable. Good surgical technique should reduce the complication rate associated with cystotomy to an acceptably low level.

Anatomy

The urinary bladder is suspended by two lateral umbilical ligaments (continuous with the uterine broad ligaments in the female) and further stabilised by a ventral umbilical ligament. The lining consists of a transitional epithelium supported by a lamina propria and then a submucosal layer. The submucosa is surrounded by a detrusor muscular layer, with the outermost layer consisting of adventitia (Figure 1).

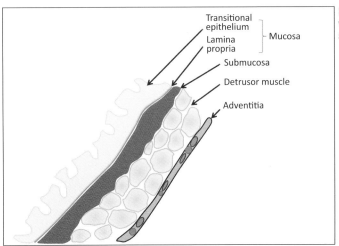

Transitional epithelium
Lamina propria
— Mucosa
Submucosa
Detrusor muscle
Adventitia

Figure 1: Layers of the bladder wall. The submucosa is the key suture-holding layer

The dominant blood supply to the bladder is the caudal vesicular artery which branches from the urogenital artery, itself originating from the internal pudendal artery. Approximately half of animals are reported to have an additional and therefore likely superfluous supply from a cranial vesicular artery. Drainage occurs into the internal pudendal veins and drainage lymph nodes are the sublumbar group as one might expect.

Indications

Indications for cystotomy include:

- Cystic calculi removal
- Cystic mass removal/biopsy
- Bladder wall biopsy
- Ureteral catheterisation
- Neoureterostomy, neoureterocystostomy.

Some of these procedures can also be performed by minimally invasive techniques using rigid endoscopy where this equipment is available.

Approach

The patient is positioned in dorsal recumbency, clipped and aseptically prepared for a caudal midline laparotomy. Prior to starting the procedure, the surgeon should check that all the equipment likely to be required is at hand and should carry out a careful swab count.

An incision extending from just caudal to the umbilicus to just in front of the pubis is made through the skin with a scalpel blade and continued through the fat to the level of the body wall. Many surgeons find that elevating the fat a little either side of the linea alba helps in identification of layers during closure.

The linea alba is identified, and rat-toothed forceps used to elevate the cranial end of the surgical site prior to careful incision with an inverted scalpel blade. A finger can then be introduced into the abdominal cavity and

passed caudally along the midline to ensure there are no adhesions, prior to careful incision of the midline fascia using a straight pair of Mayo scissors. Continued elevation of the midline and only using the distal third of the scissor blades should significantly reduce the risk of inadvertent visceral organ damage during the remainder of the linea alba incision. There should be no requirement to damage either rectus abdominis muscle belly during the midline incision. Confining the incision to the fascia should improve patient comfort postoperatively and reduce bleeding from small vessels (Figure 2). Many surgeons do not place retractors in the abdominal wall, but blunt-ended self-retaining retractors (e.g. Gelpi) can be useful in improving visibility and access.

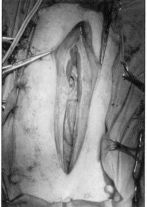

Figure 2: Ventral midline laparotomy incision. The fascia of the rectus sheath can clearly be seen superficial to the rectus abdominis muscle. Neither rectus abdominis muscle belly has been incised

The bladder can then be identified and the ventral ligament broken down if necessary (Figure 3). A 2 or 3 metric (3/0 or 2/0) monofilament stay suture with a tapercut, taperpoint or round-bodied swaged-on needle is placed at the cranial pole of the bladder. Passing the suture through the full thickness of the bladder wall twice and securing the long ends of the suture with haemostatic forceps provides a secure

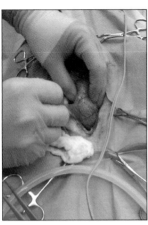

Figure 3: The avascular ventral ligament of the bladder has been identified

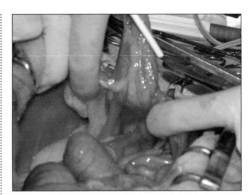

Figure 5: The stay suture in the cranial pole has been used to ventroflex the bladder through the abdominal wound and facilitate exploration of the caudal abdomen. The camera is pointing caudally and the uterine bifurcation can clearly be seen lying dorsal to the bladder

method of retracting the bladder cranially and stabilising it for the remainder of the procedure (Figure 4). If an assistant is not present, the suture can be fastened to the drapes to provide the required retraction.

Prior to retraction of the bladder, it is often worthwhile to ventroflex the bladder through the abdominal incision and carry out a logical assessment of the remaining organs (Figure 5). A full exploratory laparotomy may not be necessary – or possible through this sized approach – but the caudal abdominal viscera, ureters and dorsal surface of the bladder

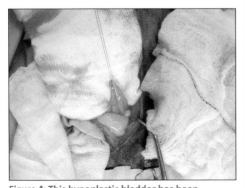

Figure 4: This hypoplastic bladder has been retracted cranially using a 2 metric polypropylene stay suture placed in the cranial pole. This dog had bilateral ectopic ureters

should be inspected. Moistened laparotomy or standard swabs can then be placed dorsal and lateral to the bladder prior to re-orientation back into the original position to give access to the ventral bladder wall.

The cranial pole stay suture can now be used to stabilise the bladder as described, and the surgeon should check that it has not become twisted at all prior to performing the cystotomy.

Cystotomy

A clean No. 11 scalpel blade is used to perform a stab incision into the ventral midline towards the cranial pole of the bladder, and a Poole or other suction tip is inserted to drain the urine and minimise spillage (Figure 6). A sharp pair of Metzenbaum scissors is then used to extend the incision caudally to the length required to perform the desired procedure. One or two stay sutures can be placed full thickness through the bladder wall either side of the cystotomy incision to allow the bladder to be held open (Figure 7).

A key principle to any surgical procedure, but of particular relevance to bladder surgery,

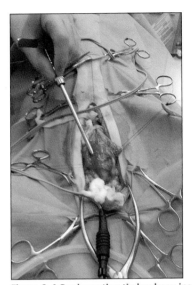

Figure 6: A Poole suction tip has been inserted through a stab incision in the cranioventral bladder wall. The incision is slightly off midline due to the presence of a bladder wall transitional cell carcinoma that was subsequently resected. There are a number of moist swabs dorsal to the bladder, of which one can be seen in the picture. Additional swabs to protect the abdominal musculature were placed before the procedure continued

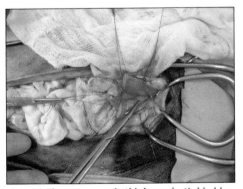

Figure 7: The cystotomy in this hypoplastic bladder has been completed to expose bilateral intramural ectopic ureters (indicated by the instrument). The bladder wall has been retracted using 2 metric polypropylene stay sutures. Two caudally positioned sets of Gelpi self-retaining retractors are being used to aid exposure

is the requirement for gentle and sympathetic tissue handling. The bladder wall incision will initially bleed relatively copiously but the surgeon must resist the temptation to swab or use diathermy on any but the largest vessels. Excessive use of swabs or diathermy has the potential to increase inflammation and can result in wall oedema that can significantly hamper the remainder of the procedure and potentially affect healing adversely. The author does not use either swabs or diathermy and maintains visualisation using gentle saline lavage and suction to remove blood and clots. The haemorrhage is self-limiting and does not present a significant problem to either patient or surgeon in the vast majority of cases.

The position of the cystotomy incision may vary slightly depending on the procedure performed, but for most cases will be positioned in the ventral midline of the bladder in a craniocaudal direction.

Closure

As in other visceral organs, the submucosa represents the suture-holding layer of the bladder and must therefore be included in any bladder closure. There are a number of methods used by surgeons, including inverting suture patterns. The author uses a one or two layer simple continuous appositional suture layer with a synthetic, absorbable, monofilament material on a swaged-on round-bodied, taperpoint or tapercut needle. The start and end of the suture is positioned just beyond the ends of the bladder incision. Sutures are placed approximately 3 mm from the wound edge and approximately 5 mm apart in a medium-sized dog (smaller bladders may need smaller sutures).

Normal or relatively thin bladder walls are closed in one layer taking care to include the submucosa, which will often result in full thickness passage of the needle. Two layer closure is usually not practical unless the bladder wall is very thickened (Figure 8) but should include the mucosa and submucosa in the first layer followed by the adventitia and muscle layers in the second.

Some surgeons place an appositional pattern (continuous or interrupted) followed by an inverting layer (using a rapidly absorbed, monofilament suture on a similar needle) in order to ensure a leak-proof closure. A well performed continuous appositional layer suture does not usually require this additional support, and often the size of the bladder can make this a little challenging, but there are no strong arguments that it is inappropriate.

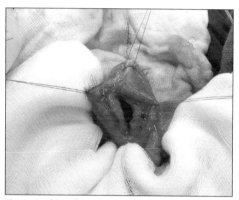

Figure 8: This Labrador's bladder wall has suffered chronic irritation from large numbers of cystic calculi. The bladder wall was approximately 12 mm thick. Closure was carried out in two layers and recovery was without incident

Non-absorbable suture material should be avoided in the bladder wall due to its potential for acting as a nidus for calculi formation. Multifilament suture material is usually not considered a good choice where wicking of fluid or bacteria can be considered a potential problem (such as during bladder closure). In addition, urease-producing bacterial infections such as *Proteus*, *Staphylococcus* and *Klebsiella* can reduce the effective strength of materials such as polyglycolic acid to as little as 48 hours.

The closure should be inspected for areas of possible leakage, particularly at either end. Placement of the ends of the suture beyond either end, and limiting the distal (or caudal) limit of the cystotomy to an area easily accessible for suturing should minimise this risk. Additional simple interrupted sutures can be placed if the surgeon is concerned, but one must avoid excessive use of suture material.

The bladder wall is considered to be capable of healing in as little as 2–3 weeks. One might consider that a particularly inflamed bladder wall would have the potential to take a little longer but selection of absorbable suture material can be based on the capacity for rapid healing. The author usually selects a material with an effective tensile strength of 3–5 weeks depending on the expected ability to heal (e.g. glycomer 631, polyglecaprone 25, polyglyconate, or polydioxanone).

A 'pressure test' is probably of limited use to the experienced surgeon but can serve as a crude test for leaks. A patient on intraoperative fluids is likely to be producing urine at a rate that will allow a small amount of pressure to be applied to the bladder with a little urine inside and the urethra gently occluded. Alternatively, additional intraluminal fluid can be supplied using a syringe filled with saline and an orange (25 gauge) needle. One must remember that any suture closure will leak if enough pressure is applied.

The suture line and surface of the bladder can then be gently lavaged with a small quantity of warm saline; unless leakage has been copious there is usually no requirement for abdominal lavage. The final stay suture can be removed from the cranial pole of the bladder and the swabs used for packing off the bladder can be removed. The omentum is draped over the suture line in order to support healing. Tacking it in position is not usually required. It is essential at this point to complete a swab count prior to abdominal closure.

The potential for seeding of transitional cell carcinoma to other tissue indicates that additional precautions are taken when dealing with lesions of this kind, including changing gloves and surgical instruments before handling any tissue other than the bladder.

Routine closure

The abdominal wall is closed using the fascia of the rectus sheath as the suture-holding layer. A simple interrupted or continuous appositional pattern is ideal, using a permanent or absorbable suture material that will provide effective support for at least 5–6 weeks (e.g. polycloconate or polydioxanone). The subcutaneous fat layer should be apposed to eliminate dead space and the skin closed in a method favoured by the surgeon. The author typically closes the fat in a simple continuous appositional pattern using a monofilament absorbable material (e.g polyglecaprone 25 or glycomer 631) and the subdermal layer in a simple continuous pattern using the same material. Skin staples or monofilament nylon skin sutures can be placed as required.

Aftercare

The patient must receive multi-modal analgesia whenever possible and the nursing staff warned that urinary incontinence may occur during the initial postoperative period.

Blood-tinged urine and occasional blood clots in the urine are also not uncommon following cystotomy and should not be a cause for concern. Cystotomy cases should not require a transurethral or cystostomy tube to be placed unless the bladder is atonic or there is a separate defined requirement for postoperative deflation of the bladder.

The performance of a cystotomy should not in itself indicate a requirement for anything more than routine perioperative antibiotic therapy. There may be an indication for an extended postoperative course associated with certain disease processes.

During the first 12–24 hours postoperatively, the clinician must ensure that accurate records are available of any urine passed in terms of quantity passed, nature of the urine and behaviour during urination. Those cases where urine is not produced in the volumes expected should be examined carefully and may require ultrasonographic assessment of residual bladder volume or free abdominal fluid that might indicate a uroabdomen. Transurethral catheterisation to empty the bladder is usually not necessary and has the potential to compromise the bladder closure unless carried out sympathetically.

The majority of cystotomy cases should recover without incident. Any case that is not recovering in the way expected by the clinician should be assessed for possible uroabdomen. ■

How to...

Get the best from liver samples

by Susana Silva

The diagnosis of most hepatic diseases relies on histopathological examination of a liver biopsy sample. However, biopsy comes at the end of a diagnostic pathway which includes a complete history, clinical examination, clinicopathological data and imaging such as ultrasonography.

Examination of liver samples is needed to achieve a 'gold standard' diagnosis, to direct therapy and to offer prognostic information. However it is important to remember that liver biopsy will produce only a small sample of the liver tissue as a whole and as such might not be a representative sample of ongoing pathology. Although in most cases biopsy is required to achieve a diagnosis, in some cases it is possible to obtain sufficient information by less invasive methods such as cytology.

To avoid frustration for clinicians and inappropriate expectations from the owners, it is very important to understand the indications, limitations and possible complications associated with each specific technique of sampling hepatic tissue.

When to consider sampling the liver

Potential situations in which obtaining hepatic tissue should be considered are:

- Evidence of hepatic dysfunction, such as elevated bile acids or jaundice of hepatic origin

- Diffuse changes in echogenicity on ultrasonography
- Discrete hepatic lesions
- Hepatomegaly of undetermined cause
- Persistently elevated liver enzymes without a detectable inciting cause
- Evaluation for the presence of a breed-specific hepatopathy.

Techniques for obtaining liver samples

There are several different techniques by which hepatic samples may be obtained. These are:

- Fine needle liver aspiration (FNA) under ultrasound guidance
- Needle biopsy
- Surgical biopsy (laparoscopic or via coeliotomy).

These techniques all have indications, advantages and contraindications (Figure 1).

Cytology samples

FNA is the least invasive technique and is usually performed under ultrasound guidance using a 22 G needle of an appropriate length; for most cases a 22 G 1.5 inch needle is appropriate (Figure 2).

Hepatic FNA can often be performed with the patient conscious, although sedation or general anaesthesia will be necessary in a

	Fine needle aspiration	Surgical biopsy		
		Tru-cut needle biopsy	Laparoscopic	Coeliotomy
Anaesthesia	+/−	+	+	+
Ultrasound-guided	+	+		
Invasiveness	−	+	++	+++
Cost	+	++	+++	+++
Experience needed	−	++	++	+

Figure 1: Practical considerations regarding the different methods of obtaining hepatic tissue

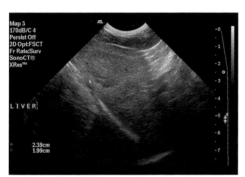

Figure 2: Example of a liver mass that could be sampled via FNA with a 1.5 inch needle; the scale in centimetres on the right side of the screen allows estimation of the depth of the nodule

nervous or less cooperative patient. As the size of the needle is small, the risk of post-FNA bleeding is minimal and therefore multiple sites can be sampled without major risk. Provided there is no evidence of haemostatic problems with previous venepunctures, it is not mandatory to assess clotting times.

The areas to be sampled should be carefully chosen so as to be as representative as possible while avoiding structures like the gallbladder and blood vessels. The needle is introduced into the liver tissue under ultrasound guidance, targeting the specific areas to be sampled. To avoid haemodilution, it is preferable to use the needle alone rather than having a syringe attached and applying

negative suction. The needle should be rapidly moved in and out of the parenchyma (a so-called 'woodpecker-like motion') and a slight twisting motion applied to maximise the cell yield. Afterwards, the cells should be carefully transferred on to a microscope slide and smeared. The spreader slide should not be pushed down too vigorously as this will increase the likelihood of cell lysis and risk non-diagnostic sampling.

Overall, liver cytology is usually the initial diagnostic test in most cases of hepatic disease. FNA yields cells without the presence of structural architecture and therefore is mainly useful in cases where a diagnosis can be obtained from individual cells (e.g. lymphoma). Criteria such as architectural changes, the presence and location of inflammation within a lobule, and location and degree of fibrosis are important when assessing a hepatic biopsy sample and are impossible to evaluate on liver cytology, thereby contributing to the rate of poor agreement between the two techniques.

Studies documenting the agreement between cytology and surgical wedge liver biopsy have shown a poor correlation between the final diagnosis. However, clinicians should not feel discouraged from obtaining hepatic FNAs as they can prove worthwhile. The suspicion of vacuolar hepatopathy and neoplasia (especially lymphoma) are the main indications for hepatic cytology, and for these specific groups of disease the agreement with liver histology is better than in cases of chronic hepatopathies or in vascular anomalies where cytology is unlikely to provide useful information.

FNA can also be used to collect bile for cytology and culture, especially in cases of feline inflammatory liver disease when bacteria are thought to be involved. Care should be taken to empty the gallbladder as much as possible to reduce the possibility of leakage; this technique is contraindicated in cases of extrahepatic bile duct obstruction. Although a transhepatic approach was previously recommended, this is no longer the case and any approach is considered reasonably safe.

If cytology does not provide or is thought unlikely to provide sufficient information, hepatic biopsy should be considered.

Histopathology samples

General anaesthesia is usually recommended to collect samples for histopathology and therefore fasting is essential; a full stomach might also interfere with sample collection. The presence of liver disease reduces the body's ability to metabolise drugs and therefore the protocol chosen for sedation and/or anaesthesia should take this into account.

It is important to assess coagulation status by evaluating activated partial thromboplastin time (APTT), prothrombin time (PT) and platelet count – ideally less than 24 hours before the procedure; a buccal mucosal bleeding time (BMBT) test should also be considered, especially in breeds predisposed to von Willebrand's disease. The liver produces all the clotting factors except for factor VIII and bleeding is indeed the most frequent complication of liver biopsy.

Liver biopsy should be avoided in patients with clotting abnormalities or severe thrombocytopenia (<80 x10^9 platelets per litre).

Even though normal clotting times make significant bleeding less likely, it is possible to have abnormalities that are not detectable by changes in PT and APTT. While it is possible to apply compression during surgical (laparoscopic and coeliotomy) biopsy this is not feasible with needle biopsy (e.g. Tru-cut), making significant bleeding a very realistic possibility.

The method chosen to acquire hepatic tissue is influenced by the size of the liver, the presence or absence of ascites, the main differential diagnoses, and the clinical condition of the patient. For example, if the liver is small it is unlikely that meaningful information will be obtained from cytology as the main differentials would be either vascular disease or a chronic hepatopathy with cirrhosis; in this instance Tru-cut liver biopsy would also be contraindicated due to microhepatica. Additionally, if there is biochemical and ultrasonographic evidence of a vascular problem such as a congenital portosystemic shunt, an exploratory surgery with portovenography ± shunt ligation and biopsy would be preferred over laparoscopic assessment and biopsy.

What constitutes a good specimen?

An ideal sample should be of appropriate size and representative of the primary hepatic pathology.

In diffuse diseases any area is likely to be representative, whilst in focal or regional disease it might be more difficult to get a representative sample and therefore ultrasonography and/or direct inspection are valuable tools. If the pathology seems focal then samples should be collected from both the abnormal-looking areas and from the normal-looking areas, as it is not uncommon for what seems normal to actually be abnormal.

Ideally two or three samples should be obtained from separate areas. As needle biopsy samples are smaller, the potential for non-representative samples is greater. Most authors suggest avoiding the use of 18 G needles, as the samples get fragmented easily and tend not to have enough portal areas to be diagnostic; the sizes most commonly used are 16 G needles for cats and small dogs, and 14 G needles for larger dogs.

Needle biopsy

There are two main types of needle used for liver biopsy; with these a small cylinder of tissue is obtained. The Menghini technique involves tissue aspiration, usually blind, using a syringe attached to a large-bore hollow needle. This technique has been largely superseded by the use of Tru-cut type needles and it will not be discussed here.

Tru-cut needle biopsy is usually performed under ultrasound guidance (Figure 3), even though it is possible to use this type of needle blindly in cases of very severe hepatomegaly. The Tru-cut needle is composed of an outer cannula and an inner notched stylet in which the specimen becomes lodged. The notched stylet is advanced first and the hepatic tissue fills the 2 cm notch. Then the outer cannula

(with sharp cutting edges) is advanced over the stylet and the liver parenchyma is cut, leaving a sample in the notch (Figure 4). Afterwards, the whole needle is withdrawn and the inner stylet is exteriorized again to expose the sample obtained (Figure 5).

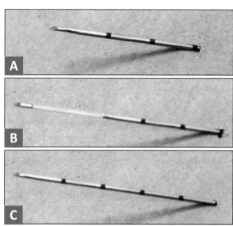

Figure 4: Step-by-step view of the Tru-cut needle as the sample is collected. Please note that this would be happening inside the organ. (A) The loaded Tru-cut needle is inserted into the organ. (B) The Tru-cut needle loaded and with the stylet advanced. Note that the stylet is extending about 2 cm deep to the initial placement site. During this step the hepatic parenchyma fills the notch of the stylet. (C) Tru-cut needle fired. The piece of parenchyma that had previously filled the notch has been cut out and is contained within the outer sheath; the needle is ready to be removed. Again note that the tip of the needle is about 2 cm deeper within the target organ than the original placement site

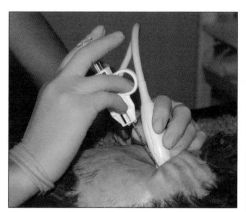

Figure 3: An ultrasound-guided Tru-cut biopsy is about to be performed on this cat, under general anaesthesia

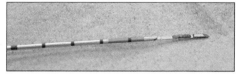

Figure 5: Core of liver tissue obtained with the Tru-cut needle; a small portion had already been cut out of the cylinder (using sterile technique) to be submitted for baterial culture

There are three types of Tru-cut needle: manual, semi-automatic, and those used with a gun-type device.

- The manual needles are difficult to control and their use is not advisable unless under direct visualization.
- The semi-automatic type needles are the most expensive ones and can be used in both dogs and cats.
- Biopsy guns fire the needle, at high speed, once the trigger is pushed. The speed at which the needle is fired makes the process of obtaining samples from a hard fibrotic liver easier. Biopsy guns are a costly piece of equipment and, while the biopsy needles used are then not very expensive, the initial cost is high; therefore this technique is most commonly used in hospitals where a large number of needle biopsies are performed. The use of an automated gun-type device is contraindicated in cats due to the potential for vagal-induced shock (often fatal) caused by the sudden impact wave in the liver.

While the automatic gun device fires both the inner stylet followed by the outer sheath, the semi-automatics only fire the outer sheath after the inner needle core is manually advanced by the operator.

If it is economically feasible to have only one type of needle, then semi-automatic Tru-cut needles have the advantage that they can be used in both dogs and cats.

The decision to perform a Tru-cut liver biopsy should be not made lightly. The potential for complications is real and bleeding from the biopsy site can be significant, especially if a main vessel is damaged. Additionally, the experience of the operator is critical to minimise the risk of complications. Tru-cut needles will advance approximately 2 cm deeper than the tip of the needle. Therefore when selecting a site for biopsy a 2 cm depth in front of the needle should be devoid of major vessels or biliary ducts.

Tru-cut liver biopsy should be avoided in patients with prolonged clotting times or thrombocytopenia. Microhepatica, significant abdominal effusion and operator inexperience are also contraindications.

Surgical biopsy

Laparoscopic biopsy

Obtaining liver samples is one of the most common indications for laparoscopy as it can be accomplished reasonably quickly and with minimal trauma to the patient. The samples obtained with the cupped forceps are smaller than those obtained via coeliotomy but bigger than those obtained via Tru-cut biopsy. Care should be taken to ensure that the sample contains not only subcapsular superficial tissue but also deeper tissue, as the former may not be a representative sample.

With this technique it is possible to inspect the liver (Figure 6) and the rest of the abdomen, to sample macroscopically abnormal areas (Figure 7) and to visualise and apply direct pressure for haemostasis caused by the biopsy. Laparoscopy requires special equipment, training and is more expensive than Tru-cut biopsy.

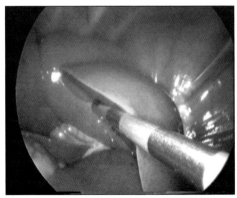

Figure 6: Inspecting the liver. Reproduced from the
BSAVA Manual of Canine and Feline Endoscopy and Endosurgery

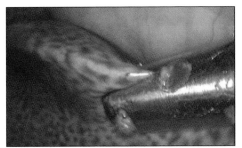

Figure 7: Biopsy of the liver. Reproduced from the *BSAVA Manual of Canine and Feline Endoscopy and Endosurgery*

Coeliotomy

A coeliotomy will also allow good visualisation of the abdominal contents but also allow more detailed investigation of the biliary tree and

vasculature. As with laparoscopy, it is important that the samples collected have sufficient tissue and that not only superficial areas are obtained; a 1 to 2 cm depth is recommended. In cases of diffuse disease, at least two areas should be sampled. If the pathology is localized then 'normal' and 'abnormal' areas should be sampled.

Conclusion

Liver biopsy is essential in the investigation of almost all hepatic diseases. There are several options available to the clinician, with various pros and cons attached to each procedure. Consideration of these points will help make the right decision for each patient and their owner. ∎

PERFORMING A TRU-CUT LIVER BIOPSY

1. Answer the following questions:
   a. Are liver samples deemed necessary?
   b. Considering your differential diagnoses, what information are you expecting to obtain by liver biopsy?
   c. Would it be possible to obtain the same information with cytology? (If so consider performing FNA prior to biopsy.)
   d. Does the patient have significant ascites or microhepatica? (If so consider other techniques.)
   e. Is a vascular anomaly one of the main differentials? (If so consider other potential techniques.)
   f. How many biopsy samples do you think are needed and what are they going to be tested for? (Check with the laboratories the requirements for special tests and make sure the containers needed are available.)
   g. How many biopsy samples do you estimate can be safely obtained in this specific case?
2. Check the clotting times and platelet count no more than 24 hours prior to the procedure.
3. If the clotting times are prolonged delay the procedure; consider administering

parenteral vitamin K1 and rechecking the clotting times 48 hours later.
4. Immediately prior to the biopsy choose the areas to sample using ultrasonography and estimate the number of potential samples that can be safely obtained; remember that representative samples are needed.
5. Make sure that you have all the equipment required (Figure 8).

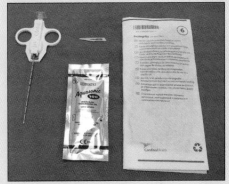

Figure 8: Equipment needed to perform Tru-cut biopsy of the liver (Tru-cut needle, scalpel blade, sterile gloves, sterile ultrasound gel) ➡

PERFORMING A TRU-CUT LIVER BIOPSY

6. Surgically prepare the skin, allowing for generous areas of clipped and scrubbed skin around the entry points.
7. Using a scalpel blade, make a small incision of the skin on the site where the needle will enter the abdomen; the use of sterile gloves is recommended. Special sterile sleeves are available for the ultrasound probes. If these are not available, the probe should be thoroughly cleaned with the scrubbing solution and the operator should be careful to avoid touching the probe with the biopsy needle.
8. Examine the Tru-cut needle for any problems and fire it once outside the patient to make sure it is working appropriately (this is also the time to make sure that you understand fully how the needle works).
9. Re-load the Tru-cut needle and it is then ready to be used (Figure 9).

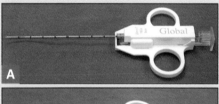

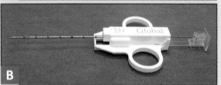

Figure 9: Semi-automatic Tru-cut needle in a neutral position (A) and in a loaded position with the fire-trigger pulled backwards (B)

10. Apply a generous amount of sterile ultrasound gel to the abdomen and, under ultrasound guidance, carefully insert the needle into the liver. Take into account that while with cytology the area sampled is the area where the tip of the needle lies, with Tru-cut needles the area to be sampled lies in front of the tip of the needle (see Figure 4).
11. Double check that there are no important structures in the 2 cm area in front of the needle.
12. Perform the biopsy and withdraw the needle.
13. Open the needle and, with the help of a sterile needle, gently ease the sample into the appropriate container.
14. Using ultrasonography, check for the presence of a significant amount of free fluid, which is likely to indicate significant bleeding, and check the liver parenchyma at the biopsy sites for evidence of active haemorrhage.
15. Repeat the procedure to obtain more samples.

It is a sensible policy to keep the animals hospitalized for a minimum of 12 hours so that the vital parameters can be monitored and, in case of suspicion of bleeding, the abdomen can be examined with ultrasonography.

If there is evidence of bleeding post-biopsy the patient should be closely monitored and the use of fresh frozen plasma should be considered to supply additional clotting factors.

It is uncommon for emergency surgery to be needed due to uncontrolled bleeding after Tru-cut biopsies of the liver unless big vessels were damaged during the procedure.

How to...

Recognise **HAC** in cats

by Andrew Sparkes

There are now published reports of more than 50 cats with spontaneous hyperadrenocorticism (HAC). The vast majority of cats (approximately 85%), as with dogs, have pituitary-dependent HAC, while the remainder have adrenal tumours. Most pituitary-dependent cases seem to arise from microadenomas; adrenal tumours may be either benign or malignant and are usually unilateral. There appears to be no sex or breed predisposition, and the average age at presentation is 10 years (range: approximately 5–15 years).

Clinical signs

The most common clinical sign in cats with HAC is PU/PD (c. 90% of cases); polyphagia, weight loss and lethargy are also common (Figure 1). The PU/PD is often seen as a result of concurrent diabetes mellitus, but some cats with HAC and without diabetes have also been reported to have PU/PD. Common changes on physical examination include an enlarged abdomen (Figure 2), alopecia and skin thinning (Figure 3), muscle atrophy, poor hair coat, hepatomegaly and fragile skin (Figure 4). Some cats with HAC develop folded pinnae.

Diagnosis

Radiography and ultrasonography may reveal unilateral (adrenal tumour) or bilateral

Clinical sign	Approximate frequency (%)
PU/PD	90%
Enlarged abdomen	75%
Polyphagia	70%
Thin skin	45%
Alopecia	40%
Weight loss	35%
Weight gain/obesity	30%
Dry/scurfy coat	30%
Lethargy	30%
Hepatomegaly	30%
Fragile skin	25%

Figure 1: Common signs reported in feline hyperadrenocorticism

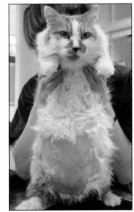

Figure 2: Hyperadrenocorticism in a cat. Note the 'pot-bellied' appearance with thinning of the skin and poor hair coat (the ventral abdomen has been clipped)

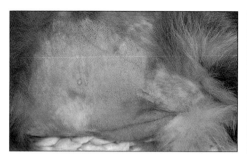

Figure 3: Ventral abdominal skin of patient seen in Figure 4. Subcutaneous blood vessels are clearly evident and the dermal thickness can be seen by looking at the skin crease by the caudal nipple. Courtesy of A. Hibbert

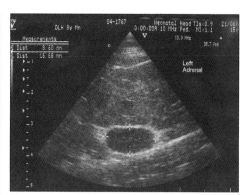

Figure 5: Adrenomegaly documented in the patient seen in Figure 2

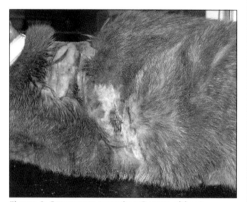

Figure 4: Cutaneous tears in a 6-year-old cat suffering from HAC. Courtesy of A. Hibbert

adrenomegaly (Figure 5), but bilateral adrenomegaly is not invariably seen in cases of pituitary HAC. Calcification of the adrenal glands is not a significant finding in cats, as many older cats can have this as an incidental change. CT or MRI may be valuable in identifying a pituitary tumour and/or adrenomegaly. Hepatomegaly is reported more commonly on radiography (c. 70%) than on clinical examination.

Routine bloodwork is often unremarkable in feline HAC, but lymphopenia is the most common abnormality seen (c. 60% of cases). A classic 'stress leucogram' is not commonly seen.

Hyperglycaemia is a common finding, with around 80% of HAC cats having concurrent diabetes mellitus, some (though not all) being markedly insulin-resistant.

Elevated liver enzymes are seen in around 50% of cases, often (though not always) in association with concurrent diabetes. Cats do not possess the steroid-induced isoenzyme of alkaline phosphatase.

The sensitivity and specificity of laboratory tests for diagnosing feline HAC have not been widely investigated and definitive recommendations and guidelines for interpretation are difficult to provide.

ACTH stimulation test

Retrospective studies suggest that the ACTH stimulation test may have a sensitivity of around 50–80% in feline HAC, with either an elevated basal cortisol and/or an exaggerated post-ACTH cortisol concentration. As in dogs, non-adrenal illness can give false positive responses in an ACTH stimulation test.

The cortisol response to 0.125 µg synthetic ACTH administered intravenously is evaluated. Optimal timing of the post-ACTH sample is difficult to determine and different studies have suggested different times. It may be that cats vary in their responses, creating difficulty in recommending a single post-injection sampling time. We commonly look at basal levels, and then two post-injection samples – one at 60 minutes and one at 120 or 180 minutes.

In healthy cats basal cortisol levels are typically <200 nmol/l, but post-injection cortisol concentrations reach up to around 600 nmol/l (most stimulating to <500 nmol/l).

Dexamethasone screening test

In cats a screening dexamethasone (DXM) suppression test is performed with a 0.1 mg/kg dose of DXM given by intravenous bolus, as there appears to be a very large number of false positive results using a 'standard' dose of 0.01 mg/kg. It has been suggested that up to 80% of HAC cats may fail to show suppression in response to 0.1 mg/kg DXM at 8 hours. However, early or mild cases of HAC may show suppression at that dose.

Dexamethasone suppression test

In cases of confirmed or suspected HAC, a high-dose DXM suppression test can be performed with a dose of 1.0 mg/kg i.v. Failure to show >50% suppression to this dose is suggestive for an adrenal tumour.

Endogenous ACTH

Measuring endogenous ACTH may be a more reliable method for differentiating adrenal from pituitary-dependent HAC. Results are typically in the upper half of the reference range or high in pituitary-dependent disease and low or non-detectable in cases of adrenal tumours.

Urine cortisol to creatinine ratio

As in dogs, measurement of the urine cortisol:creatinine ratio may be a useful screening test to rule out HAC (normal results suggest HAC is very unlikely); however, responses to non-adrenal disease probably make this an unsuitable test for confirming a diagnosis.

A diagnosis of hyperadrenocorticism in cats is most certain when there is supporting clinical and clinicopathological data and there is both an exaggerated response to ACTH and failure of suppression using 0.1 mg/kg DXM i.v.

Drug treatment

Medical therapy for HAC in cats has often been unrewarding, with very unpredictable responses.

Studies in normal cats have suggested that mitotane and ketoconazole are likely to be ineffective in suppressing cortisol synthesis. The use of mitotane in cats with HAC has generally been disappointing, although a few cats have shown suppression of cortisol responses to ACTH and improved clinical signs with higher doses (40–50 mg/kg orally, divided daily). Even when cats do apparently respond, this may take a long time, and may only be a partial response. Similarly, responses to ketoconazole (5–10 mg/kg orally q12h) have at best been partial and side effects are common.

Metyrapone inhibits cortisol synthesis. As with the previous drugs, response has generally been poor, and at best partial (doses of 65 mg/kg orally 2–3 times daily) and toxicity may occur.

Trilostane is an inhibitor of the 3-β-hydroxysteroid dehydrogenase enzyme and reduces synthesis of cortisol, aldosterone and adrenal androgens. It is commonly used to treat HAC in dogs and reports have emerged of its use in cats. From what has been published, although relatively limited numbers of cats have been involved, this appears to be a safe and effective treatment and would currently be regarded as the treatment of choice. A starting oral dose of 30 mg/cat is appropriate, but this can be administered twice daily (and at higher doses if necessary) if initial response is inadequate. Successful therapy will result in improved clinical condition, improved routine blood tests and normalisation of the

ACTH response test. Repeat evaluations at 2–4-week intervals would be appropriate, with dose adjustment as necessary until satisfactory control has been achieved.

Other forms of therapy

Irradiation of pituitary masses has been used but its limited availability severely restricts this treatment modality. It may be most appropriate for management of pituitary macroadenomas.

Unilateral or bilateral adrenalectomy has been used in many cases of feline HAC, though this is not an option to be undertaken lightly and significant perioperative mortality rates have been reported. With careful management this may be a successful form of therapy for both pituitary and adrenal HAC cases, but it should probably be reserved for cases in which trilostane has failed. Cats given

bilateral adrenalectomy will require long-term management for hypoadrenocorticism.

Successful therapy for the HAC may result in resolution of concurrent diabetes mellitus in up to 50% of cases. ■

PROGESTERONE-SECRETING ADRENAL TUMOURS

Rarely, the cause of clinical signs of HAC in a cat may be a progesterone-secreting adrenal tumour rather than a cortisol-secreting tumour. In such cases the results of functional adrenal tests may appear more like those in hypoadrenocorticism. Where clinical signs give rise to suspicion but routine diagnostic tests do not support the diagnosis, assay of serum progesterone levels should be considered. Trilostane therapy may be worth trying in these cases.

How to...

Record an **ECG**

by Nuala Summerfield

What is the ECG?

- The electrocardiogram (ECG) is a recording, taken at the body surface, of the electrical activity occurring within the heart.
- If the patient is not relaxed (e.g. muscle tremors), electrical activity occurring within skeletal muscles will cause interference with the ECG signal.
- Body conformation and body size can affect the ECG.
  - The electrical signal recorded from the body surface will be damped (decreased) in obese animals compared with thin ones.
  - QRS complexes in cats are typically of low amplitude compared with dogs.

Why record an ECG?

- Many canine and feline arrhythmias are hard to discern from auscultation alone, particularly when the patient presents in a critical state.
  - Auscultation may be difficult due to:
    - Fast heart rates
    - Muffled heart sounds
    - Extraneous noise (i.e. harsh lung sounds, panting, growling, purring).
- Arrhythmias are clinically important.
  - Arrhythmias can cause or exacerbate low cardiac output states.
  - You may not be able to resolve congestive heart failure signs without

controlling concurrent arrhythmias.
  - Arrhythmias will contribute to myocardial ischaemia.
- ***The ECG is the only way to diagnose the actual arrhythmia.***
  - N.B. Don't assume all rapid regular rates are sinus tachycardia. Sinus tachycardia cannot be differentiated from ventricular tachycardia by auscultation alone!
- But remember:
  - The ECG is not sensitive in detecting cardiac chamber enlargement (echocardiography and radiography are much more sensitive)
  - The ECG provides no information about the ability of myocardium to contract
  - The ECG provides no information about the heart valves or endocardium
  - The primary role of the ECG is for assessing heart rate and rhythm.

Clinical indications for recording an ECG

- A 'quick' lead II rhythm strip should be performed on all emergency patients to document heart rate and rhythm.
- A diagnostic ECG should be performed in the following patients:
  - If you detect an arrhythmia on auscultation, or you detect pulse deficits:
    - COUNT the heart rate when auscultating your patient, as you will

need the numbers later to judge efficacy of therapy

- Be alerted by patients with heart rates outside the normal range, i.e. too high or too low (e.g. cats in a clinic setting with heart rates <160 bpm when obviously ill or stressed. A cat presenting with CHF and bradycardia is not a good sign!)
- Try always to perform simultaneous auscultation and palpation of femoral pulse, as this will increase your chance of detecting pulse deficits.

- If you detect a heart murmur
- Cardiomegaly on thoracic radiographs
- Collapsing or fainting patient
- Drug effects or toxicities (e.g. digoxin toxicity)
- Electrolyte disturbances (e.g. hyperkalaemia caused by urethral obstruction, hyperadrenocorticism)
- Systemic diseases (e.g. thyrotoxicosis, sepsis)
- During pericardiocentesis
- Monitoring (during anaesthesia, critical care, e.g. GDV, thoracic trauma, raised intracranial pressure).

Recording the ECG

Setting up the ECG machine

- ECGs are typically recorded on special graph paper that is divided into 1 mm² grid-like boxes, with bold divisions every 5 mm in both a vertical and horizontal direction (Figure 1).
- Amplitude (measured in millivolts, mV) is represented on the y axis and time (measured in seconds) on the x axis.
- It is important to know how to adjust paper speed (Figure 2) and sensitivity (Figure 3) to optimise the quality of the ECG recording, to aid the interpretation of arrhythmias and to make it easier to measure ECG intervals accurately.
- For patients with rapid heart rates (e.g. cats), run the ECG at 50 mm/s to 'spread out' the complexes and make it easier to interpret the rhythm.
- High heart rates may obscure the irregularity of the rhythm.
- For patients with small QRS complexes (e.g. cats, patients with pericardial or pleural effusion), increase the amplitude of the ECG to twice sensitivity (20 mm = 1 mV).

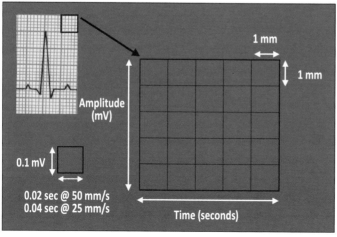

Figure 1: Understanding the ECG paper

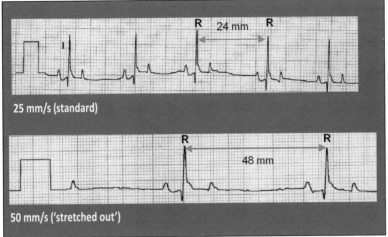

Figure 2: Choosing the paper speed

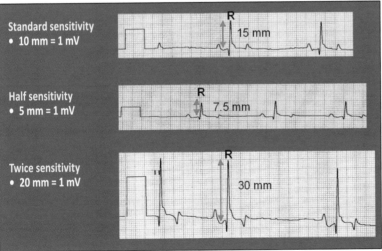

Figure 3: Setting the sensitivity (e.g. R wave = 1.5 mV)

■ For patients with large QRS complexes (e.g. dogs with left ventricular enlargement, or patients with frequent wide bizarre ventricular ectopic complexes), decrease the amplitude of ECG to half sensitivity (5 mm = 1 mV).

Calculating heart rates from the ECG

■ There are various methods that you can use:
  - An ECG ruler is easiest (Figure 4)
  - The instantaneous heart rate method (Figure 5) only works if rhythm is regular.

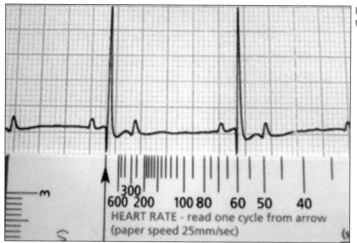

Figure 4: Using an ECG ruler to measure heart rate

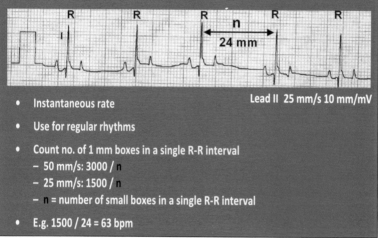

Figure 5: Counting heart rate using the instantaneous method

- Instantaneous rate
- Use for regular rhythms
- Count no. of 1 mm boxes in a single R-R interval
  - 50 mm/s: 3000 / n
  - 25 mm/s: 1500 / n
  - n = number of small boxes in a single R-R interval
- E.g. 1500 / 24 = 63 bpm

Measuring ECG intervals and amplitudes (Figures 6, 7 and 8)

- PR interval:
  - Is measured from the beginning of the P wave to the beginning of the QRS complex
  - It gives information about conduction speed through the AV node

- A prolonged PR interval can indicate that AV conduction is slower than normal (e.g. due to AV node disease/fibrosis or certain drugs such as digoxin).
- QRS duration:
  - Is measured from the beginning to the end of the QRS complex
  - It gives information about ventricular

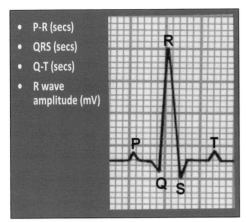

- P-R (secs)
- QRS (secs)
- Q-T (secs)
- R wave amplitude (mV)

Figure 6: Measuring intervals

Duration measured	Canine	Feline
P	<0.04 (<0.05 in giant breeds)	<0.04
PQ	0.06–0.13 (inversely related to heart rate)	0.04–0.09 (inversely related to heart rate)
QRS	<0.05 (<0.06 in giant breeds)	<0.04
QT	0.15–0.25 at normal heart rate	0.12–0.18 at normal heart rate

Figure 7: Standard canine and feline ECG durations in seconds (assumes patient in right lateral recumbency, measurements taken from lead II and no ECG filtering)

Amplitude measured	Canine	Feline
P	<0.4	<0.2
R	<3.0	<0.9
T	<25% of R wave amplitude	<0.3

Figure 8: Standard canine and feline ECG amplitudes in millivolts (assumes patient in right lateral recumbency, measurements taken from lead II and no ECG filtering)

depolarisation, i.e. the conduction speed through the ventricles
- A prolonged QRS duration can indicate delayed conduction through the ventricles (e.g. with ventricular enlargement or a bundle branch block).

■ QT interval:
- Is measured from the beginning of the Q wave to the end of the T wave
- It gives information about the time taken for ventricular depolarisation and repolarisation
- Certain physiological factors and drugs will prolong or shorten the QT interval.

■ R wave amplitude:
- The height of the R wave is measured from the baseline to the highest point of the deflection
- If the R wave is taller than normal it may be due to left ventricular enlargement, and if smaller than normal it can be due to dampening of the electrical signal due to obesity or abnormal accumulations of fluid between the heart and the chest wall.

■ P wave amplitude:
- The height of the P wave is measured from the baseline to the highest point of the deflection
- Tall P waves may be present with right atrial enlargement.

■ P wave duration:
- Is measured from the beginning to the end of the P wave
- It gives information about atrial depolarisation, i.e. the conduction speed through the atria
- A prolonged P wave duration may be present with left atrial enlargement.

Patient positioning and restraint

■ Right lateral recumbency (Figure 9) is the standard position if you want to compare measured ECG intervals with published reference ranges.

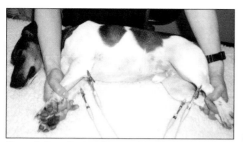

Figure 9: Standard patient positioning and restraint

- Standing or sternal recumbency (Figure 10) may be preferable and safer in stressed or dyspnoeic patients (if only concerned with rhythm diagnosis).
- Place patient on a non-conductive surface to minimise ECG artefact.
- Patient should be comfortable, to minimise struggling, that would produce artefact.
- Right arm of person restraining animal should rest over animal's neck.
- Left arm should rest over hindquarters.
- Legs should be kept parallel with each other but not touching.
- Forelimbs should be kept perpendicular to the long axis of the body.
- With calm, gentle handling, sedation is not usually necessary.

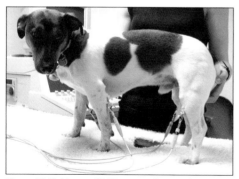

Figure 10: Taking an ECG in a standing position may be preferred in a dyspnoeic or uncooperative patient

- Some drugs (e.g. diazepam and ketamine hydrochloride) have an anti-arrhythmic effect and may mask abnormalities.
- Use flattened crocodile clips – quick and easy to apply:
  - RA attaches to right foreleg
  - LA attaches to left foreleg
  - LL attaches to left hindleg
  - N (neutral/ground lead) attaches to right hindleg.
- Correct clip position (Figure 11):
  - Just below elbows on each forelimb
  - Just below stifles on each hindlimb.
- Flatten or file the jaws of crocodile clips to prevent skin pinching (Figure 12).
- Alternatively, use a less traumatic customised clip such as Comfy Clips (Figure 13).
- Attach clips directly to the skin.
- Moisten skin and electrode.
- Use commercial conductive gel or spirit (gel may be better tolerated by cats than spirit).

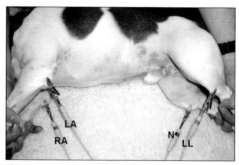

Figure 11: Position of skin electrodes

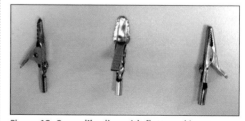

Figure 12: Crocodile clips with flattened jaws

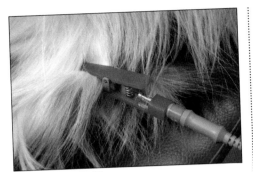

Figure 13: Comfy Clips

Identifying interference and artefacts

- Incorrect lead placement:
  - If ECG complexes in leads I, II, III and aVF are not predominantly positive, check that leads are attached to correct legs – if lead placement is correct, then an axis deviation is present (e.g. with significant right ventricular enlargement (dilation or concentric hypertrophy), deep S waves may be present in leads I, II, III and aVF which will give the QRS complexes in these leads the appearance of having a predominantly negative polarity. This suspicion should be followed up with echocardiography or radiography to confirm the ECG finding).
- Lead dislodgement.

- Muscle tremor:
  - Make sure the patient is comfortable to minimise struggling.
- Electrical interference (Figure 14):
  - Turn off all electrical equipment in the room (e.g. fluid pumps, heat blankets).
- Breathing artefacts (Figure 15):
  - Ensure no leads are resting on the chest, and that clips are attached to limbs at correct sites, away from torso.
- Purring (Figure 16):
  - Tricks to stop cats purring (if only temporarily!) include turning the tap on, blowing gently on their nose, and passing a cotton wool ball soaked in spirit under their nose. ■ © Nuala Summerfield

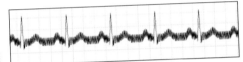

Figure 14: Electrical interference artefact

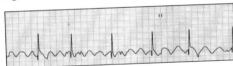

Figure 15: Breathing/panting artefact

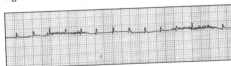

Figure 16: Purring artefact

How to...

Get the best from
fluid therapy

by Simon Tappin

I ntravenous fluid therapy is essential for many of our patients and yet often does not get as much care and attention as it perhaps deserves. Cases requiring fluid therapy fall into acute and chronic groups. Acute cases will be in circulatory shock, as a result of hypovolaemic, distributive, cardiogenic or obstructive shock. Chronic cases will be cardiovascularly stable but require therapy to restore or maintain their fluid balance.

For patients to get the most benefit from fluid therapy it is important we think carefully about why fluid therapy is required, how much is needed, which fluid would be best and what route of administration would be most appropriate.

Which fluid is best?

In almost all situations when animals are dehydrated or in shock, giving fluid of any type is better than giving none at all. The fluids available fall into two categories: crystalloids (electrolyte solutions) and colloids (containing osmotically active large macromolecules). Certain fluids are therefore better than others in specific situations; for example, colloids might be considered in hypoproteinaemic patients (<40 g/l), whilst crystalloids might be most useful in patients that are dehydrated.

Oxygen carrier fluids are most useful in anaemic patients (PCV <25%) and are not discussed further here. Care needs to be taken in some circumstances (for example, in animals with pulmonary contusion, head trauma and heart disease) as aggressive fluid therapy can cause adverse effects.

Crystalloids

Crystalloids are electrolyte solutions and are classified according to their tonicity and the electrolytes they contain (Figure 1).

Hypotonic solutions

Great care should be taken when administering hypotonic fluids, such as 0.18% NaCl and 4% dextrose, because although at administration the osmolality is fairly equivalent to serum (264 mOsm/l), the dextrose is rapidly metabolised, leaving an extremely hypotonic fluid. In essence, administration of 0.18% NaCl and 4% dextrose is effectively administration of free water. This can cause a marked drop in serum tonicity, which can lead to severe changes in electrolytes (especially hypokalaemia) and the potential for life-threatening cerebral oedema.

It is important to remember that there are specific indications for giving hypotonic fluid, such as to replace a free water deficit (e.g. hypernatraemia) or ongoing and uncontrolled free water loss (e.g. diabetes insipidus). When using hypotonic solutions to treat

Fluid	Na⁺ (mmol/l)	K⁺ (mmol/l)	Ca²⁺ (mmol/l)	Cl⁻ (mmol/l)	HCO₃⁻ (mmol/l)	Dextrose (g/l)	Osmolarity (mOsm/l)	pH
0.45% NaCl	77			77			155	5
0.9% NaCl	154			154			308	5
7.2% NaCl	1232			1232			2464	5
Ringer's solution	147	4	2	156			310	5.5
Hartmann's or lactated Ringer's solution	130	5	2	111	29		280	6.5
0.18% NaCl + 4% dextrose	31			31		40	264	4

Figure 1: The electrolyte composition of the most commonly available crystalloid solutions

hypernatraemia, the fluid administration rate should be tailored so that sodium levels fall by 0.5–1 mmol/l/h, and be closely adjusted to the patient's response (Figure 2). Apart from these specific indications, 0.18% NaCl and 4% dextrose solution is rarely used in small animal practice. It should not be administered to treat hypoglycaemia: glucose supplementation of isotonic fluids is much better suited to this purpose.

Isotonic solutions

Hartmann's solution and normal (physiological) saline (0.9% NaCl) are the

---

Change in serum sodium $= \dfrac{\text{Infusate [Na}^+] - \text{Serum [Na}^+]}{\text{(bodyweight (kg)} \times 0.6) + 1}$

This equation can be used to predict the effects of infusing various fluids

Example: A 30 kg Golden Retriever has a serum sodium level of 196 mmol/l. This needs correcting but cannot be done faster than 0.5 mmol/l/hour

Thus, using 0.9% NaCl (sodium content = 154 mmol/l): $\dfrac{[154 - 194]}{(30 \times 0.6 + 1)} = -2.2$

Each litre of 0.9% NaCl administered decreases the serum sodium level by 2.2 mmol/l

Thus infusing 0.9% NaCl at a rate of 227 [(1000/2.2) × 0.5] will reduce plasma sodium by 0.5 mmol/l/hour

Fluid	Sodium content
5% glucose solution	0 mmol/l
4% dextrose and 0.18% NaCl	31 mmol/l
0.45% NaCl	77 mmol/l
Hartmann's solution	130 mmol/l
0.9% NaCl	154 mmol/l

Figure 2: Serum sodium needs to be reduced very gradually in hypernatraemic animals. Changes can be estimated using the above equation

most commonly used isotonic solutions in veterinary practice. After volume resuscitation with isotonic solutions there is no large concentration gradient between the vasculature and the interstitum, so large water shifts do not occur. However, isotonic solutions do equilibrate with the interstitial fluid and only 25% of the infused volume remains in the vasculature after 30 minutes. These fluids are therefore referred to as *replacement* fluids, although they are also commonly used as *maintenance* fluids to maintain hydration in hospitalised patients.

One of the major differences between 0.9% NaCl and Hartmann's solution is the presence of bicarbonate in Hartmann's, which acts as a buffer. This can be useful when performing volume resuscitation in acidotic patients, as the plasma pH returns to normal more rapidly. This has particularly been shown in blocked cats with acidosis and hyperkalaemia. Traditionally, potassium-containing fluids such as Hartmann's have been contraindicated because of the hyperkalaemia; however, the amount of potassium in the solution is minimal (5 mmol/l) and studies comparing fluid resuscitation with 0.9% NaCl and Hartmann's revealed similar rates of return to normokalaemia, but with much faster resolution of the acidosis.

In addition to the lack of buffer, 0.9% NaCl is an acidifying fluid due to the high chloride content. This can be useful in patients with hypochloraemic metabolic acidosis, which is usually the result of vomiting. Lactate-containing fluids (such as Hartmann's) are useful in very young hypoglycaemic animals, which can rapidly utilise lactate as an energy source, but are best avoided in animals with liver disease and diabetic ketoacidosis because of their decreased ability to convert lactate to bicarbonate.

Potassium supplementation should be considered when using either Hartmann's or normal saline intravenously. Whilst Hartmann's

contains a small amount of potassium, this does not meet the daily needs of most patients. Daily requirements are usually achieved by the addition of potassium chloride to 0.9% NaCl (Figure 3). The same guidelines can be used to calculate the supplement to be added to Hartmann's solution, with an adjustment for the amount of potassium already present (5 mmol/l).

Serum potassium (mmol)	Amount of KCl to add to 250 ml 0.9% NaCl (mmol)
<2	20
2–2.5	15
2.5–3	10
3–3.5	7

Figure 3: Serum potassium can be supplemented by the addition of KCl to intravenous fluid therapy. Care needs to be taken not to exceed 0.5 mmol/kg/h, which can cause thrombophlebitis

Hypertonic solutions

Administration of a small volume of hypertonic saline (usually 7.2–7.4% NaCl) creates a large osmotic gradient, which draws water from the interstitial and intracellular compartments into the vasculature. This leads to a very rapid expansion of the circulating vascular volume. Use of a low volume of hypertonic saline is extremely useful when rapid volume expansion is required; for example, in giant-breed dogs where administering large volumes of crystalloid quickly can be difficult, or where the catheter site or size precludes rapid fluid administration.

Typically 4 ml/kg of hypertonic fluid is administered over a 3–5 minute period, which produces a haemodynamic effect equivalent to an isotonic crystalloid dose of 60–90 ml. Care is needed in patient selection and the administration of hypertonic saline should be avoided in those with cardiac disease, that are dehydrated and that have uncontrolled haemorrhage (e.g. pulmonary contusions). The sodium rapidly diffuses from the vasculature, with its effects reducing within 30–60 minutes. Following hypertonic fluid administration, careful and appropriate ongoing fluid therapy is needed, often at a higher level than anticipated to replace the 'borrowed' interstitial and intracellular fluid.

Numerous other beneficial effects have been associated with the administration of hypertonic saline, including: reduced endothelial cell swelling; immunomodulation via decreased leucocyte adhesion; decreased blood viscosity; and improved cardiac contractility. All may play a role in improving the outcome of patients in hypovolaemic shock.

Artificial colloids

Colloids contain macromolecules, which do not readily cross vascular barriers and therefore increase the plasma colloidal osmotic pressure (COP). This increases the osmotic gradient between the vasculature and the interstitial space. As a result fluid is retained in the vascular space, increasing the circulating volume until the molecules are broken down. Thus, colloids are more efficient than crystalloids in maintaining the circulating volume in the hours following administration (Figure 4).

There are two types of colloids available in the United Kingdom: gelatins and hydroxyethyl starches. All artificial colloids have a mixture of molecules ranging in molecular weight; this size range is more variable for the hydroxyethyl starches than the gelatins. Gelatins are produced from bovine collagen and have average molecular weights in the region of 30–35 kD (albumin by comparison has a molecular weight of 69 kD). Hydroxyethyl starches are derived from the branched plant starch amylopectin and have high molecular weights, between 200 and 450 kD depending on the product. In general the larger the size of the colloidal molecules, the longer the product remains in the circulation.

The initial action of vascular expansion after colloid administration is due to the number of molecules infused rather than their size or charge. As such, small molecules (e.g. gelatins) have a rapid effect on the COP and act quickly to hold fluid in the vascular space. However, they are excreted or extravasated within a few hours. Large molecules (e.g. hydroxyethyl starches) remain in the circulation for much longer and are removed by either the monocyte phagocytic system or broken down by plasma enzymes. Hydroxyethyl starches, which contain a range of molecules of different sizes, have an exponentially declining action on the COP, as the small molecules are cleared quickly and the larger ones more slowly.

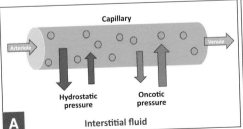
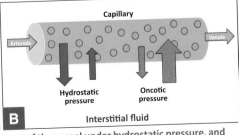

Figure 4: (A) On entering the capillary bed water moves out of the vessel under hydrostatic pressure, and returns from the interstitial space via osmotic pressure. In the normal animal the same amount of water leaves the capillary. (B) By infusing colloids the oncotic pressure within the vasculature goes up, increasing the amount of water moving into the capillary. This expands the circulating blood volume

Use of colloids has been associated with coagulation abnormalities in humans and these have also been documented in experimental studies in dogs where factor VIII and von Willebrand factor levels are reduced further than expected by dilution alone. It is controversial as to whether clinically significant effects on coagulation occur; however, most authors suggest limiting colloid usage to 20 ml/kg/day. Although generally considered very safe, all forms of colloid have been associated with anaphylactic reactions in humans; these reactions are very rare in veterinary patients.

Albumin

Human albumin, purified from human plasma, has been used to improve the COP in human patients for many years. As well as providing increased COP, albumin acts as a carrier for hormones, drugs and a wide variety of other substances such as fatty acids and bilirubin. Albumin can be provided to dogs in fresh or stored frozen plasma, and to both dogs and cats as part of a whole blood transfusion; however, the amount of albumin that can be transfused is limited due to its relatively low concentration in the plasma. For example, a unit of fresh frozen plasma (250 ml from a donor animal with a serum albumin concentration of 30 g/l) will only contain approximately 7 g of albumin, thus using plasma alone or whole blood transfusions to provide COP is very inefficient.

In contrast human albumin has been used in critically ill veterinary patients with some success. Purified human albumin is commercially available in much higher concentrations (20–25%) than is present in harvested plasma, meaning significant changes to the COP can be made (Figure 5). As human albumin is only 79% homologous to canine albumin, hypersensitivity reactions

Albumin deficit (g) = [Desired albumin (g/l) – patient albumin (g/l)] x bodyweight (kg) x 0.3

Thus, in a 20 kg dog to increase plasma albumin levels from 10 g/l to 20 g/l requires:

[20 – 10] x 20 x 0.3 = 60 g of albumin

Fresh plasma contains 30 g albumin/litre
thus, 60 g of albumin = 2 litres or 8 units of plasma

25% human albumin contains 250 g albumin/litre
thus, 60 g albumin = 240 ml of 25% human albumin

Figure 5: Albumin deficit can be calculated using the above equation and changes in response to fluid administration predicted. This example highlights that giving fresh frozen plasma is a poor way to supplement albumin

and the production of anti-human antibodies, have been reported. These adverse effects can be very serious, prompting the cautious use of human albumin in cases only where synthetic colloids have not had the desired effect.

How much to give?

How much fluid to administer depends on the requirements and clinical status of the patient.

- A well hydrated animal with good circulation will only require fluid to replace expected losses (maintenance requirements). This may be provided orally, but when intravenous fluids are used generally equates to around 50 ml/kg/day. This volume is increased appropriately to cover the increased losses during episodes of vomiting, diarrhoea, pyrexia or panting.
- Dehydrated patients that are cardiovascularly stable should have their fluid deficit estimated from clinical examination findings (Figure 6). The calculated deficit should be replaced over a 24-hour period. Generally 50% is replaced in the first 6 hours with the remaining 50% over the following 18 hours (Figure 7).

Percentage dehydration	Clinical signs
<5%	No detectable signs ↑ Urine SG
5–6%	Subtle loss of skin elasticity
6–8%	Marked loss of skin elasticity Slight ↑ in CRT Slightly sunken eyes Dry mucous membranes
10–12%	Standing skin tent Prolonged CRT Sunken eyes and protruding third eyelids Signs of circulatory shock
12–15%	Severe shock, coma and death

Figure 6: Clinical signs expected at varying degrees of dehydration

A 10 kg dog presents with a 3-day history of profuse vomiting and diarrhoea. He has a heart rate of 180 bpm, poor pulse quality and pale mucous membranes (i.e. signs of hypovolaemia). He also has tacky mucous membranes and reduced skin turgor (i.e. signs of dehydration – estimated at 7%). An emergency database shows haemoconcentration, prerenal azotemia and normal electrolytes.

At presentation he received a 20 ml/kg bolus of Hartmann's solution over 10 minutes, resulting in normalisation of the heart rate and an improvement in pulse quality.

The remaining volume to be replaced is calculated as: % dehydration x bodyweight = 700 ml.

The long term plan would be as follows:

- Replace 350 ml over 6 hrs = 60 ml/hour + maintenance = 80 ml/hour for 6 hrs
- Replace 350 ml over the next 18 hrs = 20 ml/hour + maintenance = 40 ml/hour for 18 hrs
- Remember to increase the rate to compensate for any ongoing losses
- Maintenance = 50 ml/kg/24h

Figure 7: An example fluid plan for a dog with gastrointestinal signs leading to dehydration and hypovolaemia

■ Animals that have signs of poor perfusion or circulatory shock (e.g. poor peripheral pulse quality, tachycardia, slow CRT and reduced mentation) need fluid more quickly, which leads to the concept of shock rate fluids. Historically, shock rate fluids are suggested as 80 ml/kg for dogs and 60 ml/kg for cats; these figures come from the equivalent blood volumes. However, as the primary aim of treating shock is to improve tissue perfusion, these values are not really that helpful in determining the exact amount of fluid needed to improve the patient.

An alternative approach is to infuse a bolus (e.g. 10–20 ml/kg) of crystalloid rapidly over a 10 minute period and monitor the patient closely. The response to this fluid resuscitation can be dramatic and often cardiovascular parameters improve; if they do not, a second or third crystalloid bolus can be given and the patient monitored in the same way.

If crystalloid therapy alone does not lead to an improvement, then this can be followed by boluses of colloids (5 ml/kg boluses administered over 10–20 minute periods). Once the patient is judged to be adequately volume resuscitated (based on improvement in the clinical parameters), ongoing fluid therapy can be determined. Boluses of fluid can be given quickly by squeezing the fluid bag or by using a pressure infuser, drip pump or syringe driver to give a calibrated volume.

How to give it?

Fluids can be given by a number of different routes and the method chosen will depend upon the severity and nature of the underlying clinical disorder. In well but dehydrated animals, oral fluid administration can be very successful. However, this route should not be used in animals in shock or with gastrointestinal disease, where direct expansion of the intravascular space is required.

- Subcutaneous administration of fluids is a convenient way to deliver maintenance requirements, but should not be used in shocked or severely dehydrated patients due to peripheral vasoconstriction. The subcutaneous space in both dogs and cats can accommodate relatively large volumes of fluid; the volume is limited by skin elasticity. Fairly high concentrations of potassium (up to 35 mmol/l) have been tolerated without irritation, but glucose-containing fluids should be avoided due to possible electrolyte imbalances and water shifts.

- Intraperitoneal administration allows moderately quick absorption of relatively large volumes of fluid. Only isotonic solutions should be used to prevent peritoneal fluid shifts. This route is most often used in neonatal puppies where warmed fluids can help raise the core temperature.

- Intravenous administration is preferred where possible as precise volumes of fluid can be given quickly to effect.

Several peripheral sites can be used for intravenous catheter placement, with the cephalic vein being the most common. Other sites (which are often overlooked) include the lateral saphenous vein in the dog, the medial saphenous vein in the cat and the marginal ear veins. Peripheral catheters are limited by the size that can be placed in the vein, thus administering high volumes of fluid rapidly can be difficult.

Resistance is a function of the catheter length and diameter, thus, for high flow the widest, shortest catheter should be placed and in some animals more than one catheter may be needed. Care should be taken when infusing fluids with a high osmolality (>5% glucose solution) and fluids containing high levels of potassium as these risk thrombophlebitis.

Placement of a central line (usually a jugular vein catheter) offers a number of advantages over peripheral catheters in appropriate patients. Firstly, a large bore catheter can be used, which allows high flow rates and rapid fluid administration. Secondly, catheters are available with multiple lumens, which allows the administration of multiple fluids (e.g. parenteral nutrition and maintenance fluids) as well as blood samples to be taken easily.

Thirdly, central lines terminate in the cranial or caudal vena cava and so allow measurement of central venous pressure (for example, through a dedicated channel of a multi-lumen catheter). Lastly, due to the dilutional effect of infused fluid entering a larger blood volume, higher osmolality fluids (>600 mOsm/l) can be administered safely centrally which cannot be given with confidence peripherally. Jugular catheters are usually placed using a Seldinger technique and many kits are commercially available (Figure 8). In small patients or in emergency situations (e.g. cardiopulmonary arrests) long over-the-needle catheters can be placed relatively easily for temporary venous access.

- Intraosseous is a very useful route for fluid and drug administration as fluids rapidly access the vasculature via the bone marrow sinusoids and medullary venous channels. This technique is most useful in neonatal patients and in those where peripheral perfusion is so poor that peripheral catheter placement is difficult (Figure 9). Several sites are possible, with the great tubercle of the humerus, trochanteric fossa of the femur and the ilial wing being easiest to access. Commercial kits are available, allowing placement in a similar manner to the technique used for performing a bone marrow biopsy. In very small patients hypodermic needles can be used with some success.

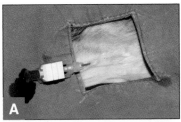

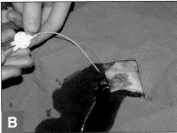

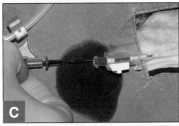

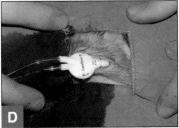

Figure 8: Jugular catheters are most often placed using a Seldinger technique. This allows a longer catheter to be placed than would be possible using an over-the-needle technique. A stylet is used to gain access to the vessel (A), through which a soft wire is placed (B). A firm conical dilator is then passed over the wire into the vessel to create a path for the catheter, which is then advanced over the wire (C). Once in position the wire is withdrawn and the catheter sutured in place (D). Reproduced from the *BSAVA Manual of Canine and Feline Emergency and Critical Care, 2nd edition*

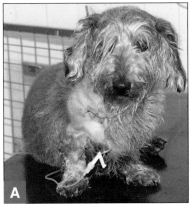

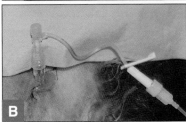

Figure 9: This dog has immune-mediated thrombocytopenia and as a result it was very difficult to place a peripheral catheter. An intraosseous catheter was well tolerated and allowed both the administration of medication and a blood transfusion

Conclusions

Administration of fluid therapy is undertaken on a daily basis in small animal practice by the majority of practitioners. By selecting the correct fluid type, administering it at the appropriate rate, and familiarising oneself with alternative methods of administration, individual patients can gain the maximum benefit from this relatively simple therapy. ∎

How to...

Perform effective cardiopulmonary resuscitation

by Simon Tappin

Unexpected cardiopulmonary arrests are generally very stressful situations; thus, good knowledge and preparation in the hope we don't ever need to use this equipment and these skills is essential. Full cardiopulmonary arrest (CPA) is defined as the sudden cessation of spontaneous and effective respiration and circulation.

Cardiopulmonary cerebral resuscitation (CPCR) provides circulatory and respiratory support, during efforts to produce the return of spontaneous circulation. Although published survival rates in veterinary patients following CPCR are low (around 5–10%), it is obvious from these studies that patients fall into two categories: those that arrest due to irreversible causes (i.e. as the end stage of their disease) and those that have reversible causes such as anaesthetic overdoses or electrolyte imbalances. Consideration should therefore be given to whether CPCR is appropriate for all patients. However, where reversible causes are present CPCR can be very rewarding.

Preparation and teamwork

Successful CPCR relies on good preparation and teamwork. Ideally there should be access to a well stocked crash box, containing all the likely equipment required to run a successful resuscitation attempt (Figures 1, 2 and 3).

Team members should have practiced the necessary techniques so that CPCR can be initiated as rapidly as possible.

To perform effective CPCR ideally at least three team members are needed: one is responsible for ventilation, a second for chest compressions, and a third for monitoring and administration of drugs. Because compressions are hard work, changing operator every 2–3 minutes is essential. It is very difficult, if not impossible, to perform

- Endotracheal tubes (all sizes)
- Laryngoscope with variety of blades
- Gauze bandage for securing endotracheal tubes
- Ambu bag or easily accessible anaesthetic machine with appropriate circuit
- Intravenous catheters and tape for securing them
- Heparinised saline
- Needles and syringes
- Urinary catheters (for airway suction and intratracheal drug administration)
- Scalpel blades, suture and sterile surgical kit
- Adrenaline, atropine and lidocaine (with doses drawn up in labelled syringes)
- Chart of commonly used drugs and doses
- Fluids and giving sets
- Alcohol and antiseptic scrub solutions
- Other drugs to consider: calcium gluconate, diazepam, mannitol, furosemide, dexamethasone
- Advanced equipment: tracheostomy tubes, interosseous needles, ECG, defibrillator

Figure 1: Basic crash box equipment

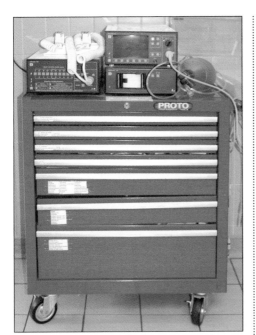

Figure 2: Crash trolley with all necessary equipment for effective CPCR

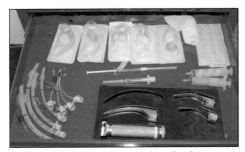

Figure 3: Equipment within crash trolley for securing an airway

effective CPCR alone, though the provision of chest compressions alone may prevent hypoxia in the short term until help arrives. Where practical, on discovery of the arrest the animal should be moved on to a suitable firm surface, in a well lit and accessible area.

Causes of cardiopulmonary arrest

There are many possible causes of cardiopulmonary arrest (Figure 4). In most cases respiratory arrest will precede full CPA. Thus, timely intervention to assist and improve ventilation (e.g. administration of oxygen, drainage of pleural fluid or pneumothorax) may prevent the development of a full cardiac arrest.

- Hypovolaemia
- Hypoxia
- Acidosis
- Potassium imbalances
- Hypothermia
- Anaesthetic overdoses
- Cardiac tamponade
- Tension pneumothorax
- Thrombosis of the coronary/pulmonary arteries
- Vasovagal syncope

Figure 4: Causes of cardiopulmonary arrest

A relatively common cause of CPA in veterinary medicine is vasovagal syncope. Although it can be easily treated, it is potentially fatal if not recognised. Brachycephalic breeds of dog in particular often have high vagal tone and slow heart rates. Physiological events such as vomiting can increase the vagal tone further, causing bradycardia and, potentially, cardiac arrest. Timely treatment with low-dose atropine (0.004–0.01 mg/kg) can increase the heart rate and prevent progression to CPA.

Basic life support

Basic life support (described by the mnemonic ABC – Airway, Breathing, Circulation) consists of establishing an airway, providing positive pressure ventilation and generating effective circulation. Alone, this may allow the return of spontaneous circulation, and once in place allows advanced life support such as drug therapy.

Airway

The first priority is to establish a patent airway. In most situations this is best achieved by the placement of a cuffed endotracheal tube (Figure 5). The tube is ideally placed under direct visualisation with a laryngoscope, as this helps reduce bradycardia induced by overstimulation of the epiglottis, and allows removal of any obstructive extraneous material. Correct endotracheal tube placement can be confirmed by visualisation, cervical palpation (i.e. the absence of a palpable tube in the oesophagus) and appropriate chest wall excursion with ventilation.

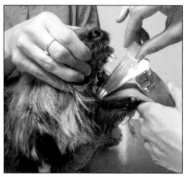

Figure 5: Intubation with a cuffed endotracheal tube is essential for positive pressure ventilation. Use of a laryngoscope ensures optimal visualisation. Reproduced from *BSAVA Manual of Canine and Feline Anaesthesia and Analgesia, 2nd edition*

A positive end-tidal carbon dioxide (ETCO$_2$) measurement suggests good tube placement; however, in CPA initial ETCO$_2$ may be very low due to poor perfusion. If laryngeal visualisation is difficult, suction may be needed to clear excessive fluid from the oropharynx. If endotracheal intubation is difficult, a stylet may help strengthen the tube or a stiff dog urinary catheter may be used to intubate the larynx and the endotracheal tube slid over the catheter (Figure 6). If intubation is impossible a tracheostomy is required, either using a 14 G needle or over-the-needle catheter as a temporary means of airway access (Figure 7) or by placement of a tracheostomy tube following surgical cut down.

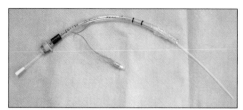

Figure 6: If intubation is difficult a stiff dog urinary catheter can be placed through the larynx and used to guide an endotracheal tube

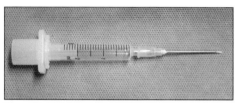

Figure 7: A wide needle attached to a syringe hub allows temporary bypass of the upper respiratory tract

Breathing

Once an airway is established, providing positive pressure ventilation with 100% oxygen is the ideal. If an oxygen supply is not readily available then room air (~20% oxygen) will be adequate for CPR. An Ambu bag (Figure 8) is a good way to provide positive pressure ventilation; however, any re-breathing bag attached to an anaesthetic circuit can be used, as long as it is purged of all anaesthetic gases before use. A ventilatory rate of 8–12 breaths/minute is appropriate in

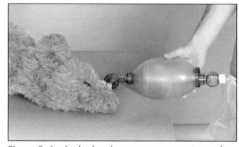

Figure 8: An Ambu bag is a very easy way to apply positive pressure ventilation

most patients, although smaller patients and those that were previously hypoxic may require a higher rate (12–20 bpm). Positive pressure ventilation should produce a normal degree of chest excursion, with even inflation and relaxation over a 2-second period.

When providing ventilation the chest wall should be seen to move; if it does not, then the endotracheal tube may be blocked, incorrectly placed or there may be thoracic disease stopping chest expansion (for example, pleural space disease). Action, such as thoracic auscultation ± thoracocentesis, is required rapidly to determine and rectify the cause. Ventilation should not be over-forceful or barotrauma of the lungs, haemorrhage and pneumothorax can occur. Overzealous (rapid) ventilation causing hypocapnia can reduce cerebral perfusion whereas prolonged long inspiratory times can increase intrathoracic pressure, reducing venous return.

If spontaneous ventilation resumes at this stage, a full CPA may have been avoided. In a respiratory arrest acupuncture of the Jen Chung (GV26) point could be considered. Insertion and twisting a 25 G hypodermic needle inserted to bone depth in the midline of the nasal philtrum below the nares, has been shown to increase respiratory rate (Figure 9). Reversal agents for drugs that cause apnoea may also be appropriate. Doxapram should be avoided as it decreases cerebral blood flow and leads to increased oxygen requirements.

Circulation

Generating circulation by effective chest compressions is an essential component of successful CPCR. Compressions aim to supply adequate perfusion to the heart, brain and lungs until the return of spontaneous circulation. Effective compressions are hard work, as the chest wall should be compressed by at least 25–33%. The aim is to provide a compression rate of 80–120/minute, with an even duration of compression and decompression. Interruptions to compressions should be avoided, as it takes time to generate forward momentum within the circulation. Thus, compressions should be continued during ventilation. Other interruptions such as to change operators or observe ECG changes, or palpate arterial pulses should be minimised as much as possible.

There are several methods for performing chest compressions. In cats and small dogs (<10 kg) the cardiac pump technique is suggested; this generates forward movement of blood by direct compression applied over the heart (Figure 10). In larger dogs, or if the cardiac pump is ineffective, the thoracic pump

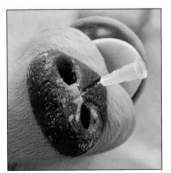

Figure 9: A needle placed in the Jen Chung acupuncture point may stimulate breathing in a respiratory arrest

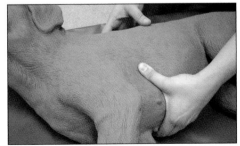

Figure 10: The cardiac pump method of chest compressions applies pressure directly over the heart and is suitable for cats and dogs up to 10 kg

technique should be used. This generates forward movement of blood by compression over the widest part of the chest, with the dog in lateral recumbency (Figure 11).

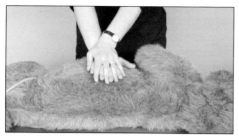

Figure 11: The thoracic pump method of chest compressions applies pressure at the widest point of the thorax and is suitable for large dogs

Open-chest CPCR is very effective in generating forward circulation and should be considered in larger dogs (>20 kg), especially if closed-chest CPCR is not generating effective forward movement of blood. It should also be considered in animals with pleural space disease, pericardial effusion or chest wall trauma. To perform open-chest CPCR a rapid left-sided lateral thoracotomy is performed in the 6th intercostal space to allow direct compression of the heart, between two hands placed within the thoracic cavity. Cross-clamping the aorta can also be considered to direct forward blood flow to the brain. In human emergency medicine there is a relatively low rate of cardiac trauma and infection after open-chest CPCR; however, if successful, it is recommended that the chest is lavaged thoroughly, samples are collected for culture and the incision is closed aseptically. Discussing with owners whether open-chest CPCR is appropriate or desired in ill patients allows this invasive procedure to be executed rapidly should the need arise.

Advanced life support

Once effective basic life support is established, more advanced and specific treatment, such as drugs and defibrillation can be considered to restore spontaneous circulation or to correct the underlying cause of the CPCR. If possible an ECG should be placed as soon as possible after CPA as it will allow identification of the underlying arrest rhythm and dictate drug therapy.

In small animals the most common arrest rhythms are:

1. *Asystole* – most commonly seen in traumatized, hypoxic or anaesthestised patients, carries a poor prognosis but should be treated with aggressive CPCR and adrenaline.
2. *Pulseless electrical activity* (PEA, previously known as electromechanical dissociation or EMD) – occurs when the ECG records normal electrical activity within the heart but there is little or no myocardial contractility. Anaesthetic overdose, acute hypoxia, acidosis, toxicity and cardiogenic shock are potential causes of PEA. Again, treatment with CPCR and adrenaline is recommended.
3. *Ventricular fibrillation* – much less common as an arrest rhythm in small animals in comparison to humans, in whom it occurs in about two thirds of arrests. Ventricular fibrillation leads to random activity within the ventricles, thus producing no propulsive ventricular contraction. Ventricular fibrillation can only be distinguished from PEA by observation of an ECG trace. Effective treatment requires defibrillation, which is best applied electrically via a defibrillator (Figure 12). This requires specialist training and equipment which is not readily available. Alternatively, in such circumstances mechanical defibrillation in the form of a forceful precordial thump over the heart base may allow the myocardium to return to a perfusing rhythm.

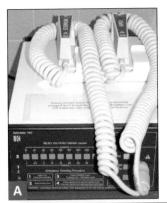

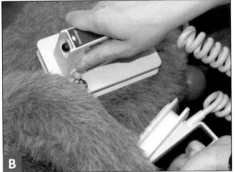

Figure 12: (A) An external defibrillator. (B) The external defibrillator paddles in place, aiming to cover at least a third of the myocardium

Drugs

Drugs can be given by a variety of routes.

1. Central venous access offers the quickest delivery to the central circulation.
2. Peripheral venous access is adequate, as long as drugs are followed by a large volume flush to move the drug into the central circulation.
3. Intraosseous uptake of drugs is very rapid and placement of an interosseous needle is relatively straightforward. These can be easier to place than a peripheral catheter in a patient with poor perfusion.
4. Drugs, with the exception of bicarbonate, can also be administered via a urinary catheter placed into the trachea through the endotracheal tube. Dosages of drugs should be doubled if this route is used and followed by a large ventilation; this helps move the drug into the alveoli, allowing uptake into the pulmonary circulation.

Where possible, drugs such as adrenaline (epinephrine) and atropine are kept drawn up in the crash box in doses appropriate for 10 kg patients (Figure 13). This avoids the

Drug	Dose	Volume required according to bodyweight					
		5 kg	10 kg	20 kg	30 kg	40 kg	50 kg
Adrenaline (low-dose) 1:10000 (0.1 mg/ml)	0.01 mg/kg	0.5 ml	1 ml	2 ml	3 ml	4 ml	5 ml
Adrenaline (high-dose) 1:1000 (1 mg/ml)	0.1 mg/kg	0.5 ml	1 ml	2 ml	3 ml	4 ml	5 ml
Atropine (0.6 mg/ml)	0.04 mg/kg	0.3 ml	0.7 ml	1.4 ml	2.1 ml	2.8 ml	3.5 ml
Lidocaine (20 mg/ml)	2 mg/kg	0.5 ml	1 ml	2 ml	3 ml	4 ml	5 ml
Bicarbonate 1 mEq/ml	1 mEq/kg	5 ml	10 ml	20 ml	30 ml	40 ml	50 ml

Figure 13: Veterinary CPR drugs

need for calculation and preparation of these drugs during stressful situations and appropriate doses can be given rapidly (Figure 14). There are no fixed guidelines for the stability and sterility of drugs once drawn up into syringes; however, replacing them every 2–4 weeks is recommended.

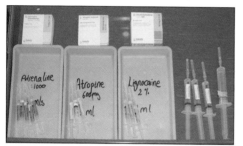

Figure 14: Drugs drawn up into 10 kg doses within the crash box

Adrenaline has effects on α-adrenergic receptors, causing peripheral vasoconstriction, increasing blood pressure and blood flow to the head, and β-adrenergic receptors increasing heart rate and contractility. Adrenaline is recommended for the initial treatment of asystole and PEA. In human medicine there is controversy as to whether high- or low-dose adrenaline is superior. High-dose adrenaline is associated with better short-term outcomes; however, it increases myocardial oxygen demand, which is detrimental when oxygen delivery is limited during, and immediately, after a CPA. In general, low-dose adrenaline is suggested in the first instance, moving to high doses if there is a lack of response.

Atropine is a vagolytic drug which is useful to treat sinus bradycardia, third-degree AV block or increased vagal tone. Cautious dosing is advised as it can cause a marked rebound tachycardia which will increase myocardial oxygen demand.

Many **other drugs** are useful in specific circumstances, such as lidocaine for

management of post-resuscitation ventricular tachycardia, sodium bicarbonate for severe metabolic acidosis and specific anaesthetic antagonists. Once heart rate and rhythm and a peripheral pulse have been restored, arterial blood flow may be maintained with dopamine.

Recent guidelines have suggested that aggressive fluid therapy during CPCR should be avoided, as excessive fluid administration can result in decreased coronary and cerebral perfusion. Thus fluid therapy is usually only given if the animal was hypovolaemic prior to the CPA.

Monitoring resuscitation

During CPCR one team member is responsible for monitoring the effectiveness of the resuscitation attempt and for the return of spontaneous circulation. ECG monitoring should always be used if available (Figure 15) and observed abnormalities dictate drug choices. Palpation of the femoral pulse is a routine technique for monitoring forward blood flow but can be misleading, as compression can generate venous pulses due to backflow of blood in the caudal vena cava. If available, a Doppler blood pressure probe placed on the lubricated surface of the eye can detect retinal blood flow (Figure 16).

If retinal blood flow is present, it suggests that there is adequate cerebral perfusion. Monitoring should also continue for other signs of effective circulation, such as improvement in mucous membrane colour, a reduction in capillary refill time and a reduction in pupil size.

The use of pulse oximetry should be avoided, as pulsatile blood flow is usually inadequate during CPCR. Measurement of $ETCO_2$ with a capnograph provides useful information. A progressive increase in $ETCO_2$ reflects the success of ventilation in moving of CO_2 from peripheral tissues to the lungs and out of the

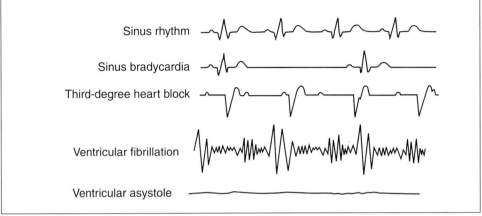

Figure 15: Examples of cardiac rhythms observed during CPCR in the dog and cat. Modified from the *BSAVA Manual of Canine and Feline Emergency and Critical Care, 2nd edition*

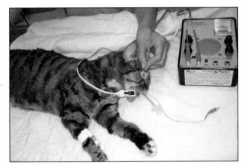

Figure 16: Use of transcorneal Doppler for detection of cerebral blood flow. Reproduced from the *BSAVA Manual of Canine and Feline Emergency and Critical Care, 2nd edition*

body in the course of the resuscitation attempt. There is no consensus as to ETCO$_2$ values as end points for resuscitation in veterinary medicine; however, documenting a reliable trace is a good indicator of successful perfusion. Ventilation should not cease immediately on return of spontaneous respiration but continue as required until the patient regains consciousness.

Post resuscitation

If the patient is successfully resuscitated, then close monitoring is essential as many animals will suffer second arrests. Particular care should be paid to oxygenation, ventilation, blood pressure and perfusion status, to avoid complications such as pulmonary oedema, renal failure and disseminated intravascular coagulation.

It is very common for neurological abnormalities, such as blindness and proprioceptive deficits, to be present after CPA. These may not become obvious immediately but develop over 12 hours, are to be expected and usually resolve after 48–72 hours. Glucocorticoids should not be administered to these patients as they may worsen outcome by causing hyperglycaemia.

Acknowledgements

companion would like to thank Sheena Warman and the Photography Department, University of Bristol, for the use of some of the pictures which accompany this article. ∎

QUICK REFERENCE GUIDE – CPCR

A – Establish airway
B – Positive pressure ventilation – 8–12
breaths/min (12–20 small dogs)
C – Chest compressions:
  Cardiac pump in animals <10 kg
  Thoracic pump in animals >10 kg
  Compress the chest by 25–33%
  Even compression and decompression time
  Aim for a rate of 80–120 compressions/min
  Try to minimise interruptions

Address arrest rhythm:
  Place ECG
  Adrenaline – indicated for asystole, PEA
  Atropine – indicated for bradycardia, third-
  degree AV block, ↑vagal tone
  Mechanical or electrical defibrillation for
  ventricular fibrillation
  If no ECG available give atropine first,
  then if no response after 1–2 minutes give
  adrenaline and repeat up for 2–3 cycles

Monitor:
  Effective blood flow
  Femoral pulse
  Retinal blood flow using Doppler probe on
  cornea
  Adequate/increasing $ETCO_2$
  Return of spontaneous circulation

Avoid excessive IVFT and glucocorticoids

How to...

Get the best
cytology samples

by Kathleen Tennant

1 Aspirate masses with a variety of needle sizes: smaller needles may gather less blood contamination but they yield fewer cells; some harder masses need a larger needle to gather a decent cell yield. Initially, a passive 'syringe off' technique can be used, redirecting the needle in multiple directions through the mass. If this results in a poor sample yield, then repeat with active aspiration using a 5 ml syringe. Active aspiration may be required to acquire samples from hard masses but may contaminate samples from well vascularised areas with blood. If aspirating, make sure that the negative pressure is released from the syringe before the needle is withdrawn or the cells harvested will shoot up into the barrel of the syringe.

2 Expel the material on to the slide and make an assessment of sample yield. If there is no visible material, re-aspirate until there is something on the slide; if there is nothing after several attempts, abandon fine needle aspiration for a biopsy technique. If there is a great deal of thick material, transfer a small amount to another slide before smearing. The aim is to produce a smear sufficiently thin that the cytologist can see through the material to the internal cell detail to make an assessment. Thick material tends to condense or cover the cells, obscuring detail and reducing the diagnostic quality of the sample (Figure 1).

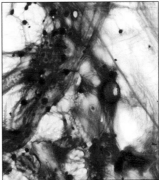

Figure 1: Cells in very thick preparations may be condensed and thus obscured

3 When collecting cytology samples by other means, roll material collected on a swab on to a slide rather than smearing and ensure that blood contamination doesn't obscure cells when making an impression smear. Dab off excess blood and make multiple impressions of the sample on different slides. Often the final slides will be the most diagnostic, as blood contamination will be minimal.

4 Smear whilst the sample is still wet using a slide-over-slide technique (Figure 2). When making the smear, spread with the upper spreader slide horizontal (parallel to the lower sample slide) unless the sample is exceptionally bloody. Resist the urge to press the slides together when spreading. There should be no downward

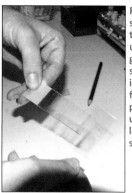

Figure 2: Slide-over-slide spreading technique. Lay the upper spreader slide gently on the lower sample-bearing slide in a perpendicular fashion. Gently but purposefully draw the upper slide along the lower to create a thin smear

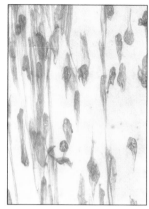

Figure 4: Overzealous and excessive downward pressure when smearing a sample results in cell rupture. These strings of nuclear material are of no diagnostic use and the cell type is impossible to determine

pressure on the upper slide, or cells and elements will tend to rupture. Lymph node aspirates and those from abdominal viscera are especially delicate and need a very light hand. Even then some cells may be ruptured while adjoining cells remain unscathed (Figure 3). It is important that only intact cells are assessed, as apparent abnormalities may appear in cells stripped of cytoplasm and disrupted. Ruptured cells and strings of nuclear material only obscure interpretation and are a waste of a well harvested sample (Figure 4). Retain both the sample slide and the spreader slide for examination. Star or 'needle-drag' techniques often leave areas that are too thick to assess.

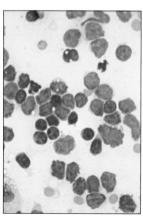

Figure 3: Only intact cells should be assessed: cells stripped of cytoplasm may appear larger and bizarre compared to the intact population

5 Allow smears to air dry, or use a hair drier. This preserves the morphology of the cells and avoids some of the artefacts generated by slow drying (e.g. red cell crenation). It is especially important to allow proteinaceous fluids such as joint fluid to dry completely before putting slides into the slide holders or stainer. Wet samples take much longer to dry once inside the slide holders, reducing cellular quality, and if slides are processed when wet, much of the sample can be washed off during staining.

6 Endeavour not to contaminate the sample with ultrasound or lubricant gel. When obtaining aspirates under ultrasound guidance, it is especially important to release the pressure on the syringe completely before withdrawing the needle. This avoids accidental aspiration of gel from the skin surface. Wiping the area of skin about to be aspirated thoroughly with alcohol can also be helpful but allow the alcohol to dry before proceeding. Contamination with gel causes two problems during assessment of cytology samples: the deeply staining crystalline material overlies and obscures the cells of interest; and the gel's affinity for the stain means that even visible cells may not stain adequately (Figure 5). Similarly, try to avoid

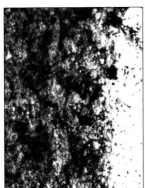

Figure 5: Heavily staining crystalline ultrasound gel causing poor cellular staining

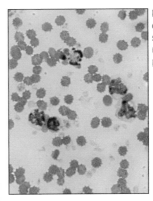

Figure 6: EDTA changes in a stored sample – cell morphology is very poorly preserved

over-generous use of lubricant gel on endotracheal tubes and urinary catheters if lavage is to be performed.

7 Always check samples obtained by nasal, tracheal or bronchoalveolar lavage for the presence of flocculent material. If the lavage fluid appears clear, then it is unlikely to be diagnostic. Remember to collect samples for cytology into EDTA tubes, and those for culture into sterile universal containers.

If the sample is not to be examined quickly, e.g. if it is to be posted, always make fresh smears at the time of sampling. When present, small pieces of flocculent material can be pipetted on to slides and a direct smear made. Often these slides are of low cellularity, but the cell morphology is better preserved when compared to those 'preserved' in saline, and they can be invaluable in achieving a diagnosis.

Body cavity fluids taken into EDTA can undergo the same kinds of cell changes seen in blood samples with prolonged exposure. Red cells become crenated and the nucleated cells disintegrate (Figure 6), so fresh smears may be of value here too.

8 Frosted glass slides are much easier to label and are therefore generally preferable. Each and every slide should be

individually labelled with the site sampled. This also indicates the side of the slide on to which the sample has been smeared. It is impossible to interpret the majority of samples if the cytologist does not know from which site the sample was obtained. Include in the history other patient factors noticed when sampling, e.g. the presence of blood streaks seen during collection of a cerebrospinal fluid sample is likely to have an iatrogenic origin.

9 Fresh cytology samples should be kept in separate bags from histopathology samples in formalin. Formalin fumes leaking from apparently sealed containers lead to a 'washed out' blue appearance on staining, rendering the cytology nearly impossible to interpret.

10 Cerebrospinal fluid (CSF) samples should ideally be collected and examined quickly, but grossly abnormal samples can still be of value after several hours. If there is going to be a very long delay (>4 hours), preparing a sedimented sample may give usable cytology samples when the original fluid would have become useless.

A tube is prepared by cutting the end off a sterile small pot, and the base attached to a slide using petroleum jelly (e.g. Vaseline) to form a watertight seal (Figure 7). The CSF is placed into the column and allowed to settle for approximately half an hour, after which the supernatant is carefully removed by pipette, leaving only the smallest amount of sediment on the slide. The column is removed, excess petroleum jelly wiped away (leaving the central sediment area untouched) and the sample left to air dry before staining or sending away.

Some more affordable cell centrifuges have become available recently and give much better concentrated samples, but be aware that the force generated can either rupture delicate cells if too high a setting is used, or squash cells together, altering their shape (Figure 8).

11 Cytological stains used in-house should be replaced regularly, or when there is a suspicion of contamination or exhaustion. Small upright jars contain a lower volume and are therefore cheaper to change regularly than a large bath. This is particularly relevant if the same pots of stain are to be used for staining skin scrape samples, which quickly contaminate them with keratinocytes, bacteria, hair and debris (Figure 9). A word of caution: spores and pollen from some plants can mimic pathogens. Keep the laboratory a plant-free environment. Even when using fresh stain solutions, slides should be thoroughly washed after staining to remove stain precipitate before examination; a large amount of precipitate makes it very difficult to look for bacteria, may mimic bacteria, and may obscure cell morphology.

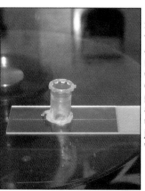

Figure 7: Sedimentation technique for CSF. A column is prepared by cutting the end off a sterile small pot and the base attached to a slide using petroleum jelly to form a watertight seal

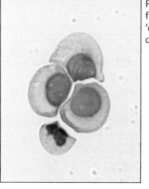

Figure 8: Cells from a CSF sample 'crowded' by centrifugation

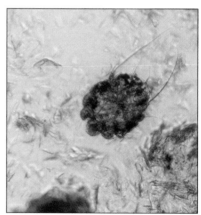

Figure 9: Debris from dermatological samples can contaminate the stains – mites are a dead giveaway!

12 Submit all smears made – the spreader slide is often omitted, but can be the one with the few diagnostic cells. Having gone to all the trouble of sampling, ensure that you give the cytologist the best possible chance of achieving a diagnosis. ■

RAPID STAINS – THE PRACTICE LABORATORY STAPLE

Diff-Quik (American Scientific products, a registered trade mark), Rapi-Diff and others are modified Wright's stains. These are convenient, user-friendly and require no complicated staining apparatus, but the trade-off is that detail, especially nuclear detail, may not be ideal. As with all stains they should be replaced regularly.

Instructions
There are many variations in recommended timings for the different solutions for optimal staining – unfortunately, as the stain becomes exhausted they will vary. The instructions below should be regarded as a very rough guide: ideally watch how the slide takes up the stain and keep going until it looks right.

- Smear slide and air dry
- Dip slide 5 x 1 second in fixative solution (pale blue). Allow excess to drain after each dip
- Dip slide 5 x 1 second in Stain Solution 1 (red)
- Dip slide 6 x 1 second in Stain Solution 2 (deep blue)
- Rinse slide with distilled water or Weise's buffer pH 7.2 (Merck)
- Air dry before examination

There is a gold-coloured scum that ends up on the surface of Solution 2 after you've used it a lot (precipitate forming) – this can and should be removed with a bit of card or paper.
If you don't have enough distilled water to rinse it off properly, run the BACK of the slide under the cold tap: better to alter the staining a little than to have lots of stain precipitate to deal with.

Top tips
- It is often easier to screen for bacteria using these stains (where nearly all stain deeply) than to use a Gram stain, where Gram-negative bacteria are pink and therefore difficult to see against what is usually a pink counterstained background
- Bacteria must be seen inside neutrophils to indicate sepsis rather than contamination
- Fungi and mycobacteria may not take up stain at all, so be sensitive to 'negative images' with unstained elements within the stained background, or, in the case of mycobacteria, inside cells

How to...

Use **progesterone testing** in practice

by Angelika von Heimendahl

P rogesterone is the most important hormone in female canine reproduction. It is easy to measure, either in-house or at a laboratory, and can be used to date ovulation and parturition, and for investigation of other abnormalities of the oestrous cycle.

Oestrous cycle in the bitch: when to mate?

Determination of the optimal breeding time of the bitch can be difficult. There is significant individual variation relating to the day on which ovulation occurs, and this is further obscured by a poor correlation between the time of ovulation and behavioural oestrus. Practically the situation is often complicated by dog breeders 'choosing' the day on which to breed, commonly using arbitrary criteria. Such criteria include having set days (e.g. 11 and 13 days after the onset of pro-oestrus) for breeding, measuring electric conductivity in the vaginal mucosa (using a 'Draminski Ovulation Detector') or looking for ferning in the saliva under the microscope.

In contrast the most useful methods employed in veterinary practice to determine the optimum mating time are measurement of the plasma progesterone levels (Figure 1) and exfoliative vaginal cytology.

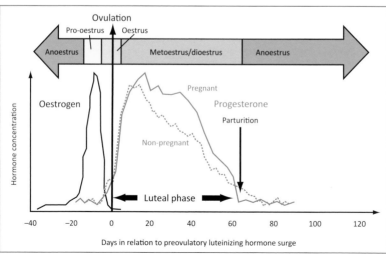

Figure 1: Different stages of the oestrous cycle in relation to changes in plasma hormone concentrations and ovulation. Adapted from the *BSAVA Manual of Canine and Feline Reproduction and Neonatology, 2nd edition*

The bitch, a spontaneous ovulator, shows a marked increase in progesterone at the time of ovulation. Prior to ovulation luteinization of granulosa cells inside the maturing follicles produce this progesterone, and following ovulation go on to form the corpora lutea, which produce progesterone for around 60 days regardless of whether the bitch is pregnant or not.

Time period	Days in relation to ovulation
Fertile period	−5 to +5
Fertilisation period	+2 to +5
Peak fertility	−1 to +4
Preferred time for natural service or fresh semen insemination	0 to +4
Preferred time for frozen semen insemination or breeding where semen quality is not optimal	+2 to +4

Figure 2: The timing of peak fertility in relation to the day of ovulation in the bitch

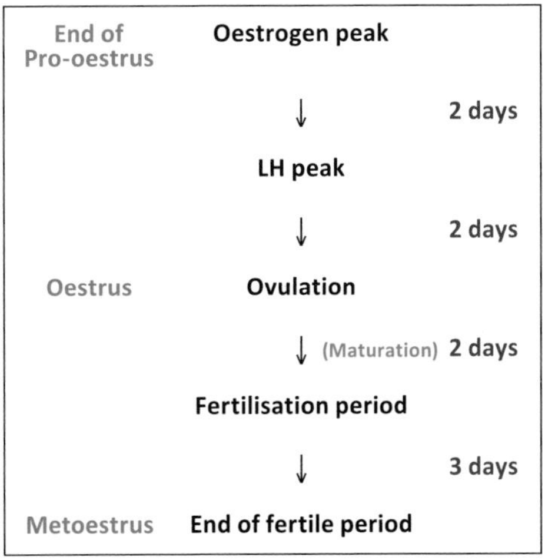

Figure 3: Occurence and timing of hormones around the period of ovulation (e.g. 2 days after the luteinizing hormone peak, ovulation occurs)

The reproductive physiology of the bitch is unusual in that the oocytes are immature at the time of ovulation and cannot be fertilised until 2 days later. Once they have completed maturation they remain fertile for 2–3 days. This results in a 3-day 'fertilisation period' that commences from 2 days after ovulation to up to 5 days after ovulation (Figures 2 and 3). Fertile matings may occur before the onset of the fertilisation period as sperm can survive for 7 days or more in the female reproductive tract.

Measuring progesterone levels

The increase in blood progesterone around ovulation follows a distinct pattern and is therefore easy to interpret. Progesterone levels double roughly every 2 days. Given that the rise is progressive, it is only necessary to take blood samples every second or third day. Longer sampling intervals decrease the accuracy of ovulation detection. Maximum concentrations of progesterone are reached between 20 and 30 days after the end of oestrus, whether the bitch is pregnant or not. These decline gradually to basal levels either just before parturition or slightly later if the bitch was not pregnant.

Progesterone concentrations may be measured by radioimmunoassay (RIA), quantitative or qualitative enzyme-linked immunosorbent assay (ELISA), or immunochemiluminescence assay. Many veterinary diagnostic laboratories offer measurement of progesterone with reporting of the results on the same day.

In-house testing to determine ovulation

There are several semi-quantitative progesterone ELISA kits available and all have a similar methodology. The results are usually obtained within 30–45 minutes of sample collection and are measured through a colour change in the wells (Figure 4).

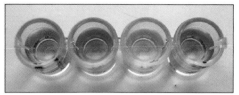

Figure 4: Results from an in-house progesterone ELISA showing colour change. Well 1 = Standard B; 10 ng/ml. Well 2 = Sample 1; ≤3 ng/ml. Well 3 = Sample 2; ≥10 ng/ml. Well 4 = Standard A; 3 ng/ml

The tests are fairly easy to run, although they require a warm room, technical accuracy when adding the substrates, and ensuring the timing is within the prescribed limits.

If the bitch is in early in pro-oestrus, the test indicator will produce a strong colour indicating low levels of progesterone. The fading of the test colour indicates rising progesterone and impending ovulation. Once ovulation has occurred, progesterone levels will further increase and remain high for the next 2 months, when the test colour will stay very pale.

In-house ELISAs can have two problems. Firstly, a rise in progesterone levels prior to ovulation is sometimes interpreted as 'ovulation imminent'. Unfortunately, the progesterone concentration can sometimes stay at this level for several days. Therefore, testing should continue and sampling should be repeated 2 days later to avoid misunderstandings with the breeder. It is important to continue testing until 'ovulation has occurred', especially as the oocyte is not fertile for the first 2 days after ovulation and matings should not be advised too early.

The second problem is that the 'window' of the test is defined by the resultant colour change and once the progesterone level exceeds 10 ng/ml the test will interpret the result as 'mate immediately' for the next 2 months of the bitch's cycle. Therefore the in-house ELISA will only give relevant results if the bitch is tested at least once pre-ovulation

and subsequent tests are interpreted in light of the result on that date. If the first test confirms that ovulation has already taken place, other methods such as vaginal cytology, will have to be used.

Laboratory testing to determine ovulation

The commercial laboratory tests are either RIA or immunochemiluminesence, and just to make things more complicated are reported either in ng/ml or nmol/l (Figure 5). Laboratory tests are more accurate than in-house tests and because of the precise value of progesterone levels, predictions can be made more easily (Figure 6). In cases where the optimum breeding time is to be determined, postage and reporting of results up to 48 hours after sampling is not a problem as the mating does not have to be performed until several days after ovulation.

Event	Progesterone level
Luteinizing hormone surge (36–48 hours before ovulation)	1.5–2.5 ng/ml (4.5–7.5 nmol/l)
Ovulation	5–8 ng/ml (15–24 nmol/l)
Fertile period	10–25 ng/ml (30–75 nmol/l)

Figure 5: Important progesterone concentrations

Plasma progesterone levels	Action/Interpretation
<1 ng/ml (6 nmol/l)	Re-test in 4 days
<2 ng/ml (6 nmol/l)	Re-test in 3 days
>2 ng/ml (6 nmol/l)	Re-test in 2 days
6 ng/ml (18 nmol/l)	Ovulation
>25 ng/mol (75 nmol/l)	Usually indicates the end of the fertile period

Figure 6: Possible testing regime

To determine the days when the bitch should be mated two factors have to be considered: ovulation and maturation. Bitches will ovulate at a progesterone concentration of around 6 ng/ml (18 nmol/l), but the time taken to achieve this concentration can vary widely between individuals with a range of 7–30 days from the onset of pro-oestrus. After ovulation the oocytes have to mature for a further 2 days before they can be fertilised. Once mature they will be viable for another 2–3 days. In order for the breeder to get the benefit of a progesterone test that will give them the right mating dates (Figure 7), even when ovulation occurs late, it is important to space the samples sensibly.

One should also consider practicalities such as weekends and bank holidays when planning matings. Normally given the predictable rise of progesterone and the time available after ovulation this system works well.

Number of matings	Days for mating
Two matings	Ovulation +1 day and +3 days
	or Ovulation +2 days and +4 days
One mating	Ovulation +2 days
	or Ovulation +3 days

Figure 7: Possible mating regimes

Determining parturition date

Given the relatively short gestation length in the bitch, it is useful to have tools to determine the physiological end of the pregnancy. Although the actual duration of pregnancy in dogs is quite constant at 61 days ± 48 hours from fertilisation, long-term sperm survival in the female reproductive tract often makes it impossible to determine the actual 'beginning' of pregnancy in relation to the mating. Furthermore, multiple matings and the unreliability of owner information can make this even more difficult.

Often vets are presented with an animal at the end of pregnancy that they have not seen before. Initially it is always useful to be given the actual dates of the mating and check for yourself in a diary, rather than relying on someone else to count out the days from possible conception. Clinical examination may not offer additional information. Clinical signs at the end of pregnancy are not specific and vary between breeds and individuals. Litter size, especially single puppy pregnancies, are also a contributing factor. An added complication with single puppies is that they are often the result of inaccurately timed matings in correlation to the time of ovulation, and do not always induce parturition.

Advising owners to measure body temperature three times a day can be useful, especially in smaller and medium-sized dogs. The temperature will fluctuate slightly in the last week but drop 2°C, typically below 37°C, 12 to 24 hours before parturition. This change in body temperature is caused by the drop in plasma progesterone 24–36 hours before parturition. Unfortunately the drop in temperature is not always so marked in larger dogs.

Progesterone testing for parturition

As mentioned above, plasma progesterone levels decline to <1 ng/ml before parturition. Measuring plasma progesterone can therefore alert to impending parturition. However, as it is important to have the results immediately, the in-house progesterone ELISA kits marketed for ovulation are preferred to postal diagnostics. It is vital to remember that the kits are designed for ovulation testing and are being used to look for the opposite result (i.e. falling progesterone) in this case. This means the test will have strong colour at parturition, when the bitch has very little or no progesterone.

When presented with a bitch with apparently non-progressive labour, progesterone testing can be very helpful. In these cases of suspected primary inertia the test can give results within 30 minutes and will confirm if parturition is underway. If the progesterone level is still high the bitch is not ready and parturition has not started. Alternatively, if the progesterone level is low, luteolysis has occurred and a Caesarean operation can be attempted. In cases of planning an elective Caesarean section (e.g. single puppy pregnancy in a Bulldog), the test can be repeated every day towards the end of gestation until the drop in progesterone is noted. Given that puppies born before 57 days post-fertilisation have poor survival rates such accurate timing of Caesarean sections is crucial.

Progesterone testing for other conditions

Progesterone testing can be useful in a range of other reproductive conditions.

'Split heats' are quite common in young bitches, but also occur in around 5% of older animals. The pro-oestrus phase is quite short and does not progress into oestrus. It is often followed by a shorter interoestrus interval. Measuring progesterone levels any time in the next 50 days can establish if ovulation has taken place or if the season was non-ovulatory.

Delayed puberty is suspected if a bitch has not shown any seasons by the time she is 2 years of age. To exclude whether a silent oestrus has taken place in the last 2 months, a progesterone level would be the first test, before further investigations are initiated.

Silent oestrus can be a big problem as some animals show no or hardly any signs of swelling or discharge during their season. In order to breed from these females testing has to start on the first day of any suspicious sign of pro-oestrus to make sure the fertile period is not missed.

Conclusion

Progesterone testing is a very useful, inexpensive and readily available tool in female canine reproduction. It can be used at different stages of the reproductive cycle and give information about the right time for mating and parturition as well as some oestrous cycle abnormalities. ■

How to...
Manage feline
urethral obstruction

by David Walker

Feline urethral obstruction is much more common in male cats than females due to the narrower, longer and more tortuous urethra. The most frequent causes of obstruction in cats are urethral plugs (mucous or mucocrystalline), urinary calculi or urethral spasm; however, regardless of the underlying cause the consequences are the same. Many cats presenting with urethral obstruction are relatively stable, but a proportion have significant electrolyte and acid–base changes and these patients demand more aggressive management.

Presenting signs and the 'minimum database'

The most common presenting sign is unproductive straining, although owners often also report perianal licking and vocalisation. If the initial clinical signs are missed then cats become anorectic, progressively more lethargic, may vomit and will eventually become comatose. Diagnosis is based on bladder palpation and this typically reveals a large, firm urinary bladder which is often painful. Cats may be clinically dehydrated and a proportion will be bradycardic due to hyperkalaemia.

In order to decide on the most appropriate management the following minimum database would ideally be obtained:

- Packed cell volume (PCV) and total solids (TS)
- Urea and creatinine
- Potassium.

It is important that cats with urethral obstruction have an intravenous catheter placed a short time after admission (from which blood can sometimes be acquired for the tests listed above) so that fluid therapy can begin. Many cats are hypovolaemic due to fluid deficits (a consequence of severe dehydration) and poor cardiac output (secondary to bradycardia and possible acidaemia leading to reduced myocardial function) which leads to poor tissue oxygenation. Clinical signs of hypovolaemia in the cat depend on the severity but can include tachycardia or bradycardia, reduced pulse quality progressing to absent peripheral pulses, mental depression, hypothermia and pale mucous membranes.

Packed cell volume and total solids evaluation may help to provide a more objective measure of the cat's hydration status, both being increased in the face of significant dehydration. Urethral obstruction leads to back pressure within the kidneys and the development of post-renal azotaemia. This azotaemia can often be quite marked (creatinine >500 µmol/l) but, assuming the urethral obstruction is successfully relieved and adequate fluid therapy is administered, this will resolve.

Any cat presenting with bradycardia or an arrhythmia should have serum potassium measured and if possible an electrocardiogram (lead II) should be obtained. It is important to note that hyperkalaemic cats can also have normal or fast heart rates and the measurement of serum potassium provides valuable information in all cats with urethral obstruction. The severity of clinical signs, including ECG abnormalities does not correlate well with the severity of the hyperkalaemia. Serum potassium increases for a number of reasons but it is primarily the result of decreased renal excretion. Hyperkalaemia may cause generalised muscle weakness but its most serious complication is its effect on the conduction system of the heart. ECG changes seen include bradycardia, decreased amplitude or absent P waves, widened QRS complexes and peaked T waves (Figure 1).

Relief of the urethral obstruction and intravenous fluid therapy (0.9% sodium chloride or Hartmann's) is often all that is required to resolve hyperkalaemia; however, cats with profound bradycardia (<80 bpm) may require more intensive management (Figure 2). Cats should not be sedated or anesthetised if they are significantly hyperkalaemic, bradycardic or arrhythmic, until action has been taken. As well as poor potassium excretion by the kidney, hydrogen ion excretion is also reduced. This can lead to a metabolic acidosis (pH <7.2, reference range 7.31–7.46) which can result in cardiac arrhythmias, decreased myocardial function and central nervous system depression.

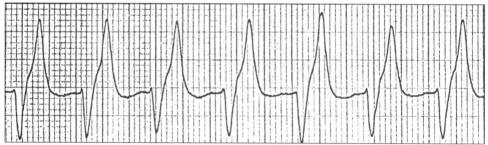

Figure 1: Lead II ECG trace (25 mm/s) from a hyperkalaemic cat showing flattened P waves, widened QRS complexes and peaked T waves. The heart rate is inappropriately low

1. Relieve the obstruction! However this may not be possible until the patient's condition has been stabilised. Consider cystocentesis.
2. Fluid therapy (0.9% NaCl or compound sodium lactate (Hartmann's)).
3. Calcium gluconate (slow intravenous injection 0.5–1.0 ml/kg 10% solution) antagonises the effects of hyperkalaemia (although the actual serum potassium value does not change, it improves the cardiac rhythm). Effects last for 20–30 minutes.
4. Insulin and glucose administration. Insulin drives potassium into cells, reducing the serum potassium concentration. Although insulin can be administered with glucose, as an intravenous infusion (0.25–0.5 IU/kg regular insulin with 1–2 g of 25% glucose/unit of insulin to prevent hypoglycaemia), this should only be done if a fluid pump is available and intense monitoring is possible. A more practical approach is to administer glucose (1–2 ml/kg of a 50% dextrose solution) and rely on the endogenous production of insulin by the patient.

Figure 2: Management of hyperkalaemia

Relieving the obstruction

Appropriate restraint is needed to unblock the feline urethra and sedation or general anaesthesia should be considered if the patient is not moribund. Patients must be stable prior to sedation or general anaesthesia, and animals with severe bradycardia (or other heart rhythm disturbances) as a consequence of hyperkalaemia should be managed appropriately. Hypovolaemia should also be corrected with fluid therapy. Boluses (10–20 ml/kg) of crystalloid (0.9% NaCl or compound sodium lactate (Hartmann's)) should be administered over 10–20 minutes and the heart rate, pulse quality, mucous membrane colour and capillary refill time reassessed.

Animals can be sedated with a combination of ketamine (2.5–5 mg/kg) and midazolam (0.25 mg/kg) given intravenously or intramuscularly (lower dose i.v.) and this will typically provide sedation for approximately 15–20 minutes. Ketamine is excreted renally and recovery can be prolonged in animals with urinary tract obstruction. In many animals sedation is inadequate and general anaesthesia is required. If the patient is not sufficiently relaxed then the risks of urethral rupture or of failing to relieve the obstruction are increased.

Urethral plugs often lodge near the external urethral orifice and the exposed distal penis should be gently massaged to loosen any obstructing material present and extrude it from the urethra. The penis is exposed by caudal pressure on the preputial skin. In some cats penile massage alone will relieve the obstruction; however, the majority of cats will require urethral catheterisation and saline flushing.

Selection of a urinary catheter

When selecting a urinary catheter an open-ended catheter is preferable to a side-ended catheter for relieving the obstruction. Many are available on the market; see also 'How to… Choose a cat urinary catheter' (page 46).

Regardless of the type of catheter used, the penis should be retracted caudally and dorsally to 'straighten out' the urethra (Figure 3) prior to catheterisation. KY jelly should be used to lubricate the catheter and

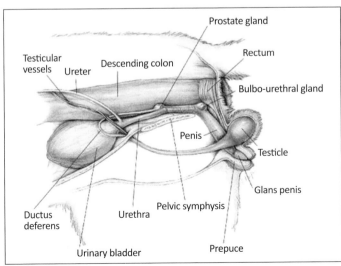

Testicular vessels
Ureter
Descending colon
Prostate gland
Rectum
Bulbo-urethral gland
Penis
Testicle
Glans penis
Ductus deferens
Urethra
Pelvic symphysis
Urinary bladder
Prepuce

Figure 3: Anatomy of the feline male lower urinary tract, highlighting the flexure in the urethra that needs to be straightened prior to catheterisation (used with kind permission from Hills Pet Nutrition™)

sterile saline to flush the urethra. Walpole's solution should NEVER be used. Walpole's is a weak acid and is likely to cause further damage to an already irritated urethra and urinary bladder. 'Pushing' of any obstruction should never be attempted as this is likely to result in the catheter traumatising the urethral wall. Once the catheter has reached the level of the obstruction gentle flushing should begin (10 ml syringe filled with sterile saline). The catheter should be gently advanced whilst flushing, if there is resistance to flushing, back the catheter out a little. This process should be repeated as frequently as is necessary to clear the obstruction.

For a comprehensive discussion regarding clearing urethral obstructions readers are referred to the article in the April 2008 edition of **companion** and for some tips when handling difficult cases to Figure 4.

- Increase the voluntary muscle relaxation: if the patient is only lightly sedated, sedate it more; if the patient is well sedated, consider anaesthesia.
- Failure to straighten the penis effectively can make the catheter difficult to pass. Some people prefer to put the cat into dorsal recumbency rather than lateral, to facilitate catheter passage. Have an assistant exteriorise the penis.
- Decompressive cystocentesis – reducing the hydrostatic pressure in the bladder may make retrograde flushing of plugs easier. Also if the obstruction cannot be relieved then this allows a short time for the patient's condition to be further stabilised before trying again.

Figure 4: Tips for difficult cases

After clearing an obstruction

Once the obstruction has been cleared, a urine sample is obtained for urinalysis (urine specific gravity, dipstick and sediment examination) and ideally urine culture. The bladder is then flushed copiously with sterile saline, generally until what you get back out is as clear as what you put in! Any particulate material can be submitted for analysis and an indwelling catheter is then placed. As before, the penis must be extended caudally to ease catheter placement. If a Slippery Sam® catheter was used for unblocking this can be used as the indwelling catheter; the soft silicone hub is very comfortable for the patient; however, this PTFE catheter is not as soft as some others on the market. If this catheter is used, a luer lock will be required to form a closed collection system. Soft red rubber urethral/feeding tube catheters are very comfortable. Silicone Tomcat catheters are also generally well tolerated; the disadvantage is the rigid catheter hub. Regardless of the type of catheter used it should be sutured in place and a closed collection system attached. This can simply be a new intravenous fluid set and an empty 500 ml or 1 litre fluid bag. Veterinary closed urinary collection systems are available; however, these will be significantly more expensive. There is no need to attach the urine collection system to the cat's tail. The urinary catheter is typically left in place for 24–72 hours. Most cats will need to wear an Elizabethan collar during this time. If the animal was 'unblocked' very easily and a good urine stream is obtained following relief of the obstruction, you may decide not to place an indwelling catheter; however, you may regret this decision later!

Cystocentesis?

The use of decompressive cystocentesis is controversial. The concern is that when the needle is inserted into the bladder there is inevitably some leakage of urine around the needle into the abdomen; however, provided the urine is sterile this is of no great consequence as it will rapidly be reabsorbed and excreted. The only occasions when urine leakage is more serious is if there is a UTI present (which is uncommon in patients with urethral obstruction), if bladder rupture occurs because the wall is severely devitalised (in which case rupture may well have occurred without cystocentesis!) or if there is subsequent urethral obstruction. Cystocentesis does not need to be performed in most patients but can be a valuable tool in very unstable patients that require sedation/anaesthesia or when relief of the urethral obstruction is proving problematic. Cystocentesis can be achieved using a 22 G needle attached to an extension set, three-way tap and syringe. The needle should enter the ventral aspect of the bladder wall and be angled caudally.

What to do next

Unless there is evidence of bacterial infection (on urine sediment examination), it is recommended that antibiotics are avoided whilst a urinary catheter is in place to avoid the development of multidrug resistant infections. Once the catheter has been removed, a 7-day course of antibiotics would be recommended; ideally antibiotic selection would be based on the results of urine culture or culture of the urinary catheter tip. Urine culture will also allow the antibiotics to be stopped after 2–3 days in those cats that don't have a urinary tract infection (approximately 50%!). Penicillins (amoxicillin, ampicillin, amoxicillin–clavulanate) and cephalosporins (cefalexin) are reasonable empirical choices. The use of fluoroquinolones or 3rd generation cephalosporins (cefovecin) is generally discouraged unless indicated by the results of urine culture and sensitivity.

Following relief of a urethral obstruction cats are often uncomfortable due to a combination of penile manipulation, urethral inflammation and urinary catheterisation. Non-steroidal anti-inflammatory drugs are generally best avoided due to the presence of post-renal azotaemia. Partial agonist opioids such as buprenorphine (0.02 mg/kg s.c., i.m., i.v. every 6–8 hours) are generally sufficient for analgesia. Prednisolone therapy is never warranted. The majority of cats will begin eating within 12–24 hours of relief of the obstruction.

Fluid therapy is mandatory following the relief of urinary obstruction. Post-obstructive diuresis often results in increased fluid requirements. Another advantage of the closed urine collection system (as well as reducing the risk of infection) is that urine output can be accurately assessed and fluid 'ins-and-outs' can be matched so that fluid rates are adequate. A balanced electrolyte solution (compound sodium lactate (Hartmann's)) is appropriate and rates of 4–10 ml/kg/h are often initially required. Urine output should be at least 1 ml/kg/h. Azotaemia usually resolves within 24 hours; it does not matter how high the creatinine concentration was – it will almost always resolve with relief of the obstruction and appropriate fluid therapy. Once the azotaemia has resolved then fluid rates can generally be decreased. Measurement of serum potassium following obstruction is useful as post-obstructive diuresis can lead to hypokalaemia. This can be addressed by the addition of potassium chloride to the intravenous fluids.

Monitoring

Ideally PCV, TS, urea, creatinine and potassium would be measured daily for the first 48–72 hours. Cats should be hospitalised after the urinary catheter is removed until they have been seen to produce a good stream of urine. If the cat cannot urinate it must be re-evaluated. A plug or stone should be detected with catheterisation; if the catheter passes easily, urethral spasm should be suspected. This can be managed by placing an indwelling urinary catheter and administering phenoxybenzamine (0.5–1 mg/kg p.o. q12h). This drug must be continued for

3–5 days before its efficacy can be accurately determined; the urinary catheter can be removed after this time.

Perineal urethrostomy

Around 30–40% of cats that have an episode of urethral obstruction (whether the result of a plug, stone or 'idiopathic') will become 'blocked' again in the future and owners should be warned of this.

The main indication for perineal urethrostomy (Figure 5) is for treatment of those cats with recurrent episodes of urethral obstruction. It must be understood that this technique (if performed well) reduces the risks of obstruction but does not prevent these cats from showing other signs of feline lower urinary tract disease. Too often this procedure is performed as treatment for FLUTD (for which it is of no benefit) or because of difficulty relieving an obstruction. It is a technically demanding procedure and the inexperienced surgeon should consider referral to a specialist. Complications of the technique include urine extravasation, stricture formation with recurrent obstruction,

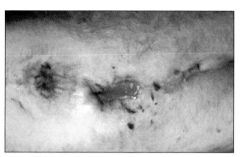

Figure 5: Male cat 2 weeks after perineal urethrostomy. This is a technically demanding procedure; although surgery reduces the risk of obstruction it does not prevent cats from showing signs of feline lower urinary tract disease (FLUTD)

recurrent UTIs, urinary and faecal incontinence, rectourethral fistula formation, rectal prolapse and perineal hernia.

Acknowledgements

Thanks go to Dr Virginia Luis Fuentes MRCVS and Zoe Halfacree MRCVS for providing some of the images included in this article. This article appeared in a longer form in the March 2009 edition of *Irish Veterinary Journal* and is reproduced with thanks. ∎

Choose a
wound dressing

by Dick White and Georgie Hollis

T he management of wounds continues to be as important a challenge for the small animal veterinary surgeon as it ever has been. Today, however, the clinician is faced with a bewildering and ever-increasing array of products for use in wound management; the most recent edition of The Formulary of Wound Products, for instance, lists more than 1500 products for topical treatment of wounds. Many of these can play a useful, and sometimes essential, role in wound management but their selection needs to be made on the basis of the needs of the individual wound rather than on the lure of attractive commercial packaging or a dogmatic 'one size fits all' approach to wound management.

Wound progression and the optimal wound environment

Wound healing is classically considered as comprising three distinct stages (Figure 1):

- Inflammatory
- Proliferative
- Remodelling.

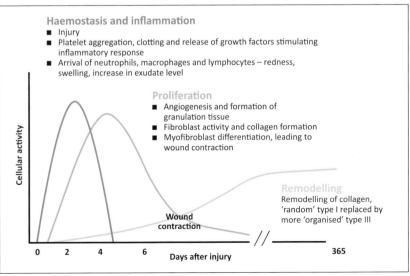

Haemostasis and inflammation
- Injury
- Platelet aggregation, clotting and release of growth factors stimulating inflammatory response
- Arrival of neutrophils, macrophages and lymphocytes – redness, swelling, increase in exudate level

Proliferation
- Angiogenesis and formation of granulation tissue
- Fibroblast activity and collagen formation
- Myofibroblast differentiation, leading to wound contraction

Remodelling
Remodelling of collagen, 'random' type I replaced by more 'organised' type III

Wound contraction

Cellular activity

Days after injury

0   2   4   6   365

Figure 1: The wound healing sequence

The processes involved in wound healing are heavily inter-related and unique to every individual, and the complex array of physiological processes cannot be supported throughout by one single product. The idea of a single dressing suiting all wound types and stages is therefore clearly flawed. The needs of the wound vary with the phase of healing; much of the research into the 'ideal' dressing recognises this and aims to optimise the wound environment so as to allow the cellular and molecular processes occurring *at that phase of healing* to progress as quickly and efficiently as possible. One key factor in this optimal healing environment is adequate tissue moisture.

The importance of the role of exudate as a crucial nutritional environment, a vehicle for cellular activity and communication, which enables the complex cascade of events that eventually lead to a healed wound, is increasingly recognised. For this reason 'advanced' wound management has embraced the principle of moist wound healing. Although the processes involved in the healing of primarily closed (e.g. by suturing) wounds are essentially similar, they are of course less apparent and wound requirements will generally progress more rapidly.

Dressings and 'advanced' wound care

The wound progression model (Figure 2) can be helpful in terms of selecting appropriate 'advanced' wound management. It presents the key observable states of the wound from presentation through wound progression and relates them to the healing cascade. Based upon the gross appearance, plotted against the level of exudate (exhibited to assist in application of the moist wound healing principle) and dressing selection, it gives a useful, though not exhaustive, guide to the topical needs of the open wound.

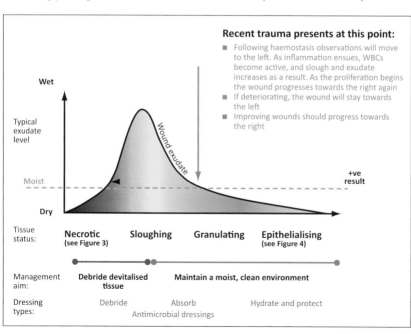

Figure 2: The open wound model

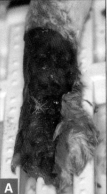
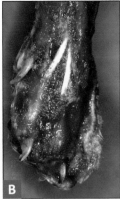

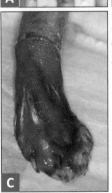

Figure 3: (A) A necrotic sloughing wound. (B) Early granulation tissue. (C) A mature bed of granulation tissue

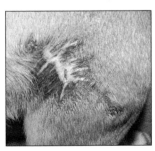

Figure 4: The final phase of wound healing, epithelialisation and contraction

Traumatic wounds may present at any stage of healing on this basis. Although some wounds may heal unevenly with several stages observable, the priority should always be to address the component furthest from the healed state.

I: HAEMOSTASIS – Problem bleeding

Haemostasis is the very first process in wound healing. Platelet aggregation at the site of injury leads to the release of growth factors, mediators and cytokines, which promote the inflammatory and proliferative phases essential for the wound response. Without this, the healing process cannot progress. Occasionally, bleeding is so problematic that haemostatic dressings may be useful.

Mildly haemostatic dressings

Calcium alginate dressings (Kaltostat, Convatec – see page 259): The haemostatic action is thought to be related to the release, on contact with blood, of calcium ions that are exchanged for sodium ions, promoting the blood clotting cascade mechanism. However, not all alginates exhibit haemostatic properties; these are dependent upon the part of the seaweed from which they are manufactured, as the guluronic and mannuronic acids responsible for haemostasis are found in the root and leaf end. Kaltostat is a typical example better known for its haemostatic properties but may be less absorbent than its non-haemostatic competitors. Surgical use of alginates is not recommended, as the structural integrity of the dressings are poor and irritant fibre loss into the wound is likely.

Collagen-based haemostatic dressings (Lyostypt B. Braun): These are woven meshes of bovine, porcine or equine-derived collagen. Their action relies on promoting the clotting cascade through thrombocyte adhesion and activation of coagulation factor XII. Collagen dressings of this type also have a role in aiding proliferation by offering a scaffold for epithelial migration (see page 262).

KEY FUNCTIONS:

- Promote coagulation in mild cases of bleeding

Dressings for major haemostasis

In the last decade dressings for major trauma patients have begun to include what are termed 'major haemostats'. These products have been developed with battlefield use in mind and provide a temporary fix for what would otherwise be a catastrophic arterial bleed. They can buy crucial time to allow critical patients to be transported or stabilised for appropriate surgical management.

Kaolin: One of the first products of this type was QuikClot (Z-Medica) composed of kaolin granules in sachet form; dressing versions are available. The first of its kind, this product has some limitations because of its exothermic action. More importantly, it requires complete and thorough removal from the wound site after haemostasis use to avoid any residue being left behind.

Chitin: This is a more recent development that has improved options significantly by using more physiologically compatible contents. Celox™ (Medtrade Products Ltd) is a flaked powder containing 100% chitin manufactured from shrimp shells. It is non-exothermic and creates a jelly-like plug in contact with blood (Figure 5) that can be removed easily after use. The chitin is applied to the source of the bleed, either as a sachet or in a swab form (Figure 6) with direct firm pressure for 3–5 minutes. Chitin is capable of stemming even femoral arterial

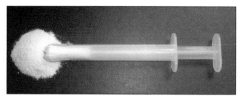

Figure 6: Celox™ applicator and powder

and aortic bleeds and achieves complete haemostasis irrespective of the presence of clotting factors. The exceptional haemostatic effect is astonishing and flushing of any visible residue is all that is required since chitin is non-toxic and is broken down by catalase in the bloodstream within 3 hours of application. Developed for military needs, its role in veterinary use may be perceived as limited; however, with a 3-year shelf life there is some comfort in having a sachet to hand just in case!

KEY FUNCTIONS:

- Promote coagulation in extreme cases of bleeding

II: WOUND DEBRIDEMENT – Supporting the inflammatory response

Much of the initial cellular inflammatory phase is directed towards debridement. The impact of devitalised tissue debris in a wound cannot be underestimated in terms of its potential for delaying wound healing. Bacterial contamination, foreign debris and non-viable tissue all require considerable cellular effort to achieve debridement by the natural inflammatory processes. Left *in situ*, this burden lengthens the inflammatory response, and when combined with bacterial load in a protein-rich environment, the risk of sepsis is significantly increased. The wound progress towards the proliferation phase will inevitably be delayed. Hence, assisting these natural debriding processes is an important principle

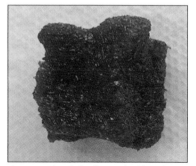

Figure 5: Blood clot formed with Celox™ powder

of early wound management; its benefits were highlighted by Hippocrates and Galen as long ago as 400 BC. Prompt and effective removal of devitalised tissue reduces what may be termed 'wound bioburden' and promotes more efficient triggering of the proliferative phase with progress towards the naturally infection-resistant granulation tissue.

Dressings for debridement

1. Mechanical
Dressings that physically attract debris and exudate from the wound surface.

Wet-to-Dry dressings are indicated in the early stages of the wound when significant bacterial contamination with inert or organic debris is present in the wound. Sterile woven gauze swabs are pre-wetted using a 0.9% saline or lactated Ringer's solution. Excess fluid is rung out of the gauze before it is packed into the wound so as to ensure close contact with the open surface. Several layers of moist swabs are placed over the 'contact' layer and these in turn are covered with dry swabs.

The dressing is anchored in placed with further layers of protective bandaging or, better, tied in place with 'bolus dressings' that provide downward pressure on the wound (Figure 7). The dressing is then allowed to dry,

drawing debris and moist exudate from the wound into the dressing away from its surface. The process of removing the dressing mechanically removes this devitalised tissue and debris. The dressing is left *in situ* normally over 12–24 hours between changes but NEVER longer to avoid bacterial maceration. Lifting the dressing may be uncomfortable and re-soaking with saline as it is removed may release its attachment to the wound.

KEY FUNCTIONS:

- Physically debride early wounds with severe contamination/debris

2. Enzymatic/chemical debridement
Enzymatic debridement has lost favour in human healthcare over the past decade. Products are perceived to be expensive in comparison to surgical and mechanical methods, being less immediate in their effect than particularly wet-to-dry methods.

Collagenase: This is harvested through the fermentation of *Clostridium histolyticum* and in cream or powder forms has the ability to digest collagen in necrotic tissue at normal physiological pH and temperature. As much as 75% of the dry weight of skin is composed of collagen, and collagenases are therefore helpful in removing dead cutaneous debris.

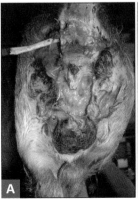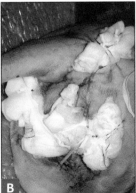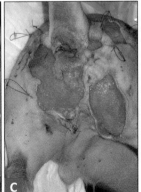

Figure 7: (A) A dirty perianal wound prior to wet-to-dry dressing. (B) A wet-to-dry dressing in place, with bolus dressing in place. (C) A healthy bed of granulation tissue

Healthy or newly formed collagen is not affected by this process and, in principle therefore, enzymatic debridement is somewhat more selective than other methods. Other examples of enzymatic debriding agents include streptokinase.

Dermisol®: This is a chemical debriding agent that contains propylene glycol with malic, benzoic and salicylic acid. Debridement is achieved by differential swelling of necrotic and healthy tissues leading to separation of the devitalised areas and embedded debris.

KEY FUNCTIONS:
- Debride later wounds by loosening, dissolving and aiding removal of necrotic tissue

3. Maggot therapy

The larvae of the common green bottle *(Lucilia sericata)* have been recognised for many years as connoisseurs of necrotic wound tissue. They secrete proteolytic enzymes capable of breaking down large proteins into shorter chains achieving an amino acid 'soup' in the wound. As they consume the protein soup they assist in cleaning the wound, a process that is not dissimilar to the natural inflammatory process that converts necrotic tissue to a semi-liquid for macrophage debridement. Larvae are now specially bred and prepared in sterile conditions for use in human medicine (Figure 8).

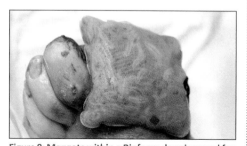

Figure 8: Maggots within a Biofoam dressing used for debridement of wound of a diabetic person's foot

The larvae also excrete important waste products including allantoin back into the wound; allantoin is known to promote cell proliferation and granulation and this is thought to be one of the additional factors contributing to the success of medical maggots in the treatment of some chronic wounds. However, maggots cannot differentiate between healthy and necrotic tissue in some species, notably rabbits, sheep and guinea pigs, which are unlikely to be good candidates as a result. Dogs and cats have been successfully treated with maggot therapy.

KEY FUNCTIONS:
- Achieves focused and highly selective removal of non-viable tissue in sloughy or necrotic wounds

4. Autolytic debridement

Hydrocolloid dressings are designed to facilitate autolytic or 'natural' debridement by assisting in the hydration of dry and necrotic tissue so that it can be removed manually without surgical intervention (Figure 9).

Granuflex® (Convatec) is one of the original hydrocolloid dressings and consists of a microgranular suspension of gelatine, pectin and sodium CMC in an adhesive polymer; it is similar in formulation to most hydrogels. The strong hydrating effect softens necrotic and sloughing tissue over several days. Several

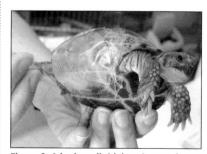

Figure 9: A hydrocolloid dressing used successfully to maintain and encourage moist wound healing for a tortoise shell injury

applications may be required before the tissue has softened to the point that it lifts away from the wound. Most hydrocolloid dressings are combined with a viral or bacterial barrier such as a thin polyurethane film, although Granuflex® includes a foam backing to provide a level of thermal insulation to the wound environment. It has been suggested that specific formulations such as Granuflex™ (Convatec) (Figure 10) also promote angiogenesis. Hydrocolloids are also used for wounds that are granulating or epithelialising that benefit from a moist environment, which they are net donators of moisture.

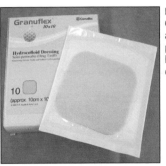

Figure 10: Granuflex™, a semi-permeable hydrocolloid dressing

III: SUPPORTING PROLIFERATION – The moist wound healing principle

Winter's research in 1962 revealed that a moist wound environment maximises the healing rate and supports optimal wound physiology in the proliferating wound; under these conditions, wounds can heal up to 30% faster. As a result, many products have been developed to help achieve this 'ideal' moist environment. The principle of advanced wound care today is therefore based on controlling the balance of exudate in the wound environment – either

absorbing excess exudate or hydrating wounds that are liable to drying.

Simple 'dry' dressings

Dry dressings are designed for wounds with low levels of exudation to prevent leakage of wound fluid and are not classed as 'advanced' dressings. They often consist of non-adherent pads for use post-surgery Melolin™ (Smith and Nephew) (Figure 11) and Rondopad™ (Millpledge). Pads with an adhesive include Primapore™ (Smith and Nephew), which has a perforated breathable cover to allow moisture evaporation (Figure 12). Leukomed T Plus™ (BSN medical) benefits from a semi-permeable film covering that acts as a viral/bacterial barrier designed to maintain moisture more effectively. Postoperative dressings over suture areas should ideally stay in place for 24–48 hours to

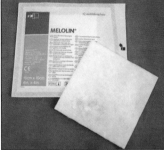

Figure 11: Melolin™, a non-adherent absorptive dressing

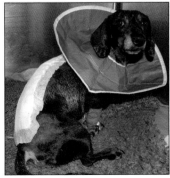

Figure 12: A Dachshund with a Primapore™ dressing in place after spinal surgery

minimise risks of any bacterial contamination breaching the fibrin seal that normally develops within the wound at 8–12 hours. For adhesive dressings designed for human skin, a 24–48 hour wear time can be challenging in the veterinary patient.

KEY FUNCTIONS:

■ Protect wounds and suture sites from mild trauma and direct contamination over short periods (24–48 hours)
■ Absorb a small amount of wound exudate post-surgery

Hydration dressings

Hydrating products act as fluid donors and are indicated primarily in the management of dry open wounds that have significant granulation tissue; they are also used for aiding debridement in fragile wounds.

Hydrogels are moisture-donating gels made of 70–95% water and variable quantities of hydrophilic polymer base such as sodium carboxymethylcellulose (CMC) or alginate. Intrasite™ (Smith and Nephew), Cutimed™ Gel (BSN Medical) (Figure 13) and Citrugel™ (Dechra Veterinary Products Ltd) are examples. They have a gel consistency comprising plant-based starch-like substances to aid in application and prevent dehydration during wear.

Some hydrogels have capacity to absorb further fluid as the polymer is able to tolerate

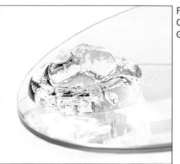

Figure 13: Cutimed™ Gel

an increase in volume while maintaining its gel form. Individual properties such as consistency, clarity of gel and ability to absorb while maintaining gel integrity vary considerably and it is the clinician's choice as to which is best suited to practice.

These differences may be marginally dependent on the brand used, but all are ideal for maintaining a healthy, bacteriostatic environment for healing. A secondary dressing is usually required to maintain their efficacy, and although they are commonly used under dry dressings a semi-permeable film-backed dressing such as a film or foam is likely to be most effective to maintain humidity and a moist environment.

KEY FUNCTIONS:

■ Hydrate dry wound tissue
■ Maintain a moist wound environment

Absorption dressings

Absorption dressings are indicated mainly in the management of wounds with excessive exudate: typically, these will be applied in the inflammatory phase.

1. Foam dressings

Foams function by drawing excess exudate away from the wound, maintaining some moisture conservation through humidity to keep the wound moist (Figure 14). A film backing will also protect the wound from outside contamination as long as a significant overlap (2 to 3 cm minimum) of the wound's edge is maintained. Typically foams are made of hydrophilic polyurethane such as Allevyn™ (Smith and Nephew) and Advazorb plus™ (distributed by Dechra Veterinary Products Ltd). Foam dressings with a semi-permeable film backing serve as a viral/bacterial barrier while allowing transfer of moisture vapour out of the dressing. Moisture vapour transfer rate (MVTR) or water vapour transfer rate may be referred to in relation to the dressing's ability

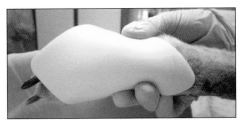

Figure 14: A foam dressing used to maintain a moist wound environment following surgery

to allow moisture to evaporate through the film membrane. It is proposed that dressings with a higher MVTR are able to handle a greater volume of exudate. However, this function will depend upon the viscosity of the exudate being produced and density of secondary dressings and bandaging over the primary dressing.

2. Hydrofibre™

Hydrofibre™ (known as Aquacel™ hydrofibre™) is a trademarked technology made entirely of strands of sodium CMC in fibre form. The sodium CMC fibres in contact with exudate form a cohesive gel which does not transfer fluid laterally across the dressing, but draws fluid in a vertical (upwards) fashion. Several layers may be applied to increase vertical absorbency, although this method can become costly if multiple sheets are to be used. Hydrofibre™ dressings are also available with ionic silver, marketed as Aquacel Ag™ (Convatec). A secondary dressing and pre-moistening is often required with Hydrofibre™ use in small animal wounds as they do not tend to exude sufficiently to prevent drying *in situ*. If hydrofibre™ is used and is found to stick to the wound bed, a saline flush should be used to remove the dressing.

3. Alginates

Alginate dressings are fine fibrous dressings derived from kelp, a seaweed rich in guluronic acid (GA) and mannuronic acid (MA) that are used to absorb excess exudate. Their properties may vary dependent upon which part of the plant is used for production, the root end being high in GA and having good haemostatic properties and the 'leaf' end being higher in MA which forms a softer gel on hydration. Most alginate dressings will combine both GA and MA in varying proportions. Alginates are thought to be a beneficial absorbent dressing which actively stimulates granulation tissue formation through the release of calcium ions. The exudate environment that is high in sodium ions causes the dressing to release calcium ions which, in turn, stimulates the degradation of mast cells releasing pre-formed growth factors. It should be remembered that this may not be considered beneficial in the equine limb wound as overgranulation will already be a significant risk. Alginates should not be used on dry wounds as they will contribute to desiccation and the fibres may cause irritation. Thorough cleansing between dressing changes is recommended to remove any gel or fibrous residue. Some brands will be promoted principally as a haemostat, such as Kaltostat™ (Convatec).

Super absorbent dressings

Occasionally, wounds become highly exudative and are therefore complex to manage; some cases may even necessitate surgical drainage if the source of the exudation is deep within the wound. However, for more superficial exudation nappies can be the most practical solution for managing such problematic wounds. These have been designed to cope with high volumes of fluid, using polyacrylate crystals, offer more convenient sizes and combine hi-tech silicone adhesives to assist in improving wearability. Eclypse™ (available through Dechra Veterinary Products) is such a dressing that can hold large volumes of fluid in relation to its size. It is one of the first products to adhere well to animal skin while offering significant fluid absorption capacity.

KEY FUNCTIONS:

- Absorb and retain high levels of wound exudate
- Enable an increased wear time between dressing changes in patients with highly exudative wounds

IV: DEALING WITH WOUND INFECTION

Wound infection is the result of bacterial proliferation in the wound environment and should not be confused with simple bacterial colonisation. Sepsis develops only when the bacterial load reaches a level that is able to overwhelm the inflammatory response. Signs include smell, redness, swelling, purulent exudate, pain and fragile tissue prone to bleeding. Debridement and bacterial sensitivity testing are likely to be the key steps in the management of septic wounds. Ongoing management with an antimicrobial dressing should aim to control the bacterial burden and also create an optimal wound environment, either debriding or maintaining moisture during wear.

Dressings for infection control

Antimicrobial dressings are designed to manage local infection in the wound and encourage normalisation of the healing cascade. They are *not a substitute for systemic antibiotics* and patients at risk or with signs of systemic infection should also be managed with suitable antibiotics.

1. Honey

Honey, following centuries of anecdotal use throughout the world, has recently re-emerged as a potential dressing for infection control (Figure 15). Manuka honey is currently the honey of choice for wound management in people, due to its superior and sustained antimicrobial effects. Honey derived from Manuka plants has been found to have an antimicrobial effect over and above that of standard honey, which is retained upon dilution, and catalyse denaturing of free radicals.

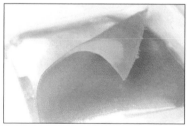

Figure 15: A honey dressing

A Unique Manuka Factor (UMF) rating will be common in association with Manuka honey, indicating the potency of the additional and sustained antimicrobial effect. A UMF of 10 or above is effective against common wound pathogens including *Pseudomonas*, meticillin-resistant *Staphylococcus aureus* (MRSA) and *Escherichia coli*. Honey products for use in wound management are prepared to meet rigorous medical standards. This involves high level filtering to remove debris and beeswax, as well as sterilising through gamma-radiation rather than the standard heat process for food-grade honey, to prevent degradation of the beneficial components and complex peptides.

2. Silver

The antimicrobial activity of silver compounds is achieved by releasing ionic silver into solution which react and inactivate molecules within the micro-organisms. Silver dressings are usually effective against common wound pathogens including *Pseudomonas*, MRSA and *E. coli* and also common yeasts and fungi, including *Candida*. These dressings have made a significant impact on wound management since the emergence of MRSA in the human hospital setting. Silver is similar in its antimicrobial effect to Manuka honey, but lacks the further anti-inflammatory and debridement properties. Several topical presentations of silver are available for use.

Nanocrystalline Silver Acticoat™ (Smith and Nephew) is unlike dressings with silver already incorporated in ionic form; the sheet form requires activation prior to use by soaking in water for 10 seconds. The manufacturers advise that saline should not be used to pre-soak the dressing as it can reduce the potency of the antimicrobial effect due to interaction with chloride ions from the salt solution.

Foams, alginates or hydrofibre are often combined with silver to incorporate the benefits of moist wound management with the antimicrobial effects; wound exudate needs to penetrate the dressings to achieve release of silver ions in these products.

Silver sulfadiazine is one of the oldest preparations of silver combined with topical antibiotic. It can be an effective cream for management of diffuse wounds and fungal conditions of the dermis. This is commonly found in the clinical setting under the brand name of Flamazine™ (Smith and Nephew).

3. Dialkyl carbamoyl chloride (DACC)

DACC dressings are a recent addition to veterinary advanced wound management with a novel method of action. This employs a physical hydrophobic interaction with a coating of natural fatty acid derivatives (DACC) which enables the dressing to 'capture' bacteria from the wound environment. In the moist environment of an infected wound the bacteria are attracted to the hydrophilic coating of the dressing and become irreversibly bound to the DACC-coated fibres. On removal of the dressing the 'captured' bacteria in contact with DACC are removed. Cutimed™ Sorbact (BSN Medical) (Figure 16) are likely to be a useful alternative to 'wet-to-dry' techniques, offering similar

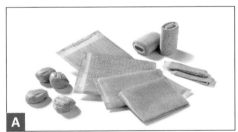

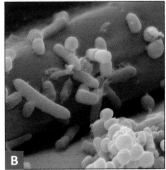

Figure 16: (A) The Cutimed™ Sorbact range. (B) Bacteria adhering to the dressing

physical characteristics to gauze while offering additional antimicrobial activity.

KEY FUNCTIONS:

- Physically removes bacteria from the wound bed
- Physical action minimises risk of antimicrobial resistance

V: FRAGILE AND PROBLEM WOUNDS

Some wounds present special problems because of failure to progress during the proliferative phase.

Dressings for protection of developing granulation tissue

Non-adherent (NA)

NA dressings are indicated as the primary contact layer to protect fragile wound tissue and are designed to minimise damage to the wound surface during dressing changes. They are usually constructed in a mesh format to allow the passage of exudate to a secondary dressing while protecting the wound surface itself. NA mesh dressings should not be left *in situ* too long since new capillary growth and fragile tissue can begin to grow through the apertures.

1. Paraffin gauze: Jelonet™ (Smith and Nephew), Grassolind™ (Millpledge UK)

White soft paraffin impregnated gauze (Figure 17) has been the mainstay of NA dressings for many years and relies on the characteristics of paraffin to prevent adherence to the wound surface. The amount of paraffin per unit area can vary considerably; excessive amounts may occlude the dressing mesh and leave a residue in the wound that is difficult to remove. For these reasons it has been largely replaced by synthetic dressings.

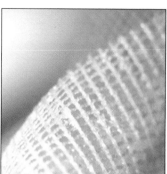

Figure 17: A Jelonet™ dressing

2. Knitted viscose: N-A™ (Johnson and Johnson)

This is now widely used in the management of granulating wounds; N-A Ultra™ is combined with silicone to reduce adherence and is easier to handle and more conformable to the wound.

3. Silicone mesh: Mepitel™ (Mölnlycke)

Silicone mesh dressings provide the least adherence of all the NA range. Although they are expensive, they can be washed and re-used on multiple occasions following resterilisation.

KEY FUNCTIONS:

- Permit drainage of exudate from wound surface
- Prevent damage and disruption to wound surface during dressing changes

Dressings to promote epithelial migration

Scaffold dressings

These work by offering a scaffold or 'matrix' for cell growth, encouraging migration across the wound bed. They require a greater knowledge of wound physiology and timing for best results. Scaffold dressings may be derived from porcine, equine or bovine collagen and are intended to be left in the wound to provide a pathway for epithelial migration. Acell™ (Genitrix) and physiological membranes such as Vet-Biosist™ (Smiths) are typical examples. Prisma™ (Systagenix) combines bovine collagen with low level silver to provide some antimicrobial support.

Scaffold dressings may be used in wounds that are prone to fragile healing and poor scar tissue formation lacking tensile strength. These products can be helpful provided the wound bed is at the right stage (granulating) for their application. Other factors underlying the wound's failure to progress should be ruled out before the use of scaffold dressings otherwise there will be some considerable expense wasted.

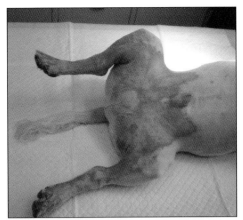

Figure 18: A superficial burn wound, which is a typical candidate for Cavilon™ spray to protect fragile tissue during healing

KEY FUNCTIONS:

■ Provide scaffold for cell migration during wound healing

KEY FUNCTIONS:

■ Protect normal tissue surrounding the wound

Dressings to protect surrounding tissues

Healthy tissue surrounding a wound can often become damaged where there is excessive exudate. Some chronic wounds can become particularly detrimental due to unusually elevated levels of tissue enzymes. Adhesives or environmental factors such as frequent contact with urine, pressure or friction will also predispose to tissue devitalisation.

Protective dressings

Protective dressings include barrier sprays and creams that protect fragile tissue, such as Cavilon™ (3M available through Dechra Veterinary Products). Cavilon™ is a useful spray application that protects fragile tissue (Figure 18) from aggravating factors that can cause wound degradation. These include excess moisture from wound fluid, urine and friction damage. When applied daily or twice daily the product appears unsubstantial on application but is extremely effective.

Conclusion

'Advanced' wound management and dressing selection should be considered as something of both an art and a science. Understanding the processes of wound healing and positively influencing their progress requires the recognition and visual perception of the wound as it presents. Debridement, moisture management and infection control are three important needs that should be assessed at the different stages of healing. Recognising the signs of progression – and regression – in a wound, whilst remaining aware of its underlying physiological needs, will ensure that your next dressing selection is appropriate. Sensitive dressing choices coupled with minimisation of many other factors that contribute to healing, including nutrition, disease, movement and cooperation, will be rewarded with a wound that heals as fast as is physiologically possible. ■

How to...
Select and carry out a
gastropexy procedure
by John Williams

A gastropexy is the surgical attachment of the stomach to the abdominal wall, most commonly as a means of preventing recurrence of gastric volvulus.

PRACTICAL TIP:
A gastropexy procedure should be performed in all cases of gastric dilatation–volvulus (GDV) or gastric dilatation (GD)

A gastropexy should always be carried out when surgery is performed in the management of gastric dilatation–volvulus (GDV). In cases of simple dilatation, which can be managed initially by gastric decompression and when surgery can be delayed, gastropexy should always be an elective procedure. When there is acute GDV the patient must be stabilised prior to anaesthesia and surgery. This is outside the scope of this article and the reader is referred to the *BSAVA Manual of Canine and Feline Abdominal Surgery*.

Given that dogs that have had one episode of gastric dilatation (GD) are at an increased risk of repeated episodes, a gastropexy aids in prevention of future volvulus. However, it does not decrease the risk of gastric dilatation.

In cases that present with GDV, recurrence rates can be as high as 80% if gastropexy is not carried out; gastropexy reduces the risk of recurrence to less than 10%. Furthermore, there is a dramatic increase in median survival in gastropexy (547 days) compared with non-gastropexy (188 days) patients. A number of gastropexy techniques have been described and are summarised in Figure 1.

Prophylactic gastropexy
Due to the success of gastropexy in preventing recurrence of GDV, it would appear

Technique	Adhesions	Advantages	Disadvantages
Simple suturing	Poor adhesions	Relatively quick	High probability of recurrence
Tube gastropexy	Adequate adhesions	Low probability of recurrence. Relatively quick to carry out	Patient interference. Increased morbidity. Increased hospitalisation
Incisional gastropexy	Strong adhesions	Low probability of recurrence	
Belt loop gastropexy	Strong adhesions	Low probability of recurrence	

Figure 1: Gastropexy techniques (continues) ▶

Technique	Adhesions	Advantages	Disadvantages
Circumcostal gastropexy	Strong adhesions (probably the most secure)	Low probability of recurrence	Technically demanding. Risk of rib fracture. Risk of pneumothorax
Incorporating (linea alba) gastropexy	Strong adhesions	Low probability of recurrence	Not generally suitable as the gastric fundus is sutured into the midline laparotomy closure. There is a risk of gastric perforation if any further abdominal surgery is carried out
Gastrocolopexy		Low probability of recurrence	Possibly higher potential for recurrence
Laparoscopic gastropexy	Strong adhesions	Low probability of recurrence	Generally not suitable for the acute case. Specialist equipment required

Figure 1: (continued) Gastropexy techniques

logical to offer prophylactic gastropexy in those breeds or lines at most risk from GDV. In bitches, such a procedure could be readily carried out at the same time as a routine ovariohysterectomy.

Clearly the risks of occurrence of GDV need to be weighed against the risk of anaesthesia and elective surgery in an otherwise healthy animal. From a surgeon's and an anaesthetist's point of view there is less risk in carrying out a planned elective procedure than performing emergency surgery on a GDV patient.

Recently the risks *versus* benefits of prophylactic gastropexy have been examined by comparing the lifetime probability (risk) of a dog dying from GDV against the expected cost-effectiveness of prophylactic gastropexy. In the group of American dogs studied, it was shown that although prophylactic gastropexy would reduce mortality from GDV, it is only cost-effective in very high risk patients. There are also ethical issues in considering carrying out such a prophylactic procedure, which are outside the scope of this article.

Belt loop gastropexy

This is the author's preferred method of creating a gastropexy as it provides excellent adhesions and is the author's technique of choice in both acute cases and for elective gastropexy. It is also technically feasible for the unassisted surgeon.

Technique

Patient positioning: Dorsal recumbency.

Assistant: Not essential, but can be useful until the surgeon becomes experienced with the technique.

Equipment extras: Balfour abdominal retractor; large abdominal swabs.

Surgical procedure

1 A routine, midline abdominal incision.

2 A tongue of seromuscular tissue is created from the stomach wall over the pyloric antrum; the author tries to incorporate at least two short gastric arteries (Figure 2).

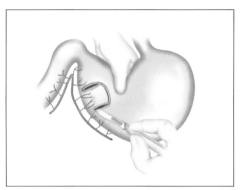

Figure 2: A tongue of seromuscular tissue is created from stomach wall over the pyloric antrum, incorporating two short gastric arteries

3 Two parallel incisions are made in the transversus muscle of the abdominal wall, caudal to the costal arch and a tunnel, wider than the flap, is created by blunt dissection with long artery forceps (Figure 3).

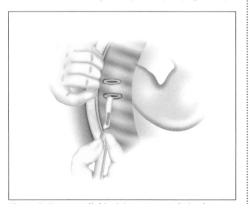

Figure 3: Two parallel incisions are made in the transversus muscle of the abdominal wall, caudal to costal arch; a tunnel, wider than the flap, is created by blunt dissection with artery forceps

4 The seromuscular pedicle is drawn gently by means of stay sutures, or Babcock forceps through the tunnel (Figure 4)

and then sutured into its original bed in the gastric wall (Figure 5).

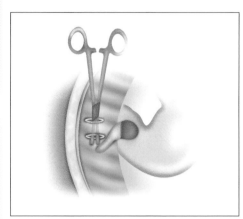

Figure 4: The seromuscular pedicle is drawn gently through the tunnel with Babcock forceps

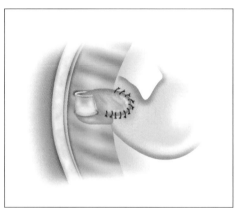

Figure 5: The flap is sutured into its original bed in the gastric wall

5 The pedicle is anchored into place with simple interrupted 2 or 3 metric monofilament synthetic suture material. Absorbable sutures such as polydioxanone, glycomer 631 or polyglyconate or non-absorbable polypropylene are suitable choices.

Tube gastropexy/gastrostomy

Tube gastropexy has the advantage of being quick to perform and allowing gastric decompression postoperatively. Though easy to place there is increased morbidity and longer hospitalisation periods associated with this technique.

Technique

Positioning: Dorsal recumbency.

Assistant: Not essential, but is useful.

Equipment extras: Balfour abdominal retractor; large abdominal swabs; long artery forceps.

Surgical procedure

1 A routine, midline abdominal incision.

2 A subcutaneous tunnel is made by means of blunt dissection with long artery forceps, from a stab incision in the skin lateral to the laparotomy wound, and caudal to the last rib on the right.

3 A Foley catheter is then drawn through the tunnel into the abdominal cavity (Figure 6).

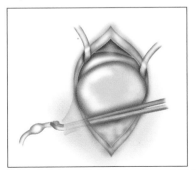

Figure 6: Foley catheter being drawn into the abdominal cavity

4 A purse-string suture of 2 metric polydioxanone or glycomer 610 is preplaced in the wall of the pyloric antrum.

5 A stab incision is made within the suture into the gastric lumen.

6 The Foley catheter is placed into the stomach (Figure 7), the balloon inflated and the purse-string suture tightened.

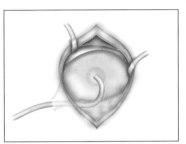

Figure 7: Foley catheter being introduced into the stomach (pyloric antrum) after preplacing a purse-string suture

7 Omentum is mobilised and wrapped around the Foley catheter (Figure 8).

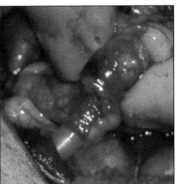

Figure 8: Omentum wrapped around catheter. © John Williams

8 Traction is then placed on the catheter to draw the pyloric antrum into firm contact with the abdominal wall and an absorbable synthetic suture material is used to suture the gastric serosa to the abdominal wall (Figure 9).

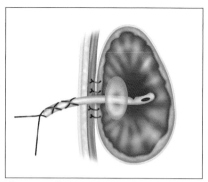

Figure 9: Relative positions of catheter, stomach and body wall

9 The catheter is fixed in place either with a Chinese friction finger trap suture pattern (Figure 10) or by means of zinc oxide butterfly tapes.

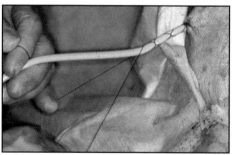

Figure 10: Chinese finger trap suture.
© John Williams

Postoperative care

The tube can be removed a minimum of 5–7 days after placement in order to allow firm adhesions to form and thus prevent leakage of gastric contents into the abdominal cavity. The bulb of the Foley catheter is deflated and the tube is pulled out. The small hole in the body wall will granulate closed in 24 hours.

Complications include premature dislodgement and inflammation around the stoma.

Incisional gastropexy

This is the simplest technique to use as it is straightforward and relies on healing between the edges of a peritoneum–transversus abdominis muscle incision and a seromuscular incision in the pyloric antrum.

Technique

Positioning: Dorsal recumbency.

Assistant: Not required, but is useful.

Equipment extras: Balfour abdominal retractor; large abdominal swabs.

Surgical procedure

1 A routine abdominal midline incision.

2 A 4–5 cm incision is made in the pyloric antrum (taking care not to penetrate the submucosa) (Figure 11).

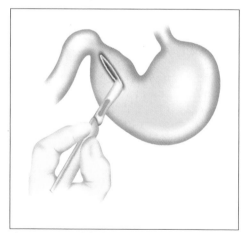

Figure 11: Partial thickness incision in the pyloric antrum

3 A similar incision is made through the peritoneum into the transversus abdominis muscle 6–8 cm from the laparotomy wound edge on the right (Figure 12).

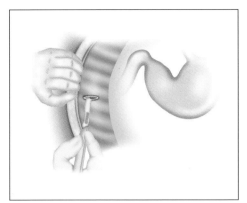

Figure 12: Incision in the right lateral body wall through the peritoneum and transversus abdominis muscle

4 Using 3 or 2 metric monofilament absorbable suture material the wound edges are sutured together (Figure 13). The two cranial incisions are closed first and then the caudal incisions.

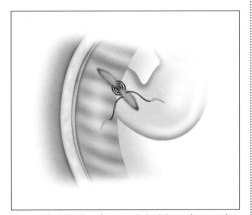

Figure 13: Suturing the gastric incision edges to the edges of the body wall incision with a simple continuous suture pattern (caudal edges are sutured in same manner)

Circumcostal gastropexy

This is a technically difficult procedure for which an assistant is essential. Though it produces strong adhesions if carried out incorrectly, there is the potential to fracture the rib and/or induce a pneumothorax. This technique is therefore more appropriate for a prophylactic gastropexy, rather than on an emergency basis.

Laparoscopic gastropexy

Laparoscopic stapled gastropexy and laparoscopic-assisted gastropexy have been described. These minimally invasive techniques offer alternatives to open abdominal surgery, but access to specialised equipment is required for these techniques and they will not be described here.

Key to success

Choose the most appropriate technique that you are most familiar with. If you are unfamiliar with gastropexy, carry it out as an elective procedure so that its use in the acute case will be straightforward.

The key to successful management of acute GDV is prompt stabilisation followed by surgery to create a gastropexy.

Failure to create a gastropexy will inevitably lead to recurrence.

Acknowledgement

Figure 1 and the line diagrams in this article have been reproduced from the *BSAVA Manual of Canine and Feline Abdominal Surgery*, edited by John Williams and Jacqui Niles. The diagrams were drawn by Samantha Elmhurst BA Hons (www.livingart.org.uk) and are printed with her permission. ∎

Index

Page numbers in italics refer to figures
